Medical Informatics in Obstetrics and Gynecology

David Parry
University of Technology, New Zealand

Emma Parry
The University of Auckland, New Zealand

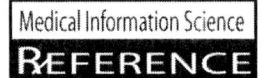

MEDICAL INFORMATION SCIENCE REFERENCE

Hershey · New York

Director of Editorial Content: Kristin Klinger
Director of Production: Jennifer Neidig
Managing Editor: Jamie Snavely
Assistant Managing Editor: Carole Coulson
Typesetter: Larissa Vinci
Cover Design: Lisa Tosheff
Printed at: Yurchak Printing Inc.

Published in the United States of America by
          Information Science Reference (an imprint of IGI Global)
          701 E. Chocolate Avenue, Suite 200
          Hershey PA 17033
          Tel: 717-533-8845
          Fax: 717-533-8661
          E-mail: cust@igi-global.com
          Web site: http://www.igi-global.com

and in the United Kingdom by
          Information Science Reference (an imprint of IGI Global)
          3 Henrietta Street
          Covent Garden
          London WC2E 8LU
          Tel: 44 20 7240 0856
          Fax: 44 20 7379 0609
          Web site: http://www.eurospanbookstore.com

Library of Congress Cataloging-in-Publication Data

Medical informatics in obstetrics and gynecology / David Parry and Emma Parry, editors.

     p. ; cm.

  Includes bibliographical references and index.

  Summary: "This book describes a number of areas within women's health informatics, incorporating a technology perspective"--Provided by publisher.

  ISBN 978-1-60566-078-3 (h/c)

  1. Obstetrics--Data processing. 2. Gynecology--Data processing. 3. Medical informatics. I. Parry, David (David Tudor) II. Parry, Emma, 1968-

  [DNLM: 1. Medical Informatics. 2. Women's Health. 3. Medical Records Systems, Computerized. WP 26.5 M489 2009]

  RG103.M388 2009

  618.0285--dc22

                         2008020897

British Cataloguing in Publication Data
A Cataloguing in Publication record for this book is available from the British Library.

All work contributed to this book set is original material. The views expressed in this book are those of the authors, but not necessarily of the publisher.

Editorial Advisory Board

Table of Contents

Section I
Introduction Chapters

Section II
Information Management Applications

Section IV
Gynecology Applications

Section V
Knowledge and Information Management and Use

Detailed Table of Contents

Section I
Introduction Chapters

Chapter I
> *Peter Stone, FRANZCOG, CmFm, The University of Auckland, New Zealand*

This chapter introduces the reader to the field of obstetrics and gynecology. The continuum of pregnancy from conception to childbirth and the postnatal period is discussed. There is coverage of the pathology that can arise within the female reproductive tract. In addition to the clinical overview; a brief introduction of the role that information technology plays in this area currently is discussed.

Chapter II
> *Premila Fade, Poole Hospital NHS Foundation Trust, UK*
> *Anne-Marie McMahon, Poole Hospital NHS Foundation Trust, UK*

Data collection is generally considered to be a benign exercise. However, once data is collected there are significant ethical and legal issues surrounding its use. In this chapter using the concept of Principlism, these issues are discussed and constructs are developed. Data and privacy laws vary from country to country; however, issues are discussed in light of the law in a number of countries.

Section II
Information Management Applications

Chapter III

David Parry, Auckland University of Technology, New Zealand

In coding and messaging, the concepts of coding health information in a structured way in discussed. The different techniques and their advantages and disadvantages are covered. Messaging looks at the types of ways or data transfer and their applicability within the health sphere.

Chapter IV

Gareth Parry, Horsmans Place Partnership, UK

In this chapter the role of IT in the setting of the primary care doctor is explored. The topics of the electronic health record and the role of IT in prevention and screening are discussed. How IT can help the primary care doctor and improve the consultation is reviewed with an emphasis on audit and artificial intelligence. Discussion around the seamless transfer of information to other parties external to the primary care doctor is included.

Chapter V

Emma Parry, The University of Auckland, New Zealand

The electronic health record has been the Holy Grail in Health Informatics for many years. In this chapter the electronic health recordis discussed from the most basic data collection through to a seamless integrated system. Pitfalls are examined within the content.

Chapter VI

Graham Parry, Middlemore Hospital, New Zealand

Imaging, with complex equipment such as ultrasound machines, has been an area of medicine full of technology for many years. In this chapter the wide diversity of computing technology use within the imaging field is discussed. Areas as diverse as booking systems and 3-D ultrasound image rendering are discussed.

Section III
Obstetrics and Neonatology

Chapter VII

Emma Parry, The University of Auckland, New Zealand

Each pregnancy is a discrete entity with a defined start and finish. It is eminently amenable to data collection and in this chapter that the potential data items and their significance are covered. The definitions of outcomes are discussed along with the potential pitfalls of data collection and analysis. Potential and real uses for data are discussed too.

Chapter VIII

Kiran Massey, University of British Columbia and BC Women's Hospital and Health Centre, Canada
Tara Morris, University of British Columbia and BC Women's Hospital and Health Centre, Canada
Robert M. Liston, University of British Columbia, and BC Women's Hospital and Health Centre, and British Columbia Perinatal Health Programme, Canada
Peter von Dadelszen, University of British Columbia and British Columbia Perinatal Health Programme, Canada
Mark Ansermino, University of British Columbia, Canada
Laura Magee, University of British Columbia and British Columbia Perinatal Health Programme, Canada

Perinatal databases are now ubiquitous in the developed world, but are often basic and not necessarily useful. In this chapter, the authors, who are part of a collaboration of maternity units, provide insights into how to develop a network of data covering a number of hospitals. This network can be used to allow continuous quality improvement and this is covered in depth.

Chapter IX

Malcolm Battin, National Women's Health, Auckland City Hospital, New Zealand
David Knight, Mater Mother's Hospital, Brisbane, Australia
Carl Kuschel, The Royal Women's Hospital, Melbourne, Australia

Part of the pregnancy continuum is the care of the neonate. A minority of neonates requires care in hospital, but those that do are usually quite sick. They require intensive input and complex care. In this chapter the role and design of neonatal databases is discussed in addition with other applications within the neonatal unit of informatics.

Chapter X

Jenny Westgate, The University of Auckland, New Zealand

The CTG provides a real-time assessment of fetal well-being. Interpretation is flawed however and over the last 15 years efforts to develop an expert system which can support clinical decision making have been developed. In this chapter the science and physiology behind this exciting development and the ultimate system are discussed.

Section IV
Gynecology Applications

Chapter XI

Liron Pantanowitz, Tufts School of Medicine, Baystate Medical Center, USA
Maryanne Hornish, Tufts School of Medicine, Baystate Medical Center, USA
Robert A. Goulart, Tufts School of Medicine, Baystate Medical Center, USA

This chapter describes how laboratory information management systems can be used to achieve an automated and seamless workflow process. The emerging role of computer assisted screening of cervical cytology and application of digital imaging to the field of cervical cytology is described, including telecytology and virtual microscopy. Finally, this chapter reflects on the impact of online cytology resources and the emerging role of digital image cytometry.

Chapter XII

Laurie Elit, McMaster University, Canada,
Susan Bondy, University of Toronto, Canada
Michael Fung-Kee-Fung, University of Ottawa, Canada
Prafull Ghatage, University of Toronto, Canada
Tien Le, University of Toronto, Canada
Barry Rosen, University of Toronto, Canada
Bohdan Sadovy, Princess Margaret Hospital, Canada

Gynecologic cancers are best managed in tertiary level units. The best surgical approach is standardized, though operating notes and ongoing health records are not. The authors describe the difficulties and solutions to these problems with standardized templates across a number of units to allow standardization of care. They provide a potential model of electronic health record for gynecologic oncology.

Section V
Knowledge and Information Management and Use

Chapter XIII

Jamila Abuidhail, Faculty of Nursing, The Hashemite University, Jordan

The author of this chapter is a nurse and has reviewed the sources of women's health information for nursing professionals. In the main part of the chapter the author has evaluated the current literature assessing the patient view of internet information.

Chapter XIV

Shona Kirtley, University of Oxford, UK

The range of information available for health professionals on the Internet is astounding. The quality is highly variable and in this chapter careful assessment is made of the current information available.

Chapter XV

David Parry, Auckland University of Technology, New Zealand

As information increases and patient expectation increases, making a decision becomes increasingly difficult. In this chapter various techniques to support decision making for both the individual and groups is discussed. Standard decision trees, Bayesian techniques, and artificial intelligence techniques are covered.

Chapter XVI

Michelle Brear, University of New South Wales, Australia

The influence of organizational factors on the success of informatics interventions in healthcare has been clearly demonstrated. Health organizations are also increasingly under-resourced due to the global downturn in government social spending, health sector privatization and aging populations.

Chapter XVII

Josipa Kern, Zagreb University Medical School, Croatia

Industry put the first demand for standards. Especially standardization is extremely important for electronics, for information and communication technology (ICT), and its application in different areas. Nowadays developing of standards is organized on global, international level, but it exists also on national level, well harmonized with international one. Its mission is to promote the development of standardization and related activities in the world with a view to facilitating the international exchange of goods and services, and to developing cooperation in the spheres of intellectual, scientific, technological and economic activity.

Chapter XVIII

Elske Ammenwerth, University for Health Sciences, Medical Informatics and Technology (UMIT), Austria

Stefan Gräber, University Hospital of Saarland, Germany

Thomas Bürkle, University of Münster, Germany

Carola Iller, University of Heidelberg, Germany

This chapter summarizes the problems and challenges which occur when health information systems are evaluated. The main problem areas presented are the complexity of the evaluation object, the complexity of an evaluation project, and the motivation for evaluation. Based on the analysis of those problem areas, the chapter then presents recommendations how to address them. In particullary, it discusses in more detail what benefits can be obtained from applying triangulation in evaluation studies. Based on the example of the evaluation of a nursing documentation system, it shows how both the validation of results and the completeness of results can be supported by triangulation. The authors hope to contribute to a better understanding of the peculiarities of evaluation.

Chapter XIX

Pirkko Nykänen, Tampere University, Finland

eHealth refers to use of information and communication technologies to improve or enable health and healthcare. eHealth broadens the scope of health care delivery, citizens are in the center of services and services are offered by information systems often via the Internet. In this chapter eHealth systems are classified on the basis of their use and their functionality and the use is discussed from the viewpoints of citizens and health professionals. Citizens are increasingly using Internet and eHealth systems to search for medicine or health related information, and they become better informed and may take more responsibility of their own health. Health professionals are more reluctant to use the Internet and eHealth systems in physician-patient communication due to power and responsibility problems of decisions. In the future the socio-technical nature of eHealth should be considered and future systems developed for real use and user environment with user acceptable technology.

Chapter XX

Nilmini Wickramasinghe, Stuart Graduate School of Business, USA

Santosh Misra, Cleveland State University, USA

Arnold Jenkins, Johns Hopkins Hospital, USA

Douglas R. Vogel, City University of Hong Kong, China

Superior access, quality and value of healthcare services has become a national priority for healthcare to combat the exponentially increasing costs of healthcare expenditure. E-Health in its many forms and possibilities appears to offer a panacea for facilitating the necessary transformation for healthcare. While a plethora of e-health initiatives keep mushrooming both nationally and globally, there exists to date no unified system to evaluate these respective initiatives and assess their relative strengths and deficiencies in realizing superior access, quality and value of healthcare services. Our research serves to address this void. This is done by focusing on the following three key components: 1) understanding the web of players (regulators, payers, providers, healthcare organizations, suppliers and last but not least patients) and how e-health can modify the interactions between these players as well as create added value healthcare services. 2) understand the competitive forces facing e-health organizations and the role of the Internet in modifying these forces, and 3) from analyzing the web of players combined with the competitive forces for e-health organizations we develop a framework that serves to identify the key forces facing an e-health and suggestions of how such an organization can structure itself to be e-health prepared.

Foreword

I am delighted to write a foreword for this book on informatics in women's health—a first for women's health. I have known Emma and Dave for 10 or more years and admire their work in this field. They are in a unique position with their combined talents to bring this collection of articles together.

What do informatics offer to women's health? How can computers improve patient care? The amazing advances in IT have contributed to improvements in many aspects of modern life. This book, a first of many, outlines the contribution of computing to women's health.

Healthcare organizations have been keen to take up some aspects of the IT industry. Administration and clerical aspects of medical care such as clinic bookings, admission, and discharge have been computerized for many years. However involving IT in directly improving the care women receive has lagged. How IT can improve the care women receive is an immense topic which is at an embryonic stage—the subject of this book. This delay is due in part to the complexity of the issues but equally because the doctor and the IT consultant come from previously unrelated fields. In order for the full potential of the computers in medicine to be realized by these two diverse groups have to interact, a new subspecialty must emerge. This text is written by some of those in the forefront of this development.

Maternity care is one of the medical specialities more suited for computerization; there are many defined events with discrete beginning and end—pregnancy. Specialities such as gynaecology with repetitive admissions and complexity are far less amenable.

Fortunately for women's health, IT offers far more than just aiding hospital administration. Data collection, the logical first small step, is well established. These datasets range from retrospectively collected variables used to produce statistical analyses and reports, to comprehensive and prospectively collected patient notes. Additional exciting uses of IT in improving patient care are outlined in this collection.

This text is the first of what will be many in this field. I hope it inspires others as it does me and enable medical professionals and those in the IT industry to work together to improve care for women.

Neil Pattison
FRANZCOG

Neil Pattison is a specialist in obstetrics and gynaecology. He has an interest in high risk pregnancy and health informatics. He was the main instigator of one of the first perinatal databases in the world and has an ongoing interest in this area. Neil introduced both of the editors to this exciting field and was supervisor to Dr. Emma Parry for her MD which had a large health informatics component.

Preface

INTRODUCTION

Women's health is composed of a broad range of both normal physiological events in a woman's life, and conditions which occur as a result of abnormality of the genital tract and pregnancy. During the last century, the field of women's health (and ill health) have rapidly changed and evolved as a clinical discipline. This is in part due to the changing roles and expectations of women. The feminist movement and newspaper articles with headlines that read "the unfortunate experiment," resulted in the medical profession realizing that high standards and an informed approach were needed.

We are now at a point where the care of women through all parts of their life, whether it is puberty, pregnancy, or menopause, is generally of a high standard throughout the developed world. Care involves screening and prevention of disease, fertility control, pregnancy care, neonatal care, and management of gynecological disease.

Within women's health expectations of good quality care are high. Health professionals working in the area have been amongst those who have responded to the challenge to provide women and their babies with evidence-based care. For example, the Cochrane collaboration is a worldwide network of interested researchers who assess quality of research and collate the best to produce meta-analyses to guide practice. The groups now cover many disciplines within medicine, but the first group's set-up (and still the majority) is from women's health.

With so much information, both about individual women and vast amounts of research, managing this data is essential. Computing power has revolutionized life in the modern world. Within health, information, communication, data storage, and decision making have all been changed immensely by computing. We are now at a point where we cannot imagine running our lives without it.

The field of health informatics has been rapidly evolving over the last 20 years. There has been an explosion of interest in all medical fields and women's health is no different. Who are the health informaticists in women's health? As is usual in a new and evolving field, initially the "experts" are self-taught with an interest, and come from a range of backgrounds such as doctors, nurses, midwives, computer scientists, librarians, information scientists, and engineers. More recently however, many teaching institutions have developed courses in health informatics and post graduate study in the area is often easily arranged via e-learning.

In tandem, a number of areas were initially developed in women's health informatics. In the 1980s a number of early informaticists started to collect maternity data on databases. In Chapter V, Parry describes the development of the early electronic health records which stored information gathered on a database. The development of the World Wide Web led to electronic communication. This allowed communication between health professionals for advice and support. It also allowed new information to be more quickly disseminated and incorporated into practice. In the 1990s many research journals started to put an electronic version of the publication on the Internet, allowing more rapid and wider access to research.

Doctors have always jealously guarded their ability to make a diagnosis and institute the correct management. Even in this area computing power has had an increasingly significant role from the early days of clinical alerts to complex assessment of the antenatal CTG, which can now outperform a human (see Chapter X).

This book describes a number of areas within women's health informatics. Clearly where technology is involved, there are commercial applications within the area. In some cases, certain applications will be referred to. These are to allow examples to be given and do not necessarily indicate an endorsement of the product by the author. As an informatics book, many references are to Internet-based sources. Apologies if these have changed following publication, however judicious use of the Internet archive, www.waybackmachine.org, may allow the resurrection of even outmoded or updated references, for the determined or those requiring academic completeness

THE CHAPTERS

The first two chapters provide some background information. In the first chapter, Stone introduces the novice reader to clinical Women's Health. For a reader coming from a non-clinical background, this chapter will provide a brief overview of the clinical area of women's health. Clearly, the reader who already has prior knowledge in this area may find that it is not necessary to read this chapter. Chapter II examines the issues around the ethics and medicolegal safety in women's health informatics. Fade uses examples to illustrate potential issues and clearly legalities, in particular, institutions will depend on the overarching national legal framework, though the ethics of women's health informatics are generally applicable. If one is planning to use data collected on women, it is imperative that he or she has a clear understanding of local regulations regarding the individuals' data.

The next section looks at technologies within women's health. In Chapter III David Parry addresses coding and messaging systems – essential for the large-scale use and sharing of information. In Chapter IV Gareth Parry examines the wealth of health informatics as it pertains to the primary healthcare setting. The primary care physician provides "cradle to grave" care and is the key individual who coordinates a woman's care. In an ideal situation he or she will have access to all the woman's health data wherever it is recorded. Chapter V examines the concept of the electronic health record and the holy grail of a parallel "cradle to grave" electronic health record which can be easily accessed by all the relevant caregivers involved in one woman's care. One of the many areas where there has been a real explosion of data storage is imaging technologies. In Chapter VI, Graham Parry describes how images from radiological tests: primarily ultrasound, are used. He looks at storage, image manipulation, also covering validity and teaching.

The next section focuses on pregnancy. Pregnancy is a discrete event with a defined end-point. This makes it ideal for the application of statistical measures. Chapter VII looks at the range of maternity information that can be gathered, and then examines the definitions which can be applied. Uses for this information are also included. In Chapter VIII, a team representing the Canadian Perinatal Network Collaboration, look at the development of perinatal databases and the more complicated challenge of networking between units. They use their own leading system in British Columbia as an example. Maternal outcomes are uniquely linked to fetal/neonatal outcomes. Neonatal databases provide the complete dataset to a pregnancy. In Chapter IX, Battin and the colleagues describe neonatal database development. The authors are practicing neonataologists in one of the biggest units in Australia and developed their own in-house database. In Chapter X, Westgate describes the role of computing to aid decision making in interpretation of the fetal cardiotocogram (CTG). This provides an eloquent example of how artificial intelligence can be better than human intelligence. For more background on this refer to Chapter XV.

Gynaecology is the area of medicine concerned with the female reproductive organs and includes areas as diverse as infertility, delayed puberty, menorrhagia, incontinence, and oncology. Cervical cytology (Pap smear) has been an important medical intervention and has resulted in a reduction in the incidence of cervical cancer by detecting the pre-malignant state which is easily eradicated before progression to invasive cervical cancer. However, as any test, cervical cytology readings can be inaccurate where there is significant human involvement. In Chapter XI, Pantanowitz and the co-atuhors from Baystate, USA, explore the role of computing to try to reduce error within this important public health area. In Chapter XII, Elit and the co-authors from Canada, describe the information gathering and storage in women undergoing surgery for ovarian cancer. This is a region-wide system and incorporates elements of Internet use for data sharing and extensive efforts to use a seamless electronic health record (see Chapter V). Although a specific area of women's health is the focus of this chapter, it provides an excellent generic framework for the development of a regional/countrywide gynecological electronic data storage and data sharing system.

For the reader who is a clinician, how many times has a patient sat down in your rooms and brought out a pile of information downloaded from the Internet? This is now a reality and knowledge is available for all, though the interpretation is often lacking. In the last section of the book, this information "overload" and its reasonable management is explored. In Chapter XIII, Abuidhail provides a broad review of the use of electronic information sources for education and support of women and their caregivers. This includes telenursing and telehealth. In Chapter XIV, Kirtley (a librarian and information scientist) provides an extensive review of the available electronic information sources in women's health for health professionals working in the field. In the final chapter, David Parry looks at decision analysis, a system of helping individuals to make decisions using computer support to make sense of the known possible outcomes of an intervention.

THE FUTURE

Who would have thought that 20 years ago a device the size of your hand could allow one to talk to a friend across the other side of the world, check the latest world news, and write, perform analysis, and submit a paper electronically! We are talking about the latest PDAs of course. The amazing explosion of computer technology over the last 20 years has been incredible. Now with the technology becoming smaller and cheaper, further amazing changes are occurring.

In the area of women's health informatics systems for data storage, image storage, data interpretation, and analysis are quickly becoming mainstream and commercial rather than home-grown. What is really lacking is a cohesive approach and universal language to allow large networks to function well. Only in the area of imaging with the DICOM system has this part way been achieved. In the future, clinicians will collaborate more, as diseases become rarer and individuals experience less. They will push for systems which can also collaborate between centers to allow data sharing. Whether this will happen we will have to wait to see.

Smaller devices mean that data is likely to be collected in a more ubiquitous way in the future with hopefully better and more extensive data capture. This coupled with cheaper devices will also hopefully translate into more use in the resource constrained setting where the majority of maternal deaths occur.

CONCLUSION

Women's health informatics is now "coming of age". It is an established area of health informatics and comprises a broad range of themes. There is currently no other book in this area and the aim of this publication is to provide interested readers with an insight into women's health informatics. We are not providing a comprehensive textbook as the margins of the field are somewhat "fuzzy" and there is no clinical role for an expert in the whole breadth of the field. Rather, this book provides an introduction for a new enthusiast, whatever field they come from, and in-depth chapters from leading authors in their respective fields. Researchers, clinical, and technical workers in this area should find this book a starting point for future work as well as an accessible introduction to those areas that they may feel uncertain in or unqualified. It is hoped that future editions will cover exciting and more importantly, clinically beneficial developments in this area. Change is constant in both women's health research and IT, and it is certain that the future developments imagined above will not be complete. The readers of this book may be those who will make the vision a reality.

Emma Parry
The University of Auckland, New Zealand

David Parry
Auckland University of Technology, New Zealand

Acknowledgment

The editors would like to acknowledge the help of all involved in the collation and review process of the book, without whose support the project could not have been satisfactorily completed. Both the editors appreciate the resources, both in time and access to scholarly articles, of their employing universities: AUT University and The University of Auckland.

The call for chapters sought experts in the field from far and wide as it was hoped to provide the audience with a global perspective. The editors thank the various professional organizations who agreed to include the call for chapters in their mail-outs. This has resulted in an international approach to the book.

The editors are indebted to the authors, without whom the project could not have succeeded. They come from different disciplines and areas of expertise and provide wide scholarly cover of the field. Many of the authors also acted as referees which is an essential component of the book development. Thanks to the authors for engaging in this process with professionalism.

Many thanks to Dr. Neil Pattison MD, who agreed to review the book and contribute the forward. In addition he introduced the authors to the exciting area of women's health informatics nearly fifteen years ago and encouraged us to research in this area.

Editing a book is an undertaking and we couldn't have done it without the support and guidance of the publishing team at IGI Global. Particular thanks go to Julia Mosemann, who patiently steered us through the editing process and kept us track!

Finally we would like to thank our daughters: Alice and Rosie, who have put up with mummy and daddy disappearing to the office at all hours to finish 'the book'. We hope you find it interesting and useful.

Section I
Introduction Chapters

Chapter I
An Introduction to Women's Health and Informatics

Peter Stone
FRANZCOG, CMFM, The University of Auckland, New Zealand

ABSTRACT

Improving women's health is a vital task for the world. The consequences of obstetric and gynecological disease are serious both for the women involved, their families, and communities. This introductory chapter introduces the reader to the field of Obstetrics and Gynecology. The continuum of pregnancy from conception to childbirth, and the postnatal period are discussed. There is coverage of the pathology that can arise within the female reproductive tract. Data collection and use has a long history in this area. In order to improve care, evidence-based medicine has been strongly emphasized and women's health has often led the way. Audit of practice, governance, and quality reviews are all areas where electronic information systems are assisting with improvements. Increasing use of e-health technologies are a major influence on the improvement

INTRODUCTION

Health informatics in Reproduction has the potential to provide the tools to lead a new revolution in the outcomes for women and their babies in the 21st century.

This may seem a bold statement but for those working in this field, it is improving outcomes in Reproductive Health that is the rationale for striving to use new ways to address health issues and indeed is the reason for this book.

The later chapters in this book will cover key topics in detail but the purpose of this chapter is to provide a context for further discussion and to challenge readers to consider the future of reproductive health and how new technologies may play a part in this future.

Societies tend to take reproduction for granted until the individual presents with a problem such as infertility, unwanted pregnancy, a sexually transmitted disease or symptoms from diseases in the genital tract. Apart from advances in science, it can be argued that progress in achieving healthier outcomes in reproductive health will require societies to refocus on valuing reproduction .

This includes not only the prevention of disease but encouraging sexual health, endeavouring to have women entering pregnancy in the best possible health, safe childbirth and valuing motherhood and childrearing. Clearly the ramifications of such statement are huge , but many of the successes in past improvements in obstetric outcomes have come as much from changed social circumstances and education as from strictly medical advances.

HISTORICAL SETTING

The improvement in maternal mortality in the western world from the 1900's has been well reviewed by Loudon (Loudon, 2000) and illustrates the impact of general health measures, new developments such as the discovery of antibiotics and the developments in blood transfusion and inversely, the adverse effects of "obstetric" or medical interventions in normal childbirth. This latter is a salutary lesson and the importance of evidence based practice is discussed later

The general measures built on knowledge previously acquired such as the description by Semmelweis in 1847 of puerperal fever and how its incidence could be reduced by handwashing saving many lives. Medical advances specifically in Obstetrics did play a role such as the use of ergot derivatives to prevent postpartum haemorrhage that J Chassar Moir pioneered in the 1930's.

Modern anaesthesia, antibiotics, blood transfusion, discovery of ecbolics, prostaglandins, structured data collection and audit, evidence based practice, new contraceptive techniques, safe abortion and ultrasound have all contributed to a revolution in the care of women and their babies, though not in all parts of the world.

DEFINING OBSTETRICS AND GYNECOLOGY

The scope of the disciplines being discussed need to be defined.

Obstetrics and gynecology and more recently "women's health" are terms to describe the science and practice of clinical care in human reproduction.

A rather narrow view would be that

- Obstetrics-the branch of medicine dealing with pregnancy, labour, delivery and the puerperium (the period from birth to the time when the changes of pregnancy have resolved- arbitrarily said to be 6 weeks)
- Gynecology-the branch of medicine dealing with diseases of the genital tract in women
- Women's health is all this in a modern context which includes the woman and family ie health is more than just the absence of disease.

The scope of these labels includes

- Physiology of reproduction
- Maternal fetal medicine
- Antenatal care, labor and birth
- Postnatal care, mother and baby
- Endocrinology of reproduction and the menstrual cycle
- Infertility - male and female
- Sexuality and womanhood
- Oncology
- Ethics "sociology" legal issues
- and many areas arising from the above –now beyond the scope of one person-hence development of "subspecialities"

From this list it is apparent that obstetrics and gynecology and women's health has a very wide scope because it encompasses everything that is involved in the human life cycle. It includes all the normal processes and events around becoming pregnant, having the baby and the "bringing up". The modern concepts of the importance of "start to life" for both the parents and the offspring include social factors as well as the fetal origins of adult disease, a new branch of science evolving from the work of Barker amongst others and loosely termed the "Barker hypothesis". A recent article clearly reviews the hypothesis (de Boo & Harding, 2006).

It is also apparent from life experience that the reproductive system does not always function normally. As described above, gynecology deals with both the disordered function (dysfunction) and defined diseases of the reproductive system in women. In infertility male reproductive disorders may also be managed by gynaecologists specialising in reproductive endocrinology and infertility.

Gynecology is the medical discipline which is involved in congenital abnormalities of the genital tract, abnormalities of puberty and the commencement of menstruation, menstrual disorders, benign and malignant tumours of the reproductive system, disorders of the lower urinary tract in women and the climacteric, the period in a woman's life as ovarian function ends. Women's Health is the part of gynecology dealing with contraception, sexual health, screening for genital and sexually transmitted diseases as well as issues of women's sexuality, social safety and domestic violence.

The challenges for modern obstetrics relate to both the science of the reproductive process and the social construct of a woman focussed society whereby appropriate health services are accessible and equitable to all women. No more is this illustrated more graphically than in the tables of lifetime risks of mortality in childbirth produced by the United Nations. Lack of basic services, simply trained personnel and unsafe

abortion practices account for the large majority of deaths in pregnancy and childbirth in the low resource developing world. Application of contemporary knowledge and practices would save over half a million lives a year.

Reproduction is a complex process in humans. In addition to difficulties of giving birth of a large headed fetus through a curved passage in a small maternal pelvis due to the erect posture, there are many aspects of pregnancy and partutrition that are incompletely understood in this species.

How labour is initiated is not known. Clearly, if it were understood how labour begins, post term and preterm pregnancy, both which cause significant special problems with adverse outcomes could potentially be modified with the aims of birth at normal term which is 37-42 weeks from the last menstrual period or 35-40 weeks (median 268 days from conception).

One of the commonest complications of pregnancy is a condition called preeclampsia or gestational proteinuric hypertension, occurring in 3-5% of first pregnancies to the current relationship. This may lead to fetal growth restriction or fetal death and serious maternal complications affecting many organ systems such as the kidney, brain, blood, liver, necessitating that the pregnancy needs to be ended for either the benefit of mother or fetus. The fundamental cause of this condition is unknown, though it is recognised to be at least in part a state of intravascular inflammation with vasoconstriction and characteristic histological changes in the placental bed.

Perhaps of even greater interest is that it is not known how the mother even tolerates the implantation and development of the fetus, who is genetically different from the mother, for the 9 months of pregnancy yet she would reject the baby's tissues after delivery.

Many fetal-neonatal outcomes are similarly unexplained. The cause of many abnormalities of fetal structure is unclear. Even more challenging is the range of neurodevelopmental problems that children may be found to manifest, such as cerebral palsy, where in only a small minority of cases is there a likely aetiological event identified.

A useful way of thinking about fetal abnormalities is to consider the broad groups of causes or associations. Four simple groups can be defined which are; genetic, chromosomal, structural and developmental. The underlying causes for many of these are not known and some basic causes can be manifest in different ways by the fetus newborn or child. Specific testing is available for some genetic disorders, chromosomal disorders, structural problems but few if any development abnormalities.

Examples of genetic disorders which may be detected before birth include thalassaemia, haemophilia, cystic fibrosis, muscular dystrophy amongst others.

Chromosomal problems include Down Syndrome (Trisomy 21 ie 3 chromosome number 21 instead of two). Trisomy 13 and 18, but there are many others.

Structural problems are surprisingly affecting up to 3-4% of babies, nearly half of these being heart abnormalities.

"Developmental" problems are such conditions as cerebral palsy, or the various learning disorders and cannot be detected before birth.

There is increasing interest in improving prenatal screening for and diagnosis of fetal abnormalities to enable parents to have information and options for pregnancy management before the baby is born. Ultrasound technologies have led the way in providing a "window" on the fetus but various measures of fetal and placental substances such as hormones which are found in the maternal blood are increasingly being used to aid in the prediction of fetal normality or fetal welfare.

In investigating the major problems of pregnancy, which are hypertensive diseases, pregnancy bleeding (antepartum haemorrhage) and fetal growth and welfare, ultrasound is currently the leading modality to enable diagnostic decisions to be made. A search through the Cochrane library will show surprisingly few studies on the efficacy of ultrasound in improving outcomes but in a number of situations including dating, diagnosing multiple pregnancies (e.g. twins) and in the use of Doppler ultrasound for fetal welfare assessment, it has clearly been shown to be of value.

Gynecology cannot be separated from obstetrics for there is great overlap in clinical conditions between pregnancies and the problems of pregnancies such as miscarriages, difficulties getting pregnant (sub fertility- infertility), although other areas such as treatment of cancers of the reproductive organs require special knowledge and skills not used often in Obstetrics. What remains important is the woman focus. An illustration of this is the prophylaxis, prevention, screening and treatments in cervical preinvasive diseases and invasive cancers in women who may wish to retain the ability to have children.

Another link between obstetrics and gynecology relates to the impact of both pregnancy and mode of delivery on pelvic floor function. Urinary and anal incontinence are both much more common in women than in men and this relates principally to the effects of pregnancy and childbirth (though also the anatomy of the lower urinary tract is also different in the female from the male). Whilst urogynecology, which is the speciality investigating and treating pelvic floor abnormalities in women is viewed as a gynaecological discipline, obstetricians are required to be able to recognise the problems the woman may present with and also be able to provide primary treatment at childbirth.

There remain many challenges in women's health such as the need for more effective and easily used contraceptives, the relationship between reproductive tract cancers and environment such as obesity and polycystic ovarian syndrome and genes that predispose to breast, ovarian and bowel cancer.

ROLES OF HEALTH CARE PROFESSIONALS IN OBSTETRICS AND GYNECOLOGY

Midwives are specialists in normal pregnancy, birth and care of women and babies in the period after birth (called the puerperium). Midwife traditionally meant "amongst women" and this describes the important supportive role midwives have in looking after woman at a very important and often vulnerable time in their lives. The International Confederation of Midwives has defined the roles of midwives in terms of training and standards which is important as they have a leading role internationally in the provision of safe care to mothers. In working with women, midwives provide the primary care and also the screening to determine which women have pregnancy problems that require medical or specialist care.

The obstetrician/OBGYN is the medical doctor trained in the management of the complications of pregnancy and also has the surgical skills required for the operative deliveries of babies.

Usually an obstetrician is trained as both an obstetrician and a gynecologist though may later concentrate on either obstetrics or gynecology.

In some countries, obstetricians may also be involved in primary maternity care.

General practitioners/primary healthcare physicians, are medical doctors who are not specialists in obstetrics but may in some places also be involved in both primary care and some of the medical complications of pregnancy but usually except in remote areas, they are not involved in the surgical aspects of childbirth.

A gynecologist is a medical doctor who has been trained in both obstetrics and gynecology. Gynecology as practised today is both a surgical and a non surgical (medical) speciality with a wide scope as described above. Gynecology as a discipline developed in the Western World in the late 19th and early 20th century when leaders in the area such as Marion Sim in the USA and Victor Bonney in Britain moved the emphasis away from the pure surgical approach to a more woman focussed one which led to the development of the Colleges of Obstetricians and Gynecologists. The modern gynecologist has as much an understanding of the endocrinology and physiology of reproduction as of the practice of surgical treatments

Doctors working in women's health may be obstetricians and gynecologists, or general practitioners/ primary healthcare physicians or may have special interests in sexual health and contraception.

AUDIT AND QUALITY

One of the lessons that the discipline of obstetrics and gynecology is learning from the history of audit (originally done for maternal and perinatal mortality) and later the challenges of evidence based medicine is that new treatments need to be well assessed before being introduced into clinical practice.

The risk to the fetus from medications was illustrated by the problems caused by thalidomide.

It took many years for it to be accepted that anterior (vaginal wall) repair was not an effective operation for urinary stress incontinence when compared with the Burch colposuspension procedure.

Obstetrics and gynecology was one of the first disciplines to be seriously challenged to defend its practices and where it could not, design and complete randomised controlled trials. The great British epidemiologist, Archie Cochrane had observed that "It is surely a great criticism of our profession that we have not organised a critical summary, by specialty or subspecialty, adapted periodically, of all relevant randomised controlled trials" (Cochrane, 1979). In 1989, Cochrane described the publication of "Effective Care in Pregnancy and childbirth" (Chalmers, Enkin, &

Kierse, 1989) as "a real milestone in the history of randomised trials and in the evaluation of care", and suggested that other specialties should copy the methods used". This subsequently led to the formation of the Cochrane collaboration which now is an internationally accessible electronic library of randomised trials. (http://www.cochrane.org/)

Of great importance and perhaps not even recognised by the triallists has been that in addition to the results, the trials themselves have provoked great discussion.

Seminal trials in obstetrics have included the Third stage trial (Prendiville, Elbourne, & McDonald, 2001) for the prevention of primary postpartum haemorrhage and the electronic fetal heart rate monitoring trial (Macdonald, Grant, Sheridan-Pereira, Boylan, & Chalmers, 1985). Arguably, the most famous randomised trial of all in obstetrics, and the source of the logo for the Cochrane collaboration was the trial of the use of antenatal corticosteroids to prevent respiratory distress syndrome (Liggins & Howie, 1972) which was published in 1972, long before the Cochrane collaboration had been formed.

One of the challenges for the many branches of gynecology is to emulate obstetrics and complete more treatment trials before the introduction of new procedures or medical treatments. The tools to do this are now available and well assessed.

EVIDENCE BASED PRACTICE

The results of treatment trials are increasingly being collated by interested groups into clinical guidelines. The professional colleges and nationally supported expert groups have developed many guidelines for practice with the aim of leading to evidence based consistent practice.

A list of useful web sites is provided at the end of this chapter. Such lists are not exhaustive but provide guidance. Use of these web sites does require that the evidence for the guideline is assessed by the reader because not all evidence is of equal quality and ultimately most guidelines are a summary expert opinion. Individual practices may on occasion differ from those recommended in the guideline and it is acceptable for this to happen provided that the clinician can defend the deviation from that which was recommended.

In reading guidelines, the quality of the evidence and the strength of the recommendations need to be considered. A typical rating system might be

Quality of evidence:

Ia. evidence from meta-analysis of randomized controlled trials
Ib. evidence from at least one randomized controlled trial
IIa. evidence from at least one well designed controlled study without randomization
IIb. evidence from at least one other type of well designed quasi experimental study
III. evidence from well designed non-experimental descriptive studies
IV. evidence from expert committee reports or opinions or clinical experience

Strength of recommendation:

a.   At least one randomized controlled trial as part of a body of literature of overall good quality and consistency addressing the specific recommendation (levels of evidence Ia, Ib)
b.   well controlled clinical trials available but no randomized trials on the topic of the recommendation (levels of evidence IIa, IIb, III)
c.   Evidence from expert committees or opinions, and/or clinical experience from respected authorities. This indicates the absence of applicable clinical studies of good quality (level of evidence IV).

As guidelines are developed by expert groups, there will almost always be need to consider a range of opinions which include the context in which the guideline was developed and for which the guideline was intended. An obvious example would be that guidelines for high and low resource environments would be expected to differ because of differing clinical resources and technologies being available.

USE OF E-TECHNOLOGIES

With this brief background to encouraging evidence based practice, where could it be expected that e-technologies might enhance the outcomes for women given the huge social and scientific challenges to be surmounted?

The very first question to be addressed is to define exactly what the question or issue is and then determine the most appropriate approaches to reach an answer. This is not to say that the answer can be preempted, for the outcome of true research can not predicted for the obvious reason that if it could, there would be little point in proceeding with the research. E-technology by its very nature has the potential to provide both the answer and /or the means to getting the answer.

A number of examples directly applicable to obstetrics and gynecology could be envisaged and are listed below. As contrasted with some of the "high tech" branches of medicine for example complex surgery, internationally, the practice of obstetrics and gynecology often occurs in remote and low technology environments where communication and transport are major factors to be considered. It is in these very settings that electronic technologies would be expected to play an increasing role in these examples.

GOVERNANCE AND STANDARDS OF PRACTICE

Obstetrics, gynecology and women's health is a branch of health care involving nursing, midwifery and medicine, which lends itself to guidelines, protocols and clinical systems. This is because much of scope of practice in reproduction involves normal processes such as birth or screening for disease and disease prevention. The traditional disease model of health care only applies to a small part of the whole such as in reproductive tract cancers. This means that reproductive health care does fit well with a systems approach to providing health care.

Example 1.

Teaching and learning	web based learning access to information and teachers
Communication	clinical conferencing, imaging
	Electronic retrieval of results
Clinical practice	structured care,eg risk assessment algorithms
	guidelines development
	Access to guidelines/protocols
	robotic surgery
	Fetal monitoring
Screening	clinical service
	Audit of screening programmes
Quality Improvement	institution of quality cycle
Decision making	decision analysis

Any system of health care provision requires governance and clinical governance may be defined as:

"a framework through which organisations are accountable for continuously improving the quality of their services and safeguarding high standards of care by creating an environment in which excellence in clinical care will flourish".(http://www.rcog.org.uk/index.asp?PageID=75)

The Royal College of Obstetricians and Gynaecologists (RCOG) has identified three groups of standards of good medical practice under the categories of professional, institutional and training. The RCOG statements and guidelines on governance and clinical standards provide a basis for the organization of care provision and the standards that should be aimed for. Whilst these were developed with in a British context, the principles are applicable generally. Well designed, accessible care, which is receptive to the needs of the women and families who are the "customers" is vital in obstetrics and gynecology. Outcomes are poor where women do not have access to care at all or where the care is deemed to be substandard for reasons as defined by the groupings above.

The leading cause of poor outcomes for women internationally is discrimination against women, recognized very early in the development of the United Nations and the history and current progress of the Convention on the Elimination of All forms of Discrimination against Women is available for all to read at http://www.un.org/womenwatch/daw/cedaw/ All health services need to have standards and a system of governance which could be compared with standards available such as those from the United Kingdom.

The purpose of audit of outcomes and comparison with accepted standards, a process termed quality improvement, is to educate and enhance outcomes for individuals and the health care system as a whole. A very effective quality improvement process for obstetricians and gynecologists, but applicable for generally is illustrated on the RANZCOG website at http://www.ranzcog.edu.au/fellows/pdfs/prcrm/Quality_cycle_050628.pdf.

Understanding this process permits both small and large quality improvement projects to be done and can be an effective audit tool.

Healthy outcomes of mother and fetus-neonate are obviously the aim and hope for every pregnant woman and her family. Unfortunately for biological as well as health care reasons this aim is not always achieved. Auditing the outcomes of mothers and babies has been a very important indicator of maternity health and many countries have detailed and often high quality reporting systems to document maternal and perinatal mortality and increasingly morbidity as indicators of quality. The reports produced by such audit systems are generally privileged, that is can not be used as legal evidence, and serve to educate and effect change with the intention of improving care. Great Britain has one of the most comprehensive and longest established systems now called the Confidential Enquiry into Maternal and Child Health (CEMACH) http://www.cemach.org.uk/.

The CEMACH Report "Saving Mothers Lives: reviewing maternal deaths to make motherhood safer (2003 – 2005)" is made accessible through a number of sites including http://www.rcog.org.uk.

The RCOG summary of the report stated

"Direct causes (deaths by pregnancy or birth)

- *Thromboembolism*
- *Sepsis*
- *Pre-eclampsia*
- *Amniotic fluid embolism*

There was a decline in deaths from haemorrhage, anaesthesia and uterine trauma.

Indirect causes (deaths from pre-existing or new medical or mental conditions aggravated by pregnancy)

- *Heart disease (there is a growing incidence of heart disease caused by poor dieting, smoking, alcohol consumption and obesity)*

The report also identifies the risk factors for maternal deaths. The links between vulnerability and social exclusion and adverse pregnancy outcomes are once again drawn. A major reason such women are more at-risk is because many do not seek antenatal care or stay in regular contact with maternity services. The range of complex non-medical problems which these women are subject to include domestic abuse (14%) and substance abuse (11%). The children of vulnerable women were also reported to have a higher risk of death or morbidity. There is therefore a need for medical and social support to be provided to these women and their children.

The report identifies avoidable factors which led to the deaths in most cases. These include a lack of cross-disciplinary team or inter-agency working, communication problems and lack of senior staff presence in the labor ward."

This report highlights some of the emerging trends that will challenge obstetrics in the future such as obesity, drug dependence which includes smoking and alcohol and other "avoidable" factors which may relate to the woman's social circumstances amongst other reasons. Previous reports and other discussion have identified the risks of the increasingly high caesarean section birth rates in many parts of the world and the implications of that for future pregnancy.

The information contained in clinical reports, which is increasingly available on line, can guide practice improvements all around the world. One of the limitations currently of electronic media remains accessibility both due to dissemination,

that is coverage of the networks and the restrictions of data handling caused by small slow internet connections. In many parts of the world such as the Pacific, e-mail and other electronic forms of data transfer can only be completed at very slow speeds such that large data files simply cannot be accessed. This has limited the ability to use the internet both for communication and as a teaching and learning tool. The lesson from this is that the implementation of "e-technologies" requires knowledge of local facilities if novel solutions to improve health outcomes are to be used.

THE FUTURE IN AN E-TECHNOLOGY ENVIRONMENT

Predicting the future shape of the traditional discipline of obstetrics and gynecology would seem to be almost an impossible or at least an unwise exercise, but research directions do inform likely directions. What then are possible future trends in obstetrics that new technologies can materially enhance? In the developed world with increasingly demanding expectations and at the same time increasingly rigorous economic demands for effective and efficient health care, risk evaluation and care tailored to assessed risk is likely to guide antenatal care. Risk factor analysis and individualizing care perhaps using neural networks to categorise patients is a distinct way forward in pregnancy management. In the developing or low resource environment, where the low risk die due to lack of basic services, structured care and protocols administered by trained health care personnel rather than traditional birth attendants would appear to be the way that maternal and perinatal mortality will be reduced and in some settings this is already happening.

In gynecology, almost anything imagined from dissemination of protocols to remote robotic surgery is feasible. In both obstetrics and gynecology there is increasing emphasis on screening and disease prevention and in women's health, screening, contraception, safe sexual practices are all activities which are occurring in the primary care community rather than in hospital and an e technology environment facilitates all aspects of these services to women.

Underpinning all the advances will be enhanced audit and quality improvement as well as evidence based practice and research led teaching training and clinical work. Use of all forms of electronic media in e-learning and in clinical medicine needs audit to ensure that the technologies being proposed best suit the applications for which they are being used. Electronic storage and retrieval not only will permit better data review and audit but will also facilitate clinical research by identifying important trends and focusing investigations appropriately.

Whilst no technology is a substitute for sound clinical practice, this introduction and the remaining chapters will illustrate how widely e technologies can play an important part in Women's Health and can improve outcomes in all settings but in different ways depending on the situation.

REFERENCES

Chalmers, I., Enkin, M., & Kierse, M. J. N. C. (1989). *Effective Care in Pregnancy and childbirth.* Oxford: Oxford University Press.

Cochrane, A. L. (1979). 1931-1971: A critical review, with particular reference to the medical profession. In *Medicines for the Year 2000.* London: Office of Health Economics.

de Boo, H. A., & Harding, J. E. (2006). The developmental origins of adult disease (Barker) hypothesis. *Australian & New Zealand Journal of Obstetrics & Gynecology, 46,* 4-14.

Liggins, G. C., & Howie, R. N. (1972). A controlled trial of antepartum glucocorticoid treatment for prevention of the respiratory distress syndrome in premature infants. *Pediatrics, 50*(4), 515-525.

Loudon, I. (2000). Maternal mortality in the past and its relevance to developing countries today. *American Journal of Clinical Nutrition, 72(suppl),* 241S–246S.

Macdonald, D., Grant, A., Sheridan-Pereira, M., Boylan, P., & Chalmers, I. (1985). The Dublin randomized controlled trial of intrapartum fetal heart rate monitoring. *American Journal of Obstetrics and Gynecology, 152,* 524-539.

Prendiville, W. J., Elbourne, D., & McDonald, S. (2001). Active versus expectant management in the third stage of labour *Cochrane Library,* (Issue 4).

ADDITIONAL READING

International Views - http://who.int/en/

Safe motherhood - http://www.unfpa.org/

safe abortion - http://www.figo.org/

International Midwifery - http://www.internationalmidwives.org

Antenatal Care-normal pregnancy - http://www.nice.org.uk

Guidance index for Obstetrics and Gynecology - http://www.nice.org.uk/guidance/, index.jsp?action=byTopic

Clinical guidelines - http://www.rcog.org.uk, http://www.ranzcog.edu.au, http://www.acog.org, Evidence based practice - http://www.cochrane.org

Heavy Menstrual Bleeding - http://www.nzgg.org.nz

KEY TERMS

Antenatal: Strictly defined means before the birth, but is taken to include the period from the confirmation of the pregnancy until the commencement of labor.

Antepartum Hemorrhage: Any bleeding from the genital tract after the gestation at which birth becomes recorded instead of miscarriage up until labor begins. Bleeding before this period is a form of miscarriage such as "threatened" miscarriage

Chromosome: The structures which hold the genes. The genes are the "goods" in the "suitcase", the chromosome is the suitcase. Humans have 23 pairs of chromosomes, that is 46 chromosomes, 23 from the mother and 23 from the father. The father provides the Y chromosome in the male fetus.

Ecbolic: A medication or drug which causes the uterus (womb) to contract (squeeze down) after the birth and delivery of the placenta. Such drugs reduce the blood loss following birth and thereby reduce postpartum hemorrhage.

Ectopic Pregnancy: A pregnancy which has implanted in any place except the uterine cavity. Most commonly, such pregnancies implant in the Fallopian tubes, which carry the fertilized egg from the area of fertilization at ovarian end of the tube to the uterus. Rarely the ectopic pregnancy may implant in other places such as the ovary, the pelvic cavity or on other abdominal organs.

Doppler Ultrasound (in Obstetrics): The use of spectral analysis of the Doppler shift obtained from blood flow in the fetal circulation to describe placenta vascular resistance or cerebral blood flow.

Infertility: Defined as inability to achieve a pregnancy after one year of unprotected sexual intercourse; a condition that may affect up to 1 in 5 couples at some stage in their relationship.

Embryo: The early baby up until 8 weeks from the last menstrual period (on a 28 day menstrual cycle) or 6 weeks from conception.

Fetus: The baby from the end of the embryonic period until birth.

Gene: The code of life, the code for the cell to manufacture proteins and other substances necessary for cellular function. There are around 20,000 genes in the human genetic code or genome.

Incontinence: The involuntary loss or passage of urine or flatus or faeces from the body

There are typically two main types of urinary incontinence:

- stress, which tends to have an anatomical basis due to changes in the bladder supports and the pelvic floor due to both pregnancy and childbirth
- urge incontinence which is usually due to an uncontrolled desire to pass urine due to an overactive or "irritable" bladder

Involution: The return of the reproductive organs and the genital tract to a non pregnant state after birth. Certain changes such as the shape of the cervix and the pigment around the nipple of the breast are usually permanent.

Labour: The process of changes in the genital tract and specifically the uterine contractions which lead to the expulsion of the conceptus (baby-fetus and "afterbirth" – placenta)from the mother.

Menopause: Strictly the time when the woman cease to have periods, i.e., menstruation. Loosely used to describe the period of time that not only the periods become infrequent and stop but also the woman has other changes due to reducing ovarian hormones as the ovaries no longer produce eggs each month. The time over which the woman undergoes the many changes related to ovarian failure including changes in mood, sleep, bone and other tissues is termed the climacteric.

Miscarriage: (no longer called spontaneous abortion as abortion has come to imply induced abortion or termination of pregnancy) Is when the early pregnancy fails to continue to grow and develop after implantation and /or after a positive pregnancy test.

- There are a number of forms of miscarriage ranging from loss of a very early pregnancy detected only by a positive pregnancy test but where an intrauterine pregnancy is never seen through to a fully formed embryo of fetus, which dies in the uterus and may or may not spontaneously miscarry. Miscarriage initially referred to the actual passage of the early pregnancy from the uterus through the genital tract and was accompanied by vaginal bleeding and cramping pains. With the advent of modern pregnancy tests and ultrasound scans, pregnancies are diagnosed much earlier hence the different categories of miscarriage nowadays.
- There are varying definitions in terms of the length of a pregnancy at which death of the pregnancy and passage of the pregnancy tissue is termed a miscarriage. Most countires in the Western world have a definition of a miscarriage which includes pregnancies up to 20 weeks (New Zealand, or 24 weeks United Kingdom for example) after which the passage of the fetus is recorded as a birth.

Parturition: The process of giving birth. Parity is the number of episodes of parturition.

Preeclampsia: Strictly means the condition which precedes eclampsia which is derived from the Greek and means a generalized convulsion related to the condition preeclampsia.

Preeclampsia is a multiorgan or multi system disorder unique to pregnancy (and for practical purposes unique to humans) which leads to generalised vasoconstriction and organ damage usually temporary. The cause is unknown but is associated with intravascular inflammation. The woman may present with high blood pressure (hypertension) protein in the urine (proteinuria) abnormal blood tests such as liver functions, kidney functions or clotting test abnormalities. There may also be fetal problems such as poor fetal growth. Often early delivery is needed as ending the pregnancy is currently the only true "cure".

Prostaglandins: Natural and synthetic hormones based on a fatty acid structure. These are potent causes of changes in the tissues in the genital tract. They cause softening of the cervix and uterine contractions. Synthetic analogues are used to induce labor, cause medical abortion and treat postpartum hemorrhage.

Pueperium (puerperal): The period of time from the birth (including delivery of the placenta) until involution has taken place. Typically taken as 6 weeks as this is when the first menstruation will occur if the woman is not breastfeeding.

Postpartum Haemorrhage: Bleeding, after delivery, from the uterus (or the genital tract) of 500mls or in severe postpartum hemorrhage 1,000mls or more. The leading cause of maternal death worldwide.

Stillbirth: This is the birth of a baby which has died in the uterus (womb). Such births are recorded at differing gestational ages in different countries, so it is important to be aware of national definitions of stillbirth when attempting international comparisons. For example, in New Zealand a stillbirth is recorded after 20 completed weeks of pregnancy or at a weight of 401 grams if the gestation is unknown. In Australia, the definition is 22 weeks or 500grams and in Britain it is 24 weeks. Clearly, New Zealand has a higher stillbirth rate simply because of a different definition than other countries.

Chapter II
Women's Health Informatics:
The Ethical and Legal Issues

Premila Fade
Poole Hospital NHS Foundation Trust, UK

Anne-Marie McMahon
Poole Hospital NHS Foundation Trust, UK

ABSTRACT

Principlism (derived from common sense morality) is the most common theory used within the health-care sphere. The elements of this theory are explored and discussed in context. A theoretical woman presenting in pregnancy is used to identify issues which can arise and explore the potential conflicts. In the second half of the chapter, health informatics and the law are discussed. Issues such as consent, confidentiality, privacy, and human rights are discussed in general. Legislation in the United Kingdom, United States, Canada, Australia, and New Zealand are discussed in detail.

INTRODUCTION

The increasing sophistication of health informatics has brought significant benefits to women's health but the increasing storage and use of confidential data has brought new ethical dilemmas. On first glance it seems unlikely that data can have a moral dimension but the way that data is collected, stored and used does. Fundamental questions like: "Do patients need to know that we are collecting data about them?", "Who does the data belong to?" and "Who decides to what uses we can put that

data?" all need to be addressed. Information and information technology are central to the overall goal of healthcare- to promote health, but the information we use has significant medical, personal, and social implications for our patients and therefore we must find a moral justification for collecting storing and using it.

We start with a sentence or two about rights because they are the currency of the day. We then follow with a brief introduction to a number of important theories of ethics and a description of an approach to medical ethics called

'Principlism'(Beachamp & Childress, 2001)which we will use to analyse the kind of ethical dilemmas which may arise in the area of health informatics and women's health. You will not find absolute answers to all the questions you might have – that is not the nature of ethics. But this chapter should provide you with an understanding of the basic principles of medical ethics and how they can be used to help you find the best answer.

The law in each country is different and therefore this chapter cannot hope to cover all aspects relevant to all readers. However the major case law and statute law within the Common Law Jurisdictions of the UK, USA, Canada and Australia will be covered as well as the European Convention on Human Rights.

HUMAN RIGHTS AND HEALTHCARE

Man lives in society and therefore must live by rules established for the good of society. To protect individuals within society they are entitled to certain rights. Rights usually entail reciprocal obligations from the State.

A number of rights have been declared universal human rights by the United Nations, in Europe they appear in statute as The Human Rights Act. Generally these rights are negative i.e. rights of non interference e.g., Article 2 the right to life. Article 2 does not establish a right to limitless health resources to prolong life but does establish that every human being has a right not to be killed (unless sanctioned by the law of the country).

The problem is that more and more often individuals couch their rights in a positive way – to demand action from the State. Such rights only have moral force if the reciprocal moral obligation on the State also has moral force. An individual cannot claim a positive right unless every other member of society is also entitled to the same

right. So an appeal to rights does not always help us establish our obligations as healthcare practitioners. A patient may say "I have a right to know" but that does not necessarily translate into a duty to tell.

The individual who claims rights must also claim his obligations (e.g., to pay his taxes and obey laws). Within the therapeutic relationship the patient has certain moral rights: to be treated fairly and compassionately, but also has reciprocal obligations: to be honest with healthcare providers and not putting others in danger. It can also be argued that being in receipt of healthcare entails an obligation to help advance the science of medicine in order for it to benefit others.

MEDICAL ETHICS

Ethics is the branch of philosophy dealing with morality and medical ethics is that branch of ethics which deals with healthcare. Four of the most influential ethical theories are: deontology (which deals with duties), consequentialism (which deals in outcomes), virtue ethics (which concentrates on moral character) and feminist ethics (which puts all of the above into the context of caring compassion and relationships).

Deontology

Deontology has its roots in the Judaeo-Christian tradition but was given a basis in reason by Immanuel Kant. Kant believed that morality could be explained by one overarching absolute rational principle which he called the 'categorical imperative' (Kant, 1785). Deontologists argue that morality may be completely explained by duty. A duty is a rule to guide action. A simple example would be the duty to always tell the truth. Generally speaking many people would agree that telling the truth is the right thing to do. Yet, it is possible to think of a scenario where telling the truth would cause harm e.g. if a violent man demands to know the whereabouts of his wife and children who are in hiding. Hence we see that duties as moral guides may conflict and therefore cannot be absolute.

Consequentialism

In contrast Consequentialists argue that duty is irrelevant because morality is located in the outcome of an action. Probably the best known Consequentialist was Jeremy Bentham who proposed 'the principle of utility'(Bentham, 1789). Every action, he claimed, should be judged; according to how much it promotes happiness – 'the greatest happiness of the greatest number'. John Stuart Mills (Mills, 1861) refined the theory to include more than just happiness in the utility calculus; he described human flourishing as the goal of utilitarianism. The main criticism of Consequentialism is that it takes no account of the moral character of the action and therefore may lead to some very counter intuitive results. For example; if a patient is ill and suffering and asks for help to end their life the right course of action, if you are a Consequentialist is to help them to die (in fact it would be morally wrong not to kill the patient) because death will end to their suffering.

We expect the state and government to treat us all equally and therefore consequences often seem to acquire more moral force when more people are involved. Duties are important as guides for individuals but on a population basis utilitarian arguments are much more significant. For example the duty not to kill has less moral force the more lives are at stake (Smart & Williams, 1973). And, when a Government considers whether or not to fund health prevention programmes or expensive cancer drugs it must consider the overall health benefits of each alternative course of action.

Virtue Ethics

But, any conception of morality seems empty without a description of moral character. Aristotle (Aristotle, 350 B.C.) first expounded the idea of virtue. For Aristotle virtue was midway between two extremes of action and inaction e.g. courage is the mean between cowardice and recklessness. In order to decide rationally what is the virtuous action the agent must use reason. Virtue ethics has been updated since Aristotle (MacIntyre, 1985) but a major problem remains - it does not provide answers to moral questions. However, the idea that professionals should cultivate certain character traits - integrity, compassion, veracity, wisdom and fidelity is powerful. Professionals have knowledge which their clients or patients do not have; therefore the relationship is unequal and must be governed by certain rules of conduct and behaviour which we call professional ethics.

The Feminist Ethic of Care

To treat all men equally is a fundamental rule of egalitarian society but when it comes down to the individual it is uncomfortable to believe that we should not show preference for our loved ones. Traditional moral theory has concentrated on universal moral principles which apply equally to all moral agents but it is unrealistic to expect an individual not to take more account of his own or his family's happiness and wellbeing when deciding on the right course of action. This partiality that humans have for family, friends, themselves and members of their social group is addressed by the feminist ethic of care theory, which argues that rationality alone cannot adequately explain or guide our actions, and that caring, compassion and relationships must be taken into account in moral decision making (Tong, 1998). Humans live in social groups and show partiality for family and friends. If this did not happen society would disintegrate and therefore moral theory must take account of this reality.

Principlism

Common sense morality (i.e. moral intuition) which takes a little from every theory mixed in with cultural and religious factors may be good enough to guide an individual through most ethical dilemmas. However when moral intuition does not give an acceptable answer some kind of structure is necessary to understand what is morally important in one situation and link it to another situation. There are various ways in which this can be done but since no single theory of morality seems adequate to the task I am instead going to use the 'Principlism' approach of Beachamp and Childress (Beachamp & Childress, 2001) to examine a few of the ethical dilemmas posed by health informatics in women's health.

Principlism is not a theory of ethics; it is a form of applied ethics derived from common morality which gives us a structure to look at real problems, to identify the morally significant factors and to weigh up the pros and cons of various options. It allows us to take into account duties and consequences and also individual and relationship factors which play a part in real life moral dilemmas. Principlism is not without its critics; it is argued that the principles are too broad to provide any real guidance and that they can be used to justify any conclusion. Beachamp and Childress counter this by arguing that the principles take moral shape though specification; a process by which moral rules are formed to create a coherent moral universe. Although not a comprehensive moral theory (but then no one theory seems to provide all our answers anyway), Principlism is nonetheless a useful tool to use to work through moral dilemmas

First we need to explore the principles and understand how they should be applied. Central

to this approach to medical ethics is the idea of professionalism or professional virtues. The principles in themselves have no guiding force unless interpreted with wisdom, compassion and integrity. Nor are they understandable unless we have a belief in our professional duty to our patients. Central to the therapeutic relationship are veracity (truth telling) trust (confidentiality), and fidelity (loyalty). The four principles are: respect for autonomy, justice, nonmaleficence and beneficence. There is no ranking of the principles; they have equal moral status.

RESPECT FOR AUTONOMY

Autonomy essentially means self rule. This is a fundamental tenet of western society –that man is free to pursue his own goals, to live his life as he chooses and to have jurisdiction over his own body. It does not mean merely freedom or liberty; it also means the exercise of reason and choice. However our autonomy is limited everyday – we limit it ourselves by making foolish decisions (e.g. when drunk), it is limited by society for our protection (e.g. wearing seat belts) and it is limited by society for the protection of others (e.g. the criminal justice system).

Within the sphere of medicine we show respect for autonomy by involving patients in decision-making, this means telling the truth and giving them the information necessary to make informed choices. Autonomy is not absolute; patients cannot demand healthcare which is not clinically indicated. However, they can refuse healthcare and are free to make (what we may consider to be) unwise or foolish decisions.

Justice

There are three components to justice in medical ethics: lawfulness, rights and fairness.

1. **Lawfulness.** Professional ethics requires all healthcare professionals to act within the law.
2. **Rights.** Certain rights are believed to be universal (e.g. the right to life), while others vary dependant on social and cultural environments (e.g. privacy laws in different countries). Most individuals attach significant moral force to the concept of rights but in general rights only have a negative value (a right to non interference) and do not impose a positive duty on another (person, persons or profession) or on the state to provide help or resources. The right to healthcare is not universal and not unfettered even where healthcare is free at point of need.
3. **Fairness.** When considering any ethical dilemma the notion of fairness demands that the healthcare professional give thought to the interests of society in general and other individuals in particular (if those other individuals are intimately involved in the situation). Generally, these interests will be outweighed by the professional's duty of care to their patient but they are an important consideration particularly in public health policy and where other person(s) are at risk of significant harm through the action or inaction of the patient. Further whenever we use healthcare resources we must consider how our practice impacts on the whole health economy.

Beneficence

Our primary motivation as healthcare professionals is 'the good' or 'the benefit' of our patients. However it cannot be the only principle governing our actions. In the past doctors have been accused of paternalism; of considering they always knew what was best for the patient. But, what we consider to be good for the patient may not be what the patient considers to be in their best interests.

So, beneficence has to be constrained by respect for autonomy which can only be achieved by involving patients as fully as possible in medical decision making. Beneficence for our patient must also be balanced against the interests of society. If doing good for our patient will cause harm to others (direct or indirect) this must be taken into account in deciding the correct course of action. Beneficence also includes a consideration of the wider good – it can be argued that the benefit to society of increasing medical knowledge or improving medical practice morally outweighs the loss of privacy of the individual when their health information is used for audit or research.

Nonmaleficence

Nonmaleficence is the obligation not to cause harm. The obligation not to cause harm is generally considered more stringent than the obligation to help prevent harm but healthcare professionals have a legal and ethical duty of care to their patients which includes not causing and preventing harm. To do no harm has equal but not more moral force than beneficence. Often the treatment we prescribe has harmful effects as well as benefits. Although statistically the benefits outweigh the harms, for the individual concerned we do not know which will predominate. Only the fully informed patient can decide if the benefits outweigh the harms of the treatment. Each individual will have different priorities and may weigh up the facts differently. Beneficence to our patient may also need to be balanced against nonmaleficence to other patient(s):- If treating our patient and respecting their confidentiality will cause harm to another person(s) then the benefit to our patient has to be weighed against the harm to the other person(s). If the harm outweighs the benefit then the duty of confidentiality may have to be broken.

To highlight a number of the ethical dilemmas around consent, confidentiality and ownership of data in health informatics we are going to consider what issues might come up during an antenatal clinic visit. Our hypothetical patient is called Susan.

CONSENT AND DATA COLLECTION

Susan a 35 year old pregnant female attends her first antenatal clinic. The doctor tells her he is going to take some blood for some routine tests and asks Susan if she would like an HIV test. Susan asks why she needs to be tested; she does not consider herself to be at risk of HIV. The doctor explains that HIV screening is offered to all women in pregnancy.

HIV screening is now offered to all pregnant women in many countries. This is because research has shown the potential health benefits of screening to both the mother and child. The research involved unlinked anonymous testing of antenatal women in the 1990's (Nicoll et al., 1994) using blood from routine antenatal blood tests to ascertain the prevalence of HIV in pregnant women. The women were not consented or told that their blood would be tested for HIV. The data was stored anonymously, women and their caregivers had no access to the data, and the data was unlinked, so even if access had been permitted no individual would have been able to get their result. Cases of HIV were diagnosed but not assigned to an individual. The rationale for this approach was that information was needed on prevalence to calculate the cost benefit analysis of routine screening.

Screening programmes are public health programmes; their ethical justification is the overall health benefit to the community. In order to justify a screening programme for HIV in pregnancy certain criteria must be met:

1. The screening test must be sufficiently sensitive and specific;
2. Effective treatment must be available;
3. Screening must be cost effective.

In order to ethically justify unlinked anonymous testing we must be satisfied that the moral significance of the loss of autonomy of the individual is insignificant compared to the potential benefits to the community of the knowledge gained. There is no benefit accrued by the individual taking part in anonymous unlinked screening, and there is no physical harm as long as there is genuine doubt as to the benefits of screening. However, the issue of harm is more complex; individual liberty is compromised every time something is done to us without our permission even if we are unaware of it. Our privacy is compromised if data is collected about us. This deprivation of privacy can only be justified if the overall benefit to society (justice) significantly outweighs the harm to the individual. Clearly this argument is only valid if testing is anonymous, unlinked, and solely for the purpose of determining whether a benefit exists. It would not be ethically justifiable to hold data about an individual which significantly affected their health and not tell them about it under any other circumstances.

HIV infection is a diagnosis with enormous social and health implications. However the medical justification for testing is strong: If a woman is HIV positive the chance of passing HIV to her foetus is up to 30% without intervention but with intervention it may be reduced to 1% (Giles, Mijch, Garland, Grover, & Hellard, 2004). Because the benefits of treating women in pregnancy are now well established routine screening is offered to all pregnant women in most countries. Specific consent is required for HIV testing because of the social implications of a positive diagnosis. The significance attached to consent correlates to the seriousness of the decision the patient must make. In contrast the assumption of consent is made for certain other tests, including hepatitis B and syphilis, both of which have serious health implications but less social stigma attached to them. The logic of implicit consent lies in the reasonable expectations of a pregnant woman seeking healthcare; to protect herself and her baby from harm.

Consent is important because it is a way of showing respect for the patient's autonomy. Informed consent requires the patient to be given all the information they require, in a way they can understand and must be free from undue influence from third parties. Sometimes this can be extremely challenging if the woman does not speak English or comes from a male dominated culture. It may be the issue cannot be raised on the first antenatal visit and it may be that novel ways of imparting information and communicating confidentially need to be devised. The challenge is to show respect for your patient and their culture, whilst at the same time endeavouring to maximise the chances of a successful pregnancy (beneficence). It may be that getting an HIV test is less important than gaining the trust of the pregnant woman and her family so that they maintain contact with healthcare services throughout the pregnancy (nonmaleficence).

Appropriate consent for an HIV test must include an explanation of why the test is necessary and what the implications of a positive result are for the patient, her unborn baby and any sexual partners. When Susan is consented for an HIV test she should be also reassured that her test result will remain secure and confidential. Health information such as HIV status is particularly sensitive and must therefore be treated and stored with extra vigilance. Specific consent also needs to be granted by the patient before sharing this information with others including other healthcare providers. Sharing of patient data for the purposes of patient care is often routine – the potential benefits to the patient greatly outweigh any possible harm but, where the information is particularly sensitive, explicit consent should be sought (see below) because the risk of harm to the patient from unauthorised access to this data is much greater.

Data Storage

The doctor then asks Susan if she has had any previous pregnancies or any other significant past medical problems. Susan tells the doctor she had an abortion age 16 but asks him not to document this in the antenatal notes because her family and partner are not aware of the abortion.

Information taken from a patient in the course of a consultation is routinely documented in the healthcare record. In general consent to recording of information is implied by consent to the consultation. Often antenatal notes are held by the patient. Other information e.g., blood tests results and x-rays may be available on hospital IT systems. All of this data must be stored securely and treated confidentially because confidentiality is central to the therapeutic relationship between patient and healthcare provider. Patients will only tell us all we need to know about them if they trust us and we promote their trust by keeping their confidences. So we see the duty of confidence is derived from the principle of beneficence- in order to act in the patient's best interests we must respect their confidentiality. Patient information should only be shared within the healthcare team where it is necessary to do so for the healthcare needs of the patient. Electronic storage must be password protected with different levels of access depending on professional need.

Some information is considered to be especially sensitive (e.g., HIV status, sexually transmitted diseases and psychiatric notes). This information is often held separately from the patient record to ensure confidentiality. This can have significant implications for the healthcare team which may not have all the relevant healthcare information they require to make the right clinical decisions. For example data on termination of pregnancies (TOP) is considered sensitive and is usually stored separately from the rest of the healthcare record to ensure patients' privacy. This data is therefore not available automatically to the doctor in antenatal clinic. This information is important because previous TOP increases the risk of preterm labour. Women often attend antenatal clinic with their current partner and may be reticent to discuss previous terminations or may not see them as relevant to the current pregnancy.

There is a tension between doing what we consider best (beneficence) for our patient (which relies on having available all the relevant information) and respecting their privacy. Even inadvertent loss of privacy by allowing sensitive information to be available in the healthcare record where others can see it may have catastrophic personal consequences for the patient (e.g. if a partner finds out about a previous termination of pregnancy) and significant implications for the therapeutic relationship. If there is a loss of trust the patient may decide not to access healthcare in the future or may choose not to be honest about their medical history, both of which may compromise their future health (nonmaleficence).

On balance it is better to encourage communication in a safe environment where the patient can be open about their medical history rather than risk the confidentiality of sensitive information by making it more widely available. It would be prudent to reassure Susan that information about her TOP will not appear on her healthcare record nor will it be divulged to anyone outside the healthcare team.

Sharing Data

Susan notices a poster on the wall of the antenatal clinic which advises that anonymized patient data may be used for audit and clinical governance purposes. However, she is not told that details of her age and pregnancy are being logged for a prospective audit of hysterectomy rates in the hospital.

Data which is recorded for one reason is often used for another. All healthcare institutions have a duty to promote best practice and clinical ex-

cellence. This can only be done by using patient information to measure actual practice against gold standards. Patients are often unaware that data about them will be used for this purpose. Research in the UK into patients' knowledge of how their data is used and attitudes towards use of their data showed that most were comfortable with health professionals having access to their data but felt that information used for purposes other than healthcare should be anonymized (NHS Information Authority, The Consumers association, & Health Which, 2002). Interestingly patients are generally more concerned about who uses their data rather than what it is used for: patients trust health professionals to treat their data confidentially but are less trusting of clerical workers, administrators and managers (Whiddett, Hunter, Engelbrecht, & Handy, 2006).

Consent for this sharing of data is generally regarded as implicit to the provision of healthcare, but the justification for considering it to be so is not clear. Patients generally understand that we do tests to find out what is wrong with them therefore we do not need to ask for specific consent for all tests. However, since it is clear that patients are not always aware that information about them (their information) will be used for purposes other than their healthcare, respect for our patients' autonomy suggests we should ask their permission to use their data.

The ethical issues become clearer if we use the principles: First, nonmaleficence. – No harm is done to the individual by using their anonymized data as long as it is only used for the advancement of healthcare. Second, beneficence. – The patient has nothing to gain directly from the use of their data but they do gain (better healthcare) from the use of patients' data in audit and research. Third, justice. – As we said earlier individuals have rights (e.g. the right to receive healthcare) and obligations, one of which could be a duty to promote the advancement/ improvement of healthcare by allowing their data to be used for this purpose. Sharing of data could be seen as part of an implicit therapeutic bargain that patients make when they access healthcare. Finally, autonomy. – Respect for our patients' right to self determination suggests we should ask their permission to use their data. Autonomy does not automatically trump the other principles but our previous discussions on autonomy have demonstrated the importance of consent.

The use of Susan's anonymized data for audit and research is ethically justifiable but she should be informed that information about her pregnancy may be used for these purposes. It is unclear whether patients read posters but the empirical evidence suggests many patients are not aware of how their data is stored and used. If extra data (not required for the purposes of her healthcare) is required purely for research purposes, then explicit informed consent should be taken.

Genetic Information

Susan asks the doctor if she needs antenatal testing for genetic disease. Her estranged sister recently had a late termination but she does not know why. She is not aware of any family history of inherited disease.

Genetic information is at the same time individual and shared. When an individual attends a genetic clinic a comprehensive family tree is devised. The patient gives information about their extended family often without the family members' explicit consent. So although the information given is not all personal to the individual and can not be said to be owned by the individual, the data gathered during the consultation and information from genetic tests are governed by the rules of confidentiality. Therefore the healthcare professional is bound by this duty not to disclose information to a third party unless there is an overwhelming imperative to do so, usually couched in terms of significant risk of serious harm. This is a high threshold and involves a careful risk assessment. Some ethicists have argued that the way round this problem is to view genetic

information as different and therefore not subject to the usual rules of confidentiality. Parker and Lucassen (Parker & Lucassen, 2004) talk about a 'joint account' of genetic information where the default position is that genetic information should be shared with family members unless there is a good reason not to.

In the UK guidelines developed by The Joint Committee on Medical Genetics (Royal college of Physicians, Royal College of Pathologists, & British society for Human Genetics, 2006) state that information on a family pedigree does not belong to one person and can be shared between health professionals treating different members of the family without explicit consent. This is because the information one family member gives may highlight that another family member is at significant risk of being affected by or of being a carrier of genetic disease. It is good practice to inform patients that the information they give may be shared in this way. Confidentiality does however govern the use of specific test results which cannot be passed onto other family members or their physician without their permission. If permission is not forthcoming then this duty of confidentiality can only be broken if there is significant risk of serious harm. The guidelines suggest that when consent is obtained for genetic testing it should be obtained for sharing the results with other family members so that the issue of breaking confidentiality is avoided as much as possible. It is essential that patients understand the full implications of genetic tests including the issue of paternity. As in all other areas of medicine communication and information are the benchmarks of good practice.

Susan's obstetrician has a duty to avoid harm to her and her baby and to act in her best interests. Susan should be encouraged to talk to her sister and other family members. It may be the abortion was performed for a chromosomal abnormality rather than an inherited genetic condition. Susan's obstetrician will need to consult her sister's doctor; who will have to make a decision on how much information to divulge after assessment of the risk to Susan's baby and after consultation with Susan's sister. Justice requires confidentiality to be broken if there is a significant risk of serious harm to Susan's baby.

PATIENT ACCESS TO OUTCOME DATA

Susan is nervous about having an amniocentesis because a friend had a miscarriage after having the procedure. She asks to see data on the doctor's miscarriage rates before she will agree to the procedure

All hospitals collect data on clinical outcomes (e.g., length of stay and mortality). This data can be analysed in a number of ways including (e.g., by age of patient, by principle diagnosis, or by attending physician). The primary purpose of this data collection is financial - to ensure the hospital is paid for the work it has done. But in several countries Freedom of Information Acts mean this data is now available to the public. League tables have been devised showing variations in length of stay, hospital acquired infection rates and mortality rates between hospitals. It is argued that, in order for patients to make a choice about healthcare they should have access to all this data.

The real challenge is making this choice meaningful. To make an informed choice patients need to have access to outcome data that is meaningful. Outcome data is influenced by patient selection. A surgeon who chooses only to operate on low risk patients will have better outcome figures than a surgeon who specialises in high risk procedures. Complication rates are often presented as a percentage e.g. for amniocentesis the accepted miscarriage rate is 1%(Tabor et al., 1986) above the background rate. But this can vary due to pure chance or due to case mix – if an obstetrician does more high risk pregnancies (rate of chromosomal anomalies) then the risk of

miscarriage is higher because the background risk is higher.

To comply with professional registration and regulation Doctors are required to show evidence of good practice in line with standards drawn up by their professional associations. This includes monitored practice, feedback from colleagues and patients and benchmarking statistics which compare individuals' practice and outcomes. This data could also be used to inform patient choice. Some professional bodies have already decided to publish patient survival data. For example the UK Society for Cardiothoracic Surgery in conjunction with the UK Healthcare Commission have developed a website where survival rates for individual units and surgeons (adjusted for case mix) can be viewed by the public (Healthcare Commission, 2007).

A number of important questions arise:

- Should this data also be available to all patients to inform their choice?
- Do the health professionals have any rights over how this information is used?
- If all outcome data is available to patients how can we be sure they will be able to understand and interpret it correctly?
- Does this entail another duty to our patients – to explain the data?
- How will we train colleagues and what effect will being a trainer have on our outcome data?

Allowing a patient to access outcome data in order to make an informed choice about healthcare maximises autonomy, but only if the data is robust and fully understood by the patient. Choice is generally good but only if the patient feels guided and is not overwhelmed with information. If data is published it must be explained in easily understandable lay terms. Information is not a substitute for trust. Not all patients wish to make choices, but they do all want good healthcare. A healthcare professional's duty of care involves not only giving information but also giving advice. This advice already includes interpreting evidence based medical data, so it is not fair to extrapolate that advice to include interpretation of other outcome data.

It is important to not be swayed wholly by the autonomy argument – the other principles are equally important considerations in healthcare. It would perhaps be better to ensure all healthcare professionals achieve a minimum acceptable standard with rigorous professional monitoring rather than publication of crude figures which are open to statistical manipulation. However some professional groups may consider publication of their data if they are allowed to decide what data is relevant and control the analysis of the data.

Healthcare professionals have a right to be treated fairly so any data published about them must be accurate and put into the appropriate context. It would not be fair to publish raw data without showing how case mix and other factors impact on outcome. Justice also requires us to think about the overall 'good' for our health services – the next generation of specialists need training and research and innovation are essential. Any data collection and publication must not stifle either process.

Susan should be advised that the doctor doing the amniocentesis is appropriately trained and his/her practice appropriately monitored.

HEALTH INFORMATICS AND THE LAW

There are now greater demands than ever for more integrated health information systems to support rapid advances in epidemiological and health economics research. In response to those demands, increasingly sophisticated technology is evolving to support the collection, processing and management of personal (and often sensitive) clinical data. However, as technology evolves and the ability to access information

is opened up, the risk of inappropriate access (whether intentional or accidental), the manner in which information is processed, or the nature or context in which it is used (or even disposed of) may pose a threat to confidentiality rights, civil liberties and human rights. This opens up not only an ethical dilemma for the clinician and all those involved in the processing of data, but also a legal dilemma in terms of responsibilities and constraints on practice. There are national and local guidelines, policies and protocols in place in each jurisdiction to govern and regulate practice, but more importantly there are statutory regulations by which we must abide. Before we look at statute law we should understand the legal foundations of consent and confidentiality which are fundamental to any discussion of the doctor-patient relationship, medical practice generally, and our handling of patient information.

Consent

Anything we do to patients including recording their personal information can only be done with their consent. Our ethical duty to respect self determination is echoed in the law: "*Every human being of adult years and sound mind has a right to determine what shall be done with his own body; and a surgeon who performs an operation without his patient's consent commits assault...*" Judge Cardozo 1914 ("Schloendorff v New York Hospitals", 1914) This respect for self determination over rides the principle of the sanctity of life ("NHS Airdale Trust v Bland," 1993) and applies not only to bodily integrity but also to freedom of thought and mind. It is generally agreed that a person's personal information belongs to them and should therefore only be shared with their consent unless there is an overwhelming reason to disclose the information without consent (i.e. the public interest) – for more detailed discussion see next section.

The law recognizes two forms of consent: implied and express. The form consent takes should be proportional to the gravity of the consequences of the action. Implied consent is generally acceptable for routine medical consultation including the recording of personal information, general physical (but not intimate) examination and routine investigations. Consent is implied by the cooperation of the patient.

Express or explicit consent is required for more invasive investigations and treatment, intimate investigations and, investigations or treatments with significant social consequences e.g. treatment for sexually transmitted diseases or testing for HIV. For express consent to be valid the person giving consent must be adequately informed, have the capacity to consent and be free from duress or undue influence (M. Stauch, K. Wheat, & Tingle, 2006a).

It is argued that implied consent is enough for the routine recording of personal data. However, implied consent only covers what is reasonable for the patient to understand and is implied by their co-operation. It is reasonable to expect that a patient will understand that their personal data will be used for their healthcare but it is we know unreasonable to expect a patient to know that her data may be used for other purposes (Beachamp & Childress, 2001; Tong, 1998).

Consent only applies to confidential data, once data is processed and anonymous, it no longer belongs to the individual, and therefore the legal requirement for consent no longer applies. Therefore it is lawful for healthcare organizations to collect health-care data on length of stay, diagnosis and mortality etc without patients' consent as long as the data collected does not have the characteristics of confidential information (see next section).

As we will see later most data protection and privacy laws require consent, but what is not entirely clear is the form this consent should take. UK NHS guidelines make it clear that explicit consent must be sought for *"using their personal information in ways that do not directly contribute*

to, or support the delivery of, their care."(NHS, 2003).

CONFIDENTIALITY

The categorization of data as confidential is dependent on the quality of information (e.g. patient identifiable data), and the way in which the information is obtained and subsequently managed. The various laws in each country afford protection for the subject of the data or information, but also give guidance and provide safeguards for those involved in the process of health informatics. This is because if legal constraints were too onerous, the efforts of researchers, practitioners and data managers would be severely hindered by an unhealthy culture of caution.

It is generally understood that when a patient seeks advice and treatment from health care professionals she consents to the process of collecting, documenting and sharing of her personal information for the purpose of her healthcare. It is also recognised that because such information is of a sensitive nature the patient should enjoy the privilege of utmost confidence. Therefore a duty of confidence is imposed on all persons involved in the collection, processing and management of confidential data. The justification for this duty is well articulated by Raanon Gillon (Gillon., 1986):

"The commonest justification for the duty, of medical confidentiality is undoubtedly consequentialist: people's better health, welfare, the general good, and overall happiness are more likely to be attained if doctors are fully informed by their patients, and this is more likely if doctors undertake not to disclose their patients' secret. Conversely if patients did not believe that doctors would keep their secrets then either they would not divulge embarrassing but potentially medically important information, thus reducing their chances of getting

the best medical care, or they would disclose such information and feel anxious and unhappy at the prospects of their secrets being known."

The legal duty of confidentiality is clearly defined by Lord Goff: *"I start with the broad general principle... that a duty of confidence arises when confidential information comes to the knowledge of a person (the confidant) in circumstances where he has notice, or is held to have agreed, that the information is confidential, with the effect that it would be just in all the circumstances that he should be precluded from disclosing the information to others."* ("AG v Guardian Newspapers (No. 2, 1990, p. 281).

Lord Keith added that a duty of confidentiality arose out of certain relationships including the doctor patient relationship (AG v Guardian Newspapers No. 2, 1990, p. 255).

The obligation of confidentiality is neither easily defined nor absolute. In basic terms, there are three justifications in law for the disclosure of confidential information: patient consent, public interest or statutory requirements. In situations where a public interest is at stake, the duty of confidence may be broken (e.g. reporting an outbreak of a communicable disease for the health and safety of the public). The public interest argument is a utilitarian one and is stated clearly by Lord Goff: *"...although the basis of the law's protection of confidence is that there is a public interest that confidences should be preserved and protected by law, nevertheless that public interest may be outweighed by some other countervailing public interest which favours disclosure."* ("AG v Guardian Newspapers, No. 2, 1990, p. 282).

In the UK a number of statutory provisions positively require disclosure of confidential information in the interests of public health (e.g. the Public Health Act 1984); or to allow the administration of justice (e.g. the Road Traffic Act 1998.) Furthermore, section 60 of the Health and Social Care Act 2001 allows the Secretary of State to make regulations *"requiring and*

regulating the processing of prescribed patient information for medical purposes as he considers necessary and expedient: (a) in the interests of improving patient care; or (b) in the public interest;" whilst the Health Service Regulations 2002 allow for the creation of disease databases e.g. cancer registries which include confidential patient information (M. Stauch, K. Wheat, & Tingle, 2006b). Such provisions are likely to be similar in other jurisdictions.

Privacy

Some confusion arises between the specific duty to respect a confidence and the somewhat broader duty to respect individual privacy. The obligation to preserve privacy is arguably more onerous as it overlaps with human rights. Almost every country now includes and describes a right to privacy in its constitution or legal system. There is no absolute right to privacy in UK law but provision for privacy is made within domestic interpretation of the European Convention on Human Rights (ECHR)(European Court of Human Rights, 2007) via the Human Rights Act (1998) – namely the 'right to a private life' (Article 8). This legislation applies to the handling of medical and personal information. In the USA the general right of privacy is recognized in common law and the Fourth and Fifth Amendments of the Constitution. In Canada both the Constitution and Charter of Rights and Freedoms do not recognize an explicit right to privacy (Canadian Charter of Rights and freedoms, Part 1 of the Constitution Act, 1982, Schedule B to the Canada Act 1982(United Kingdom), 1982) but privacy is regulated at both federal and provincial levels with personal health information being incorporated into privacy laws in 2002 (Federal Privacy Act and Personal Information and Electronic Documents Act (PIPEDA) 2001, 1982). Australian privacy laws allow individuals to exercise rights and choices about handling of data in the public and private sector (The (Commonwealth) Privacy

Act 1988 (as amended by the Privacy Amendment (Private Sector) Act 2000, 1998), and in New Zealand similar provisions for privacy are incorporated within The Privacy Act.

Human Rights

A chapter on the law and ethics of health informatics would not be complete without a discussion about human rights. Article 12 of the United Nations Universal Declaration of Human Rights 1968 states that: *"No one shall be subjected to arbitrary interference with his privacy, family, home or correspondence, nor to attacks upon his honour and reputation. Everyone has the right to the protection of the law against such interference or attacks."*

Gross violations of human rights have in the past occurred during research and experimentation. Particularly horrifying experiments occurred in the Nazi concentration camps. At the Nuremburg trials the Judges articulated a set of ethical principles (The Nuremburg Code) to prevent such abuse of human rights from occurring again. This was followed in 1964 by the World Medical Association's Declaration of Helsinki (amended 2000). Most countries now have in place a mechanism for the rigorous ethical review of all proposed research. Further consideration of research ethics is beyond the scope of this chapter but Human Rights will be considered in relation to health informatics generally.

Firstly it is important to realise that few rights are absolute. It would be inaccurate to claim that there are no circumstances in which interference can be justified in the interests of the state. Most of the core rights are subject to limitation and qualification. For simplicity, within this text, human rights are considered in relation to the European Convention on Human Rights (ECHR). Confidential information is protected by Article 8 of the ECHR:

(8.1) Everyone has the right to respect for his private and family life, his home and correspondence

(8.2) There shall be no interference by a public authority with the exercise of this right except such as in accordance with the law and is necessary in a democratic society in the interests of national security, public safety or the economic well-being of the country, for the prevention of disorder or crime, for the protection of health or morals, or for the protection of the rights and freedoms of others

Essentially, there is an obligation not only to refrain from interference, but also to provide effective respect for a private life, and therefore failure to recognize the nature of confidential information or support patient privacy may constitute a breach of the Convention Right. A fair balance must be struck between competing interests of the community. Disclosure of personal information without consent by State authorities will amount to a breach of right to respect for a person's 'private life' unless the conditions in Article 8(2) are satisfied. There is a reasonable expectation of privacy where information is obviously private or, where, as in the opinion of Lord Hope disclosure would be *"highly offensive to a reasonable person"*. [a] In Z v Finland ("Z V Finland," 1998) the European Court of Human Rights stated clearly that *"the protection of personal data, not least medical data, is of fundamental importance to a person's enjoyment of his or her right to respect for private and family life as guaranteed by Article 8 of the Convention."*

However, healthcare practitioners may be consoled by the fact that there is legal protection if data is sufficiently anonymized and its' use is strictly controlled. The Department of Health (UK) produced guidelines which suggested that disclosure of anonymous patient data to a third party would still breach the duty of confidentiality. This was successfully challenged in the Court of

Appeal by 'Source Informatics'. 'Source Informatics' purchased anonymized patient prescribing data from GPs for commercial reasons (to obtain information on doctors' prescribing habits to sell on to pharmaceutical companies). The Court of Appeal ruling concluded that because the data was anonymized patient identity was not revealed and therefore a privacy right was not violated.[b]

What if an individual requests right of access to personal data held on them by the State? Data protection and privacy statutes guarantee rights of access to the individual. The Access to Health Records Act 1990 (UK) was a direct result of a challenge in the ECHR.[c] The applicant was a man who had been brought up in the care of a local authority. On reaching adulthood he sought access to childhood case records because he wished to sue the authority for negligence in their child-care duties. The local authority permitted him access to 65 documents (out of a total 352). He successfully asserted that refusal to allow access to the remaining files constituted a breach of his Article 8(1) rights to privacy.

DATA PROTECTION

There is considerable overlap in terms of the legal provisions between the jurisdictions. There are a number of core principles that apply generally and directly to data in terms of its use, collection and dissemination. The Organization for Economic Co-operation and Development (OECD) Guidelines have been influential in shaping many of the data protection laws.[d]

The OECD Guidelines set out eight basic principles:

1. **Collection:** Data should only be collected for a defined purpose.
2. **Quality:** Consent should be obtained for data collection. Data collected should be accurate.

3. **Purpose:** Data subjects should be informed of the purpose for which information will be used. Researchers must adhere to specific guidelines concerning the process of data collection, use and dissemination.
4. **Use:** Data should be used for a legitimate purpose in line with legislation. Data should be kept for the minimum period necessary. Data should be destroyed if no longer required.
5. **Security:** Where possible data should be anonymized or names substituted for unique identifiers with a secure code held separately. Data must be secure, password protected and only accessible to healthcare professionals for the purpose of clinical care, audit or research which has been granted ethical approval. Rules of access must allow individuals to apply to see information kept about them.
6. **Openness:** Data should be processed and used fairly.
7. **Individual participation:** Individuals involved in data collection have a responsibility to adhere to principles of practice laid down in legislation;
8. **Accountability:** Member countries are expected to incorporate the recommendations within domestic law and appoint data commissioners or information officers to oversee compliance with obligations.

HEALTH INFORMATICS AND LEGISLATION

UK

The European Directive 95/46/EC on Data Protection was adopted by the Council of Europe in October 1995 for implementation by October 1998. One of its more important purposes was to safeguard 'the fundamental rights of individuals'

Figure 1. Key principles of the DPA 1998

SCHEDULE 1

1. Personal data shall be processed fairly and lawfully and, in particular shall not be processed unless:
   (a) at least one of the conditions in Schedule 2 is met, and
   (b) in the case of sensitive personal data, at least one of the conditions in Schedule 3 is also met.
2. Personal data shall be obtained only for one or more specified and lawful purposes and shall not be further processed in any manner incompatible with that purpose or those purposes.
3. Personal data shall be adequate, relevant and not excessive in relation to the purpose or purposes for which they are processed.
4. Personal data shall be accurate and, where necessary, kept up to date.
5. Personal data processed for any purpose or purposes shall not be kept for longer than is necessary for that purpose(s).
6. Personal data shall be processed in accordance with the rights of data subjects under this Act.
7. Appropriate technical and organisational measures shall be taken against unauthorised or unlawful processing of personal data and against accidental loss or destruction of, or damage to, personal data.
8. Personal data shall not be transferred to a country or territory outside the European Economic Area unless that country or territory ensures an adequate level of protection for the rights and freedoms of data subjects in relation to the processing of personal data.

in line with provisions of human rights legislation. The Directive requires that Member States establish a set of principles and incorporate them into domestic legislation thereby providing a mechanism of regulation for users of personal information. In essence, the legislation obliges users of personal information to comply with provisions, confers rights upon individuals to gain access to information held about them, and makes provision for the supervision and enforcement of the legal obligations via the appointment of a Data Protection Officer (or Commissioner).

The UK implemented the Directive via enactment of the Data Protection Act 1998 (DPA) and the main provisions came into force 1 March 2000. The 1998 Act covers manual and electronic records and includes all health records thereby incorporating the more stringent provisions on the processing, storage and disposal of sensitive personal data. There are additional provisions

and rules concerning the transfer of personal data outside the European Community territory.

The DPA contains 8 key principles within Schedule 1 (Figure 1) that are applicable to maintenance of electronic personal data. Schedule 2 (Figure 2) provides conditions relevant for the purposes of the first principle (i.e., processing of personal data) and Schedule 3 relates to processing of sensitive data (The Data Protection Act, 1998). 'Personal data' relates to living persons who may be identified as a result of that data, whereas 'Sensitive Personal Data' includes information on racial or ethnic origin and physical or mental health of the data subject. Accordingly, there are more stringent and detailed provisions on the processing of sensitive personal data that focus on the rights and freedoms of the data subject.

Current UK guidance says that any legislation which sets aside the obligation of privacy must be compatible with the Human Rights Act

Figure 2. Relevant conditions for purposes of processing of any personal data (DPA 1998)

SCHEDULE 2. (abbreviated by the author)

1. Consent to the processing of data is given by the data subject.

2. Processing is necessary –
    a.   for performance of contract to which data subject is a party or,
    b.   where at the data subject request steps are taken with a view to entering a contract.

3. Processing is necessary for compliance with legal obligations to which the data controller is subject (excludes contractual obligations).

4. Processing is necessary to protect vital interests of the data subject.

5. Processing is necessary for:
    a.   administration of justice
    b.   exercise of function conferred on persons by or under any enactment
    c.   exercise of any functions of the Crown, Minister of the Crown or government Department
    d.   exercise of any functions of a public nature – exercised in the public interest by any person.

6.1 Processing is necessary for the pursuit of legitimate interests by the data controller, a third party or parties to whom the data is disclosed. Exceptions are if processing is unwarranted by reason of prejudice to rights, freedoms or legitimate interests of the data subject.

6.2 Secretary of State may specify circumstances in which this condition (6.(1)) is, or is not, considered satisfied.

and therefore must: pursue a legitimate aim, be considered necessary in a democratic society and be proportionate to need.

USA

In the USA The Health Insurance Portability and Accountability Act (1996), better known as HIPAA, addresses many areas of the healthcare data processing including data storage and recovery. The primary goal of the legislation is to assure proper protection and allow a flow of health information for the purpose of promoting health. HIPAA covers all personally identifiable health information. This includes information received or stored in electronic, paper, or even oral form and there is no limitation period for the protection.

Key safeguards are summarised below (Figure 3). The legislation categorises provisions relating to administrative, physical and technical responsibilities. The HIPAA Privacy Rule additionally requires health care providers and healthcare professionals to comply with its standards and to ensure contingency plans for recovery of lost data and protection from malicious software systems. Furthermore, encryption and decryption mechanisms are required (Office for Civil Rights, 2006). The Privacy rule is enforced by the Office for Civil Rights [OCR] of the Department of Health and Human Services (HHS). Enforcement of the Privacy Rule began April 14, 2003. Over the last four years, HHS has improved the privacy practices of covered entities through its enforcement program.

Figure 3. Key HIPAA Data Security Rules

(Summarised by author)

1. **Access to medical records** - Patients generally should be able to see and obtain copies of their medical records and request corrections if they identify errors and mistakes. Access to records is generally within 30 days of request.
2. **Notice of privacy practices** - Health care providers (under HIPAA) must provide a notice to their patients on how they may use personal medical information and their rights under the new privacy regulation.
3. **Limits on use of personal medical information** – Personal health information (PHI) may be shared among providers to provide quality treatment. Generally, information should not be used if not in relation to health care without consent.
4. **Prohibition on marketing** - Restrictions and limits on the use of patient information for marketing purposes. Pharmacies, health plans and other covered entities must first obtain an individuals specific authorization before disclosing their patient information for marketing.
5. **Stronger state laws.** – State law requiring disclosure in public interest will override the federal protection.
6. **Confidential communications**- A reasonable compliance with the principle of confidentiality is required.
7. **Complaints** - Formal complaints may be filed directly to the provider and information regarding the process of filing such complaints should be included in the notice of privacy practices.

Canada

There is both federal and provincial regulation of privacy within Canada: the 1982 Federal Privacy Act and the 2001 Personal Information and Electronic Documents Act (PIPEDA) (Personal Information and Electronic Documents Act (PIPEDA), 2001). Health information was excluded from the provisions of PIPEDA until January 2002 and in January 2004 provisions were extended to all organizations that collect, use or dispose of personal information. There are 10 overarching principles to consider here (summarised in Fig. 4) reflecting the OECD Guidelines.

Additional professional guidance in specific relation to the matter of health informatics is given by COACH (Canadian Organization for Advancement of Computers in Health) COACH was established in 1975 and is dedicated to promoting clearer understanding of health informatics within the Canadian health system. Although not within the legislative framework, it affords some very relevant guidance and provides professionals with a framework to minimize risk, maximize integrity and protect privacy for all personal health information. Most recent guidelines for protection of health information were published in 2007.

Australia

In Australia the Australia Privacy Act 1988 focuses solely on protection of personal information. There are 11 principles which regulate each stage of the information cycle starting with initial collection of personal information and ending with its erasure or disposal.

The OECD Guidelines form the foundation for the Information Privacy Principles (IPPs) and the National Privacy Principles (NPPs) set out in the Privacy Act. The IPPs cover the public sector and the NPPs cover the private sector.

Figure 4. The 10 Overarching principles of PIPEDA

```
1. Accountability – Appointment of a Privacy Officer and development of information
   policies outlining privacy protection clauses
2. Identifying purposes – Consent must be obtained from the data subject and a
   reasonable rationale for collection of information should be documented.
3. Consent – Must be meaningful and 'informed'
4. Limiting collection – No indiscriminate collection of data and avoidance of deceitful
   or misleading techniques to obtain data.
5. Limiting use and disclosure – Data must have a purposeful use and disclosed only in
   accordance with guidelines on privacy. This includes destruction and anonymization
   of data that no longer holds a 'useful' purpose.
6. Accuracy – Information must be accurate and updated where appropriate.
7. Safeguards – Technical and administrative considerations should ensure access and
   security is safeguarded by policies and procedures.
8. Openness – Policies should be easily understood and made readily available.
9. Individual access – Individuals must be allowed access to records and such requests
   documented.
10. Challenging complaints – Fair and impartial investigative procedures must be
    documented and handled sensitively by appropriately trained personnel.
```

New Zealand

New Zealand's Privacy Act was enacted in 1993 and amended several times most recently in 2002. It regulates collection, use and dissemination of personal information held by any agency and includes both public and private sectors. There are 12 privacy principles based on OECD guidelines and Australia's Privacy Act. The Act is primarily concerned with personal information handling practices.

The Privacy Commissioner of New Zealand has published a guide which explains the provisions of the Health Information Privacy Code (adopted in 1994) (New Zealand Privacy Commissioner, 1994). The guide is designed to assist health agencies in dealing with personal health information, whether they collect, hold or use personal data. Especially useful are the chapters on disclosing information to third parties.

A summary of the key legislation, websites and some of the case law cited in the text with some additional resources are included for quick reference in Figure 7.

CONCLUSION

Each person involved in health care, in every jurisdiction, region, hospital, clinic, pharmacy and community health programme has a responsibility for the protection of health information, and for the protection of the information systems that enable us to deliver quality health services. A number of rules and principles are common to all data protection privacy laws. There are also safeguards in place for practitioners and those involved in the overall process of health informatics. Confidentiality and security issues should pose concerns for researchers and information technology support staff. Clinicians must be aware of their obligations to the patient whenever they ask for, receive, document and use patient information. More attention should to be paid to the issue of consent for the taking, using and recording of patient data. Where ethical dilemmas arise they can be analyzed by reference to the four principles: beneficence, non maleficence, justice and respect for autonomy. Where the principles conflict (which, as we have seen they often do)

Figure 5. Australia Privacy Act principles

1. **Collection:** How and when personal health information may be collected, purposes of collection, consent.
2. **Use and disclosure:** How and when personal health information may be disclosed, consent.
3. **Data quality:** Completeness and accuracy of personal health information.
4. **Data security and data retention:** How and for how long records must be kept, destruction of records.
5. **Openness:** Providing advice to consumers regarding privacy arrangements and consumer rights.
6. **Access and correction:** How consumers may access information in their health record and responsibilities for incorporating corrections.
7. **Identifiers:** Issues about the use of record numbers, Medicare and DVA numbers etc.
8. **Anonymity:** Consumers have a right to request anonymous consultation "where it is lawful and practical".
9. **Trans border data flows:** Regulates transfer of personal health information to locations that may have less privacy protection for consumers than Victoria.
10. **Transfer or closure of the practice of a health service provider:** Provisions that ensure practice patients are adequately advised of changes to the situation of the practice where previously available healthcare will no longer be available.
11. **Making information available to another health service provider:** Regulates disclosure of personal health information to another healthcare provider on request of the patient.

Figure 6. New Zealand Privacy Act principles

Principles 1-4 - Govern the collection of personal information. This includes the reasons why personal information may be collected, where it may be collected from, and how it is collected.

Principle 5 – Storage of personal information must be designed to protect personal information from unauthorised use or disclosure.

Principle 6 - Individuals have the right to access information about themselves.

Principle 7 - Individuals have the right to correct information about themselves.

Principles 8-11 - Place restrictions on how people and organisations can use or disclose personal information. These include ensuring information is accurate and up-to-date, and that it isn't improperly disclosed.

Principle 12 - Governs how "unique identifiers" – such as IRD numbers, bank client numbers, driver's licence numbers and passport numbers – can be used.

Figure 7. Key legislative provisions and electronic sources relating to privacy laws and data management

General Information on Privacy laws:

Organization for Economic Cooperation and Development (OECD) especially the Report on the Cross Border Enforcement of Privacy Laws at: http://www.oecd.org

---

UK and Europe

Legislation:
Freedom of Information Act 2005
The Health Service (Control of Patient Information) Regulations 2002 SI 2202 No.1438.
Health and Social Care Act 2001
Human Rights Act 1998
Data Protection Act 1998
Access to Health Records Act 1990
European Directive 95/46/EC

Professional Codes and Guides:
Confidentiality NHS Code of Practice November 2003

Websites:
http://www.echr.coe.int/ECHR/EN
http://www.dh.gov.uk/en
http://www.freedomofinformation.co.uk/
http://heartsurgery.healthcarecommission.org.uk

Case law
Campbell v Mirror Group Newspapers Lt [2004] 2 AC 457, [2004] 2 All ER 995
R v Department of Health ex parte Source Informatics Ltd [2000] 1 All ER 786;
(2000) 52 BMLR 65; [1999] 4 All ER 185; (1999) 49 BMLR 41
Z v Finland (1998) 25 EHRR 371
AG v Guardian Newspapers (No 2) [1990] AC 109
Gaskin v United Kingdom (1989) 12 EHRR 36; [1990] 1 FLR 167 ECtHR

USA

Legislation:
Health Insurance Portability and Accountability Act (1996) (HIPAA).
Standards for Privacy of Individually Identifiable Health Information, 45 CFR Parts 160 and 164 (promulgated under HIPAA 1996, PL 104-191

Websites:
http://www.hhs.gov/ocr/hipaa/privacy.html
http://www.hhs.gov.foia/ (US Department of Health and Human Services Freedom of Information page)

Canada

Legislation:
Personal Information and Electronic Documents Act 2001 (PIPEDA).
Canadian Charter of Rights and Freedoms , Part 1 of the Constitution Act 1982, Schedule B to the Canada Act 1982 (United Kingdom) 1982 c.11,s.8.
Federal Privacy Act 1982.

continued on following page

Figure 7. continued

Websites:
http://laws.justice.gc.ca/en/charter
http://www.coachorg.com   (Canadian Organization for Advancement of Computers in Health (COACH) established 1975
http://www.privcom.gc.ca (Privacy Commissioner of Canada homepage)

Commonwealth of Australia

Legislation:
The (Commonwealth) Privacy Act 1988 (as amended by the Privacy Amendment (private Sector) Act 2000).
Australia Privacy Act 1988

Websites:
http://www.privacy.gov.au
http://www.health.gov.au/healthconnect

Case law:
Australian Broadcasting Corporation v Lenah Game Meat Pty Ltd (2001) 185 ALR 1;

New Zealand

Legislation:
Health Information Privacy Code 1994.
The Privacy Act 1993
Bill of Rights Act 1990

Websites:
http://rangi.knowledgebasket.co.nz/gpacts/public/text/2002/an/073.html
http://privacy.org.nz

a balancing process has to take place. The principles are designed to be used as a structure to allow ethical dilemmas to be compared and moral rules constructed.

Finally it is worth restating the idea conveyed earlier in the chapter: The principles in themselves must be interpreted with wisdom, compassion and integrity, and healthcare professionals must maintain an unwavering dedication to the virtues of professionalism.

REFERENCES

AG v Guardian Newspapers (No 2), 109 1990.

Aristotle. (1999). *Nicomachean Ethics*. Hackett Publishing Indianapolis.

Beachamp, T. L., & Childress, J. F. (2001). *Principles of biomedical ethics 5th edition* Oxford University Press.

Bentham, J. (1789). *The principles of morals and legislation.*

Canadian Charter of Rights and freedoms, Part 1 of the Constitution Act, 1982, Schedule B to the Canada Act 1982(United Kingdom) 11 (1982).

The (Commonwealth) Privacy Act 1988 (as amended by the Privacy Amendment (Private Sector) Act 2000 . (1998).

The Data Protection Act. (1998). from http://www.opsi.gov.uk/acts/acts1998/ukpga_19980029_en_1

European Court of Human Rights. (2007). The European Court of Human Rights. Retrieved 1st June 2008, 2008, from http://www.echr.coe.int/echr/en/bottom/contact/

Federal Privacy Act and Personal Information and Electronic Documents Act (PIPEDA) 2001., (1982).

Giles, M. L., Mijch, A. M., Garland, S. M., Grover, S. R., & Hellard, M. E. (2004). HIV and pregnancy in Australia. *Australian & New Zealand Journal of Obstetrics & Gynaecology, 44*(3), 197-204.

Gillon, R. (1986). *Philosophical Medical Ethics* (p. 108). Chichester: John Wiley.

Healthcare Commission. (2007). *Heart surgery in the United Kingdom.* Retrieved June 2008, from http://heartsurgery.healthcarecommission.org.uk

Kant, I. (1785). *Groundwork of the metaphysics of morals*

MacIntyre, A. (1985). *After Virtue, 2nd edition.* Duckworth Press

Mills, J. S. (1861). *Utilitarianism.*

New Zealand Privacy Commissioner. (1994). Health Information Privacy Code 1994. Retrieved June 2008, from http://www.privacy.org.nz/health-information-privacy-code-1994/

Confidentiality NHS Code of Practice (2003).

NHS Airdale Trust v Bland 1993).

NHS Information Authority, The Consumers association, & Health Which. (2002). *Share and Care! Peoples views on consent and confidentiality of patient information.*

Nicoll, A., Hutchinson, E., Soldan, K., McGarrigle, C., Parry, J. V., Newham, J., et al. (1994). Survey of human immunodeficiency virus infection among pregnant women in England and Wales: 1990-93. *Communicable Disease Report. CDR Review, 4*(10), R115-120.

Office for Civil Rights. (2006). Office for Civil Rights - Privacy of Health Records. Retrieved June 2008, from http://www.hhs.gov/ocr/hipaa/privacy.html

Parker, M., & Lucassen, A. (2004). Genetic information: A joint account? *BMJ, 329*, 165-167.

Personal Information and Electronic Documents Act (PIPEDA), (2001).

Royal college of Physicians, Royal College of Pathologists, & British society for Human Genetics. (2006). *Consent and confidentiality in genetic practice: Guidance on genetic testing and sharing genetic information. Report of the Joint Committee on Medical Genetics.* London: RCP, RCPath, BSHG.

Schloendorff v New York Hospitals. (105 NE 92 1914).

Stauch, M., Wheat, K., & Tingle, J. (2006a). *Text, cases and materials on medical law 5th Edition* Routledge Cavendish .

Stauch, M., Wheat, K., & Tingle, J. (2006b). Chapter 5. In *Text, cases and materials on medical law chapter 5th Edition 2006*: Routledge Cavendish.

Smart, J., & Williams, B. (1973). *Utilitarianism: for and against.* Cambridge University Press.

Tabor, A., Philip, J., Madsen, M., Bang, J., Obel, E. B., & Nørgaard-Pedersen, B. (1986). Randomised controlled trial of genetic amniocentesis in 4606 low-risk women. *Lancet, 1*(8493), 1287-1293.

The Knowledge basket. (2002). The Privacy Act 1993. Retrieved June 2008, from http://gpacts.

knowledge-basket.co.nz/gpacts/public/text/2002/
an/073.html

Tong, R. (1998). The ethics of care: A feminist virtue ethics of care for healthcare practitioners. *Journal Medicine and Philosophy, 23*, 131-152.

Whiddett, R., Hunter, I., Engelbrecht, J., & Handy, J. (2006). Patients' attitudes towards sharing their health information. *International Journal of Medical Informatics, 75*(7), 530-541.

Z V Finland, 371 (EHRR 1998).

ENDNOTES

[a] See : *Campbell v Mirror Group Newspapers Ltd* [2004] 2 AC 457, [2004] 2 All ER 995 and the reasoning of Lord Hope based on the concept from *Australian Broadcasting Corporation v Lenah Game Meats Pty Ltd* (2001) 185 ALR 1 cited in: *Mason & McCall Smith's Law and Medical Ethics* J K Mason & G T Laurie   (7th edition) Oxford University Press (p. 262-263)

[b] *R v Department of Health, ex parte Source Informatics Ltd* [2000] 1 All ER 786, (2000) 52 BMLR 65 [1999] 4 All ER 185, (1999) 49 BMLR 41

[c] *Gaskin v United Kingdom* (1989) 12 EHRR 36, [1990] 1 FLR 167, ECtHR

[d] See especially : Report on the Cross Border Enforcement of Privacy Laws at: http://www. oecd.org

Section II
Information Management Applications

Chapter III
Coding and Messaging Systems for Women's Health Informatics

David Parry
Auckland University of Technology, New Zealand

ABSTRACT

Recording information about symptoms, observations, actions, and outcomes is a key task of health informatics. Standardization of records is vital if data is to be used by different groups, and transferred between organizations. Originally, coding focused on causes of death and other outcomes. Such systems include the international classification of diseases (ICD). However, more recently the need to allow communication between health organizations has encouraged the development of standards such as health level seven (HL7). Further work has focussed on vocabularies such as systematic nomenclature of medical terms (SNOMED), which allow standardised recording of any health-related information. Coded data is necessary to allow computers to assist in decision making and for audit purposes. With the rapid development of computer networks and the Internet, there has been a growing effort to include semantic information with computer data so that the meaning of the data can be bound to the data store. The chapter discusses these standards and the areas that are undergoing rapid development.

INTRODUCTION

"We need three types of clinical information standards: document structuring standards; term lexicons; and ontologies"(Gardner, 2003)

Coding and messaging systems allow the standardisation and systemisation of information storage and transmission in healthcare. They al-
low the accurate and structured representation of information which can be used to impart a common understanding. The aim of this chapter is to introduce some of these systems along with the theory that underlies them and the uses to which they are put. These approaches are particularly important in women's health informatics for a number of reasons:

- In pregnancy it is common for women to be cared for by a number of healthcare professionals, and communication between them should be precise and efficient
- Past outcomes and complications often have a great influence on the care plans for women in subsequent pregnancies, and this information is much more effective if standardised. Information recorded in previous pregnancies may be useful for risk prediction if presented in a suitable format.
- Government agencies and healthcare organisations require accurate and extensive information in order to fulfil their information needs. Information relating to births has been collected for centuries, and improvement in morbidity and mortality can only be noted with standardised recording.
- Funding and fee for service are often related to the case mix of the institutions providing the care.
- Health Surveillance and audit of outcomes is particularly important for screening programmes and also to understand long-term trends such as the general rise in operative deliveries.
- Research in the area of women's health often requires re-examination of clinical records generated in the past. Accurate coding allows the selection of suitable records and patients for research studies as well as linkage between history, intervention and outcomes.
- An exciting area of research is the development and use of decision support tools that use historical data to provide patients and clinicians with guidance concerning the likely outcome of clinical decisions and the natural history of disease. This sort of decision support is covered in more detail in Chapter XV.

For all these reasons, coding of clinical events, diagnoses and interventions is an important part of an information system designed to support women's health.

At it's heart, coding is a systematic and reproducible method of recording pertinent information for the improvement of management of healthcare. Messaging involves the transmission of healthcare information in a standardised and efficient format within and between information systems that are involved in the care of people.

In terms of system efficiency, coding can dramatically reduce the amount of data stored, and also increase the usefulness of this data for analysis. However the coding process is demanding and requires care and understanding of the principles of the coding system being used.

The next section of this chapter gives some background to the development of modern coding and messaging system. The main varieties of coding systems in use currently (ICD, READ, DRG) are described in the coding systems section. Messaging systems are then described including health level 7 (HL7) and Digital Imaging and Communications in Medicine (DICOM). More complex and complete systems for recording information including some controlled vocabularies such as SNOMED and ontologies are then described. Finally a discussion of the state of the art, and some future areas of development is contained in the final section.

BACKGROUND AND HISTORY

Medicine has grappled for many years with the need to have efficient means of communicating data about patients, diseases and treatments. From the time of Hippocrates, writing down clinical information has been a major part of health care. Comparison between patients, and agreement on diagnosis and symptoms requires agreed recording and communication standards. Medical language has been sometimes seen as a barrier between professionals and lay people, but precision and flexibility are vital even if a private language appears to be in use. Precision and comprehensibility are not mutually exclusive. When computers are involved the need for standards becomes even more important despite valiant efforts over many years in attempting to teach computers to understand natural language (Rosenfeld, 2000). Indeed medical work can be seen as concerned primarily with information communication, storage and transformation. Unambiguous and precise communication of information is vital and a major issue in healthcare (Coiera & Tombs, 1998).

Coding clinical observations has a long history in women's health, for example the "Bishop Score" (Bishop, 1964), derived as a scoring system using various observations in order to aid decision making in induction of labor.

A very precise and often formalised natural language, including a large number of specialised words and compounded terms is taught to clinicians in training. This allows precise description of anatomical features, symptoms etc. and also the construction of new descriptors by combination of existing ones. Although this process is dynamic, for example the term "Gestational proteinuria and hypertension" has recently replaced "Pre-Eclampsia" in many units it does not usually cause difficulties in communication. However, the general tendency as in many fields is to avoid ambiguity rather than encourage standardisation. Thus, a great many synonyms are used and often the preferred term is different in different specialities or countries. This issue makes data processing related to medicine difficult, and for that reason a large number of coding systems have been proposed and a number are currently in use. Ultimately, any coding system is based around an ontology – although this may not be made explicit to the user of the system.

There are 3 main types of coding system:

1. Hierarchical systems with fixed codes or terms determined by some central body, for example the International Classification of Disease version 10 (ICD10) (World Health Organization, 2001). In most cases these systems allow a patient to have membership of more than one code simultaneously, although many systems, such as Diagnostic related groupings (DRG's) require the identification of a Primary ICD diagnosis code. Sometimes membership of more than one lowest level code in the same branch is not allowed. Medical Subject Headings (MeSH) are another example of this type of coding system (U.S. National Library of Medicine, 2001).

2. Format-based systems, that specify the allowed format without giving a complete lexicon of the terms – for example the health level 7 (HL7) messaging system. Interestingly the 3rd version of this standard is beginning to include semantic information and standards. (Health Level Seven Inc)

3. Vocabulary systems such as SNOMED that allow the construction of descriptors from primitive elements (American College of Pathologists, 2000).

Often only type 1 is given as a "true" coding system. However, such systems are less useful than the others at communicating a dynamic status, for example in the case where a patient's diagnosis is not yet definitive, or when symptoms may or may not be significant.

Semantics of Coding

Ultimately all coding systems attempt to represent clinical information in a way that can be understood by humans and/or computers. The job of coding involves a standardised representation of a particular significant piece of information. However coding systems are beginning to go beyond the concept of simply being controlled vocabularies or dictionaries, and instead focussing on the importance of meaning, and use. Much of this work can be linked to the concepts of "the semantic web"(Berners-Lee, Hendler, & Lassila, 2001), although work in the medical domain actually preceeded this initiative. As defined on the WWW consortium website (http://www. w3.org/2001/sw/) "The Semantic Web is about two things. It is about common formats for integration and combination of data drawn from diverse sources, where on the original Web mainly concentrated on the interchange of documents. It is also about language for recording how the data relates to real world objects". The semantic web, then involves being able to extract the useful data from complex documents that are generated from heterogeneous sources, and provide a method to allow this data to be analysed and made useful. It also allows data to be related to the real world.

In terms of practical implementation, sematic web research involves the manipulation transfer and analysis of documents written in a suitable format across the Internet.

In the context of healthcare, this means that all records, messages and documents can contribute to a picture of the state of the patients, without the need for overarching single electronic health record. The key to semantic interoperability is that the definitions for what things mean are common, if this is done then every piece of information around the patient can in theory be accessed as-

suming there are suitable procedures, controls and interfaces. In the case of the semantic web, this common understanding has been built on the basis of standard data type diagrams (DTD's) for XML documents, and some approaches such as HL7 level 3 are implemented in XML(Dolin et al., 2001).

A general model of the role of coding and semantics is shown in Figure 1.

Because observations can be converted to a standard form or code, many observations can be represented in a single document, and assuming that the mapping between observation and code is consistent, then a collection of documents can be represented within a world model.

Coding, Messaging and Workflow

By allowing consistent formatting and transmission of information, the process of transferring information between systems and users can be simplified. Coding of diagnosis for example, allows protocols to be set up that distribute information in a way that supports appropriate patient care. Thus coded data about symptoms, diagnosis or treatment can act as metadata to a fuller description of a current patient state, their likely prognosis and the protocols that need to

Figure 1. Data to knowledge

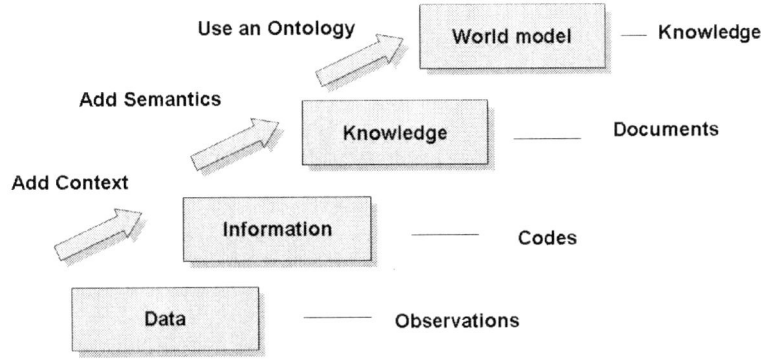

be followed to ensure appropriate care. For these reasons, early, accurate coding is important.

Traditionally coding has been a post-event activity, often based around the discharge summary, and performed by trained clinical coders. Associations of clinical coders such as the Professional Association of Clinical Coders PACC-UK (http://codeinfo.org/paccuk/index.html), and the American Association of clinical coders and auditors (http://codeinfo.org/paccuk/index.html). Post-event coding has the advantage that the diagnoses and procedures are more likely to be certain at this stage, and there may be written artefacts to guide the coder. This approach is particularly attractive when coding is primarily a source of information for reimbursement to the treating institution, as it allows a holistic view to be taken of activity, along with income from that activity. However the disadvantages of this approach include the fact that coded data is then not available to the clinical team during the

event, that mistakes or misunderstandings can be generated by the need of coders to interpret non-coded information, often from a wide variety of sources, and the disruption to clinical practice of having paper records being sent to the coding department.

As electronic health records have become more common, coding at the point of care, or near to the point of care has become attractive. This obviously reduces the time taken to produce codes, can reduce data storage requirements in clinical records, and can allow the codes to be used immediately in decision support applications such as PRODIGY(Wilson, Purves, & Smith, 2000) (now known as CKS). Disadvantages of this approach include the need to train clinical users in often complex coding schemes, the lack of time in many clinical encounters and the danger of propagating uncertain diagnoses through a system.

Accuracy of coding by non-experts can be improved by using specific paper templates or elec-

Figure 2. Choice of appropriate code

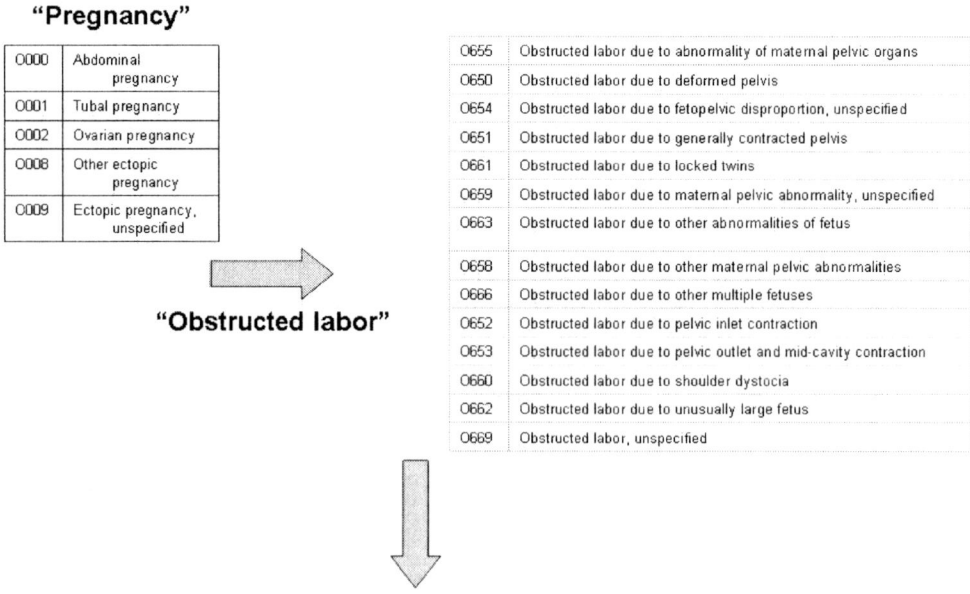

"Pregnancy"

O000	Abdominal pregnancy
O001	Tubal pregnancy
O002	Ovarian pregnancy
O008	Other ectopic pregnancy
O009	Ectopic pregnancy, unspecified

"Obstructed labor"

O655	Obstructed labor due to abnormality of maternal pelvic organs
O650	Obstructed labor due to deformed pelvis
O654	Obstructed labor due to fetopelvic disproportion, unspecified
O651	Obstructed labor due to generally contracted pelvis
O661	Obstructed labor due to locked twins
O659	Obstructed labor due to maternal pelvic abnormality, unspecified
O663	Obstructed labor due to other abnormalities of fetus
O658	Obstructed labor due to other maternal pelvic abnormalities
O666	Obstructed labor due to other multiple fetuses
O652	Obstructed labor due to pelvic inlet contraction
O653	Obstructed labor due to pelvic outlet and mid-cavity contraction
O660	Obstructed labor due to shoulder dystocia
O662	Obstructed labor due to unusually large fetus
O669	Obstructed labor, unspecified

O653 - Obstructed labor due to pelvic outlet and mid-cavity contraction

tronic systems to support selection of the correct code. These have been shown to produce results comparable with that of expert coders(Silfen, 2006). The time taken to code can also be reduced by using cascading menu approaches, where the user navigates through the hierarchy that is present in many codes such as Read or ICD10, for example choosing first the system or site and then being presented with intermediate context-sensitive choices. By using this approach, decisions on coding and the required precision can be made more easily with less risk of grossly inaccurate codes and a better understanding of the subtle differences between them (see Figure 2).

Users of Information

Clinical staff actually treating the patient are major users of information. In addition, there is a need for communication between hospital staff and community care professionals including GP's, Pharmacists and family planning professionals. Non-clinical cares including social services may also require information. Insurance companies, charity funders and governmental organisations require data in the form of activity reports and for statistical purposes. Obviously the patients themselves can use their own information Efficient and effective coding allows large scale databases to be constructed, which can be anonymised to allow statistical analysis, for example in terms of prescribing trends. An example of such a database is the UK General Practice Research Database (Walley & Mantgani, 1997). Similar databases can be used as sources of recruitment for clinical trials, or for audit purposes.

In the US a major user of coded information is the Medicaid system, and this has used Diagnostic Related Groups (DRG's) to identify the severity and hence expected cost of treatment of patients. Software –GROUPER – is used to convert diagnosis and procedure information into a DRG, in this case a case mix index. (CMI). Health care facilities can then calculate their actual costs,

compared to the reimbursement derived from funding sources.

Along with clinical and research uses coding assists with accurately describing the mix of patients being seen, auditing of the outcomes compared with other centres and estimation of effort. Other scoring systems measure the likelihood of survival in intensive care – for example APACHE, and have been shown to be good at predicting outcome (Beck, Taylor, Millar, & Smith, 1997), fortunately, although not specifically designed for women's health. There are a number of systems to measure nursing intensity or worklaod – for example the therapeutic intervention scoring system (TISS)(Keene & Cullen, 1983), although these systems are not necessarily very useful for calculating nurse/patient ratios (Adomat & Hewison, 2004).

Clinical staff can use historical coded information to audit their practice, as well as comparing their Casemix with other professionals and linking input to output. Pregnancy care is particularly interesting in this regard- especially in terms of the decision to intervene. The problem is difficult to analyse because outcomes for mother and baby are usually good whatever the decisions made. Essentially, if an intervention is made, comparison with a group where intervention has not been made is difficult because the outcome set is very unbalanced, with good outcomes in the vast majority of cases. By looking at large series of deliveries and analysing the decisions made, then there has been some understanding of the decision making process, but this remains an area of active research (E.C. Parry, Parry, & Pattison, 1999).

CODING SYSTEMS

Coding systems in medicine exist to remove ambiguities, simplify representation, assist with audit and outcome analysis and support decision making as well as having a major role in administration of healthcare systems. Historically, the coding of disease and especially cause of death has been intimately linked to the collection of statistics. Coding systems can trace back their origins to at least the "Bertillon Classification of Causes of Death," which was introduced at the end of the 19th century. Generally, coding occurs at the end of an episode, for example the method of delivery of a baby is coded after the baby is delivered.

ICD10

The international classification of diseases is currently in its tenth version (World Health Organization, 2001). This system is administered by the World Health Organisation and is free to use. ICD10 covers a vast range of diagnoses as well as procedures and modifiers. IC-10-CM (clinical modification) which is used for diagnosis includes alpha numeric codes that are 1 to 7 digits long, based largely around anatomical site, followed by disease process and then modifiers. ICD-10-CM is available from the Centres for disease control (http://www.cdc.gov/nchs/about/otheract/icd9/icd10cm.htm) and contains over 68,000 codes in the July 2007 release. Pregnancy codes begin with an 'O' and the modifier generally relates to the trimester.

Gynaecologic disorders do not have their own initial letter but are classified according to the site or type of illness. ICD10 PCS (procedure coding system) is as the name suggests a means of coding procedures. Previous releases of ICD combined the procedures and the clinical descriptions but these are now separate. There are over 86,000 procedures listed in the July 2007 release. Some examples of codes relating to obstetric procedures are shown in Table 2.

ICD codes are designed so that they are increasingly precise from left to right so that when searching for particular diagnoses, one can use select a portion of the code to give the correct degree of precision. For example, looking at Table 1 it can be seen that a search for O104.1* would give all the secondary hypertension patients no matter which trimester they were in.

Read

Read codes were developed for the primary care sector by Dr. James Read in the UK and version 3 was delivered in 1995 (O'Neil, 1995). Read codes are not free to use, but many countries have purchased a licence for use in their healthcare system. Their use is widespread in the UK and has enabled the general practice research database to be built up, containing anonymised data about eight million people(Walley & Mantgani, 1997). This large dataset has been used for investigations into women's health issues, for example (Bromley, Vries, & Farmer, 2004) on the use of hormone replacement therapy. Read codes come in a number of varieties but are generally related to an hierarchy in which successive characters of the code identify the anatomic location or the

Table 1. Examples of ICD-10-CM codes with descriptions

ICD10 Code	Description
O104.11	Pre-existing secondary hypertension complicating pregnancy, first trimester
O104.12	Pre-existing secondary hypertension complicating pregnancy, second trimester
O104.13	Pre-existing secondary hypertension complicating pregnancy, third trimester
O104.19	Pre-existing secondary hypertension complicating pregnancy, unspecified trimester

Table 2. ICD 10 procedure codes

ICD10 Code	Description
10D07Z3	Extraction of Products of Conception, Low Forceps, Via Natural or Artificial Opening
10D07Z4	Extraction of Products of Conception, Mid Forceps, Via Natural or Artificial Opening
10D07Z5	Extraction of Products of Conception, High Forceps, Via Natural or Artificial Opening
10D07Z6	Extraction of Products of Conception, Vacuum, Via Natural or Artificial Opening
10D07Z7	Extraction of Products of Conception, Internal Version, Via Natural or Artificial Opening

condition or the procedure more precisely. In many countries Read codes are being superseded by SNOMED CT.

Diagnostic Related Groups (DRG)

DRG's were originally developed to compare casemix between hospitals, so that health providers with more complex cases were not penalised compared to those with simpler workloads. Because of this role, DRG's are linked closely to values for cost of care and length of stay. DRG's comprise a much smaller list of categories than other coding systems- for example in the Austalian DRG system there are only 17 Obstetric codes and 20 Gynaecological ones. Perhaps surprisingly, this reduced granularity and focus on severity of illness or difficulty of treatment can make coding difficult as the code use terms such as "catastrophic" or "severe" complications, which may be difficult to impliment. Recent work in Australia has shown wide variations in the reporting of DRG's (Coory & Cornes, 2005), and this has implications for the idea of paying standard fees per DRG, rather than the calculated cost of service. Similar problems exist if using DRG 's to measure quality of outcome, or level of care. In the obstetric domain, a particular problem is that there is not always a causal link between the risk to mother and baby, the procedure performed, or the outcome of the procedure. For example, a "ceasarian section with catastrophic complications" (O01A) can occur in a pregnancy

that is assessed as low risk, whereas an "Vaginal Delivery without Catastrophic or Severe complications" (O60B), can occur after extensive efforts in pregnancy evaluated as being at high-risk of complications.

The DRG system grouper can accept ICD10 codes as an input. Recently work in Taiwan (Yang & Reinke, 2006) has demonstrated that a severity score comparable to DRG can be calculated directly from the ICD10 values.

MESSAGING SYSTEMS

Role of Messaging Systems

Messaging systems allow transfer of information between health information systems. It is very common to have multiple organisations dealing with the care of a woman, during a particular episode. Communication between organisations, and hence between information systems is therefore vital. Such communication occurs in many domains outside healthcare, and is seen as an important factor in increasing efficiency (H.R.Johnston & M.R. Vitale, 1988). Messaging systems allow information to be transferred between systems by using interfaces rather than a common system. Therefore if one part of the system changes, then only the interface needs to change rather than the whole system. However, it is attractive to extend the role of messaging systems to become document storage and management systems., and this expansion has occurred in the case of the most commonly used system – Health level 7(HL7).

HL7

HL7 is so called because it sits at the top of the International standards organisation (ISO) Open system interconnect (OSI) standard . This means that HL7 is associated with the *application* layer, which is the highest one of the model. This corresponds to the application layer of the TCP/IP protocol. In practical terms this means that HL7 messages can be transmitted by any system that is OSI compliant HL7 is administered by the HL7 organisation (http://www.hl7.org/) and is an American National Standards Institution (ANSI) standard. Originally HL7 was a simple messaging protocol, designed to encapsulate clinical information by providing standardisation of formats and minimum data sets. In this approach it has been very successful, with large-scale adoption across many countries and systems, particularly in the area of pathology results and pharmacy orders. Within the message format the vocabulary used is dependent on the application but the Logical Observation Identifier Names and Codes (LOINC) Vocabulary (Huff et al., 1998) is often used.

Health level 7 version 3 has been developed since 2001 to incorporate a clinical document architecture based around XML representations of clinical notes (Dolin et al., 2001). This representation is much more semantically rich than previous approaches and has caused some debate as to whether this will improve the standard or reduce its applicability.

OTHER SYSTEMS

Medical Subject Headings (MeSH)

Medical subject headings (MeSH) are the index terms used by the National library of Medicine (USA). MEDLINE covers more than 11 million journal articles, published since the 1960's and beyond. Historically, MEDLINE can trace its heritage back to the work of Dr. John Shaw Billings (1838-1913) who served as a surgeon in the American Civil War and the director of the National Library of Medicine between 1865 and 1895. During this time "INDEX Medicus" was first published (1879). Index Medicus is an expanding, regularly updated, bibliography covering many medical journals, containing information about author, source, subject and often an abstract of the article. MEDLINE has acted as a successor to this effort. Around 500,000 articles are added to MEDLINE every year, from more than 5000 journals. MEDLINE is accessible via a number of sites including "PubMed" and "Ovid". MEDLINE is available via CD ROM and via the Internet in the PubMed format at no cost to users. Other related databases such as CINHAL (mostly nursing–related) and PSYCHLIT are available from the National Library of Medicine.

MeSH codes are of the form <A00.000...> where A represents an alphabetic character and 0 is a digit between 0-9. As the name suggests MeSH is a hierarchy, with branches being represented by adding 3 digit combinations separated by full stops. Up to 4 extra XXX digit sets can be included.

It is important to note that MeSH is a bibliographic indexing scheme rather than a coding system for describing disease. Thus the choice of index terms is driven by the need to categorise documents, rather than clinical activity. Although arranged as a hierarchy, terms can occur in multiple locations, which raises issues with the disambiguation of terms if MeSH is used for the analysis of documents or ontology construction (D. T. Parry, 2006).

DICOM

Digital Imaging and Communication in Medicine (DICOM) is a standard that was jointly

Table 3. Root headings for terms taken from MeSH

Code	Description
C13	Female Genital Diseases and Pregnancy Complications
A16	Embryonic Structures
A01.673	Pelvis
A16.378	Fetus
A16.254	Embryo
A16.759	Placenta
A16.950	Zygote
A16.631	Ovum
C02.800	Sexually Transmitted Diseases
C13.371	Genital Diseases, Female
C13.703	Pregnancy Complications
E04.520	Obstetric Surgical Procedures
F03.600	Mood Disorders
F03.800	Sexual and Gender Disorders
G08.520	Reproduction
M01.438	Multiple Birth Offspring

developed by the American College of Radiologists and the National Electrical Manufacturers Association(NEMA) in the early 1980's. Currently NEMA holds the copyright for the standard – available from its website http://medical.nema.org/, and although the standard is version 3 the latest revision is known as the 2007 version. DICOM covers the representation, transport and storage of images, originally mostly X-rays, but now extending to ultrasound, MRI, waveforms and other data. DICOM at its simplest level is a file format, which combines patient and other data with the image. In essence the clinical information and patient information are inseparable from the image. This approach is used to avoid non-identifiable images, or wrongly identified images, being produced. Each DICOM file has only one image, but this can be composed of a number of frames which allow for the production of Cineloops. The DICOM standard allows a number of image formats including JPEG, MPEG and lossless

JPEG to be used in the file. In terms of transporting the data, DICOM 3 supports transport over TCP/IP, and there are a number of HTTP based approaches, so that conventional web services can be used. DICOM can also deal with files that are transferred or stored on CD's DVD's and other physical transfer media. Some work has been done on assessing the image quality of images compressed using lossy and non-lossy methods(E. C. Parry, Sood, & Parry, 2006),in the context of transfer of obstetric ultrasound images via cheap memory sticks.

The DICOM standard includes "structured reporting", so that the radiology report is included in the file. Recent work (Zhao, Lee, & Hu, 2005) has shown that this can be represented in a XML format, thus increasing the portability and verifiability of the reports.

Because of its origins, DICOM is an extremely precise standard, designed to allow accurate reproduction of images in various formats.

Unified Medical Language System (UMLS)

UMLS is an extremely large repository of concepts and related terms for use in biomedical science. Developed by the National Library of Medicine (NLM), it includes not only its own subject hierarchy (MeSH), but also the metathesaurus, which incorporates ontologies from other sources (Nelson, Schopen, J., & N., 2001). These have lead to the identification of currently over 800,000 strings, with about 330,000 unique concepts. The NLM is to be congratulated for not only providing an extremely large lookup table for these concepts (MRCON), but also providing a list of the relations between them (MRREL). The UMLS also contains the SPECIALIST lexicon, of medical and non-medical terms and the semantic network, that allows complex semantic relations to be checked and constructed. The recent releases of UMLS (Anantha Bangalore, Karen E. Thorn, Carolyn Tilley, & Lee Peters, 2003) have incorporated a new object model and implementation of the system using Java and XML.

Ontologies

An ontology acts as guide to the relationship between concepts in a domain, which may or may not themselves represent physical objects. An ontology is useful for purposes of knowledge sharing and reuse, in fact an ontology can "express formally a shared understanding of information" (Noy et al., 2001) page 60. That is, by understanding the relationships between objects then the interaction between objects, the operations that can be performed on them, and the appropriate position of new objects becomes easier. Tacit ontologies seem to exist in everyday life, as people generally appear able to share knowledge of relations in normal activities. An ontology employs a richer set of relations than a hierarchy, which normally just consists of "is-a" relations. For example one can say in a anatomi-

cal ontology that the uterus is **contained within** the abdomen, and that the fetus is **contained within** the uterus in normal pregnancy. Hence the fetus is **contained within** the mother's abdomen. However other relations are possible – so for example the uterine artery can be said to be **supplying** the fetus **via** the placenta. Many ontologies have extremely rich sets of relations available e.g. Unified Medical Language System (UMLS), WordNet, PROTÉGÉ. The relations for UMLS are described in Chapter 2. There has been a great deal of interest recently (Musen, 2001) in the construction of ontologies for representing medical knowledge. In many ways an ontology is similar to an XML document, or a class in an object-orientated programming language (Ensing, Paton, Speel, & Rada, 1994). The representation encodes a hierarchical structure, with inheritance of properties from root to branch, with additional attributes at each level. The advantage over the fixed hierarchy of say ICD10 is that such ontologies can be modified with the inclusion of new branches or leaves, and the location of such a new item can give information about it even to users that are not aware of the new terms used. This approach has been encoded in XML, for use in clinical guidelines (Harbour & Miller, 2001) and anatomy. Effectively an ontology allows the users to agree on quite complex relationships between items, and what the consequence of those relationships are – thus in the relationship above, if an item supplies another item then if the original item is disrupted, this may affect the final one – so reduction in blood flow in the uterine artery leads to reduction in blood supply to the fetus.

Systematized Nomenclature of Medicine-Clinical Terms (SNOMED CT)

SNOMED CT is a clinical vocabulary currently administered by the international health terminology standards development organisation (IHTSDO) http://www.ihtsdo.org/. Member countries are; Australia, Canada, Denmark, Lithuania, The Netherlands, New Zealand, Sweden, United Kingdom and United States. SNOMED CT (Systematized **No**menclature of **Med**icine-**C**linical **T**erms) was originally developed by the American College of Pathologists, and contains more than 600,000 concepts. SNOMED is organised as an "is-a" hierarchy. Exploring the SNOMED hierarchy is a very good way to begin to understand its power and browsers such as cliniclue (www. cliniclue.com) and SNOB are freely available within the countries that are part of IHTSDO. Synonyms for concepts are also included, and there are concepts that link concepts, across the hierarchy. Concepts are futher categorised into observable entities, diagnoses etc. For example "Pregnancy" code 289908002 is an observable entity and lies below " Female genital tract functions" (289907007) in the hierarchy. Conceptual Relations to other concepts – including disorders of pregnancy etc. are also available. As a vocabulary SNOMED can be used to generate documents using standardised terms – just like natural language, two parties need to use the same vocabulary in order to understand each other.

Evaluation of coverage(Penz JF, 2004) has demonstrated that SNOMED-CT was able to code 90% of previously unresolved narratives, using automated tools. Other recent work has shown that by using SNOMED, coding of free-text clinical documents may be amenable to automation (Patrick, Wang, & Budd, 2007). This demonstrates that the coverage and arrangement of SNOMED concepts is sufficient to allow understanding, and opens the prospect of electronic health records that combine the ease of use of free-text by humans while storing data that can be analysed by machine.

DISCUSSION

Coding and messaging systems can be seen as part of a continuum of semantic richness, begin-

ning with controlled vocabularies and ending with complex semantically rich documents. The essential role of coding and messaging systems is to enable sharing of both information and understanding. This is particularly important in the area of women's health where patients are often cared for by a wide variety of clinical workers, sometimes coming from different organisations. Conversion between systems will remain an important function for informaticians for the foreseeable future, along with extension and refinement of such systems. Perhaps most importantly the choice of the correct standards to use will continue to challenge system developers and health providers. With the replacement of READ by SNOMED CT in the UK as part of the major "connecting for health" initiative, a more stable landscape seems to be emerging.

Efficient and effective coding and messaging offer the vision of a "world minimum dataset" sharing information between the national and regional datasets that exist around the planet. International comparisons, but more importantly use of such data to identify and support best-practice may lead to improved care especially for particularly rare conditions or combinations of them. However tt should always be remembered that the woman is at the centre of women's health and these tools, while useful, should not mask the individual. Perhaps there is a role for "coding for clients", so that the experiences of women can be recorded and given the attention it deserves. Coding does not replace care, but it can support it.

FUTURE RESEARCH DIRECTIONS

Undoubtedly there has been an enormous effort in the fields of coding and messaging. Two challenges still exist, the need for organizations to adopt and use these standards and agreement on the combination of standards to use. HL 7 appears to be the strong front-runner in the messaging field, and with version 3 seems to be merging into the world of web services and the semantic web. Similarly SNOMED CT appears to be the future of controlled vocabularies, although world-wide adoption relies on governments joining the standards organization, which may be a rate-limiting step. The example of the WHO maintaining and developing ICD may be an example of the way forward in the future. Moving from proprietary to open standards is a theme across computing, and with the development of the semantic web and interoperability, health care will move the same way. Indeed if women are to control the use of their health data, means of coding and decoding health information for consumers of health may be a major issue in the next few years.

REFERENCES

Adomat, R., & Hewison, A. (2004). Assessing patient category/dependence systems for determining the nurse/patient ratio in ICU and HDU: A review of approaches. *Journal of Nursing Management, 12*(5), 299-308.

American College of Pathologists. (2000, 2000). About SNOMED. Retrieved January 11, 2002, from http://www.snomed.org/about_txt.html

Bangalore, A., Thorn, K. E., Tilley, C., & Peters, L. (2003). *The UMLS Knowledge Source Server: An Object Model For Delivering UMLS Data.* Paper presented at the AMIA Annual Symposium, Washington.

Beck, D. H., Taylor, B. L., Millar, B., & Smith, G. B. (1997). Prediction of outcome from intensive care: A prospective cohort study comparing Acute Physiology and Chronic Health Evaluation II and III prognostic systems in a United Kingdom intensive care unit. *Critical Care Medicine, 25*(1), 9-15.

Berners-Lee, T., Hendler, J., & Lassila, O. (2001). The Semantic Web. *Scientific American,* (May 2001), 29-37.

Bishop, E. H. (1964). Pelvic Scoring for Elective Induction. *Obstet. Gynecol., 24*(2), 266-268.

Bromley, S. E., Vries, C. S., & Farmer, R. D. T. (2004). Utilisation of hormone replacement therapy in the United Kingdom. A descriptive study using the general practice research database. *BJOG: An International Journal of Obstetrics and Gynaecology, 111*(4), 369-376.

Coiera, E., & Tombs, V. (1998). Communication behaviours in a hospital setting: An observational study. *British Medical Journal, 316*(7132), 673-676.

Coory, M., & Cornes, S. (2005). Interstate comparisons of public hospital outputs using DRGs: Are they fair? *Australian and New Zealand Journal of Public Health, 29*(2), 143-148.

Dolin, R. H., Alschuler, L., Beebe, C., Biron, P. V., Boyer, S. L., Essin, D., et al. (2001). The HL7 Clinical Document Architecture. *J Am Med Inform Assoc, 8*(6), 552-569.

Ensing, M., Paton, R., Speel, P. H., & Rada, R. (1994). An object-oriented approach to knowledge representation in a biomedical domain. *Artificial Intelligence in Medicine, 6*, 459-482.

Gardner, M. (2003). Why clinical information standards matter. *BMJ, 326*(7399), 1101-1102.

Harbour, R., & Miller, J. (2001). A new system for grading recommendations in evidence based guidelines. *British Medical Journal, 323*(11 August), 334-336.

Health Level Seven Inc. (2001). HL7 Version 3 (Draft). Retrieved 11 January, 2002, from http://www.HL7.org/Library/standards_non1.htm

Huff, S. M., Rocha, R. A., McDonald, C. J., De Moor, G. J. E., Fiers, T., Bidgood, W. D., Jr., et al. (1998). Development of the Logical Observation Identifier Names and Codes (LOINC) Vocabulary. *J Am Med Inform Assoc, 5*(3), 276-292.

Johnston, H. R., & Vitale, M. R. (1988). Creating Competitive Advantage with Interorganizational Information Systems. *MIS Quarterly, 12*(2), 153-165.

Keene, R., & Cullen, D. (1983). Therapeutic Intervention Scoring System: Update 1983. *Critical Care Medicine 11*(1), 1-3.

Musen, M. (2001). *Creating and using Ontologies: What informatics is all about.* Paper presented at the Medinfo 2001, London.

Nelson, S., Schopen, M. J. S. & N., A. (2001). *An Interlingual Database of MeSH Translations.* Retrieved October, 2003, from http://www.nlm.nih.gov/mesh/intlmesh.html

Noy, N., Sintek, M., Decker, S., Crubézy, M., Ferguson, R., & Musen, M. (2001). Creating Semantic Web Contents with Protégé-2000. *IEEE Intelligent Systems*(March/April), 60-71.

O'Neil, M. P., & Read, C. J. (1995). Read Codes Version 3: A User Led Terminology. *Methods of Information in Medicine, 34*(1/2), 187-192.

Parry, D. T. (2006). Evaluation of a fuzzy ontology based medical information system. *International journal of Health Information Systems and Informatics, 1*(1), 40-49.

Parry, E. C., Parry, D. T., & Pattison, N. (1999). Induction of labour for post-term pregnancy: an observational study. *Australian and New Zealand Journal of Obstetrics and Gynaecology, 38*(3), 275-279.

Parry, E. C., Sood, R., & Parry, D. T. (2006). Investigation of optimization techniques to prepare ultrasound images for electronic transfer [Abstract]. *Ultrasound in Obstetrics and Gynecology, 28*(4), 487-488(482).

Patrick, J., Wang, Y., & Budd, P. (2007). *An automated system for conversion of clinical notes into SNOMED clinical terminology.* Paper presented at the Conference Name.

Penz, J. F., Carter, J.S., Elkin, P.L., Nguyen, V.N., Sims, S.A., & Lincoln, M. J. (2004). *Evaluation of SNOMED coverage of Veterans Health Administration terms.* Paper presented at the Medinfo. Amsterdam.

Rosenfeld, R. (2000). Two decades of statistical language modeling: where do we go from here? *Proceedings of the IEEE, 88*(8), 1270-1278.

Silfen, E. (2006). Documentation and coding of ED patient encounters: An evaluation of the accuracy of an electronic medical record. *The American Journal of Emergency Medicine, 24*(6), 664-678.

U.S. National Library of Medicine. (2001, 15 November 2001). Medical Subject Headings. Retrieved 11 January, 2002, from http://www.nlm.nih.gov/mesh/

Walley, T., & Mantgani, A. (1997). The UK General Practice Research Database. *The Lancet, 350*(9084), 1097-1099.

Wilson, R. G., Purves, I. N., & Smith, D. (2000). Utilisation of computerised clinical guidance in general practice consultations. *Studies in health technology and informatics, 77*, 229-233.

World Health Organization. (2001, 14 November 2001). ICD-10: The International Statistical Classification of Diseases and Related Health Problems, tenth revision. Retrieved 11 January, 2002, from http://www.who.int/whosis/icd10/

Yang, C.-M., & Reinke, W. (2006). Feasibility and validity of International Classification of Diseases based case mix indices. *BMC Health Services Research, 6*(1), 125.

Zhao, L., Lee, K., & Hu, J. (2005). Generating XML schemas for DICOM structured reporting templates. *Journal of the American Medical Informtics Association, 12*(1), 72-83.

ADDITIONAL READING

Biomedical Informatics: Computer Applications in Health Care and Biomedicine (Health Informatics) by Edward H. Shortliffe and James J. Cimino

HL 7 Web site: www.hl7.0rg

IHTSDO Web site: www.ihtsdo.org/

Chapter IV
Women's Health Informatics in the Primary Care Setting

Gareth Parry
Horsmans Place Partnership, UK

ABSTRACT

Women's health in primary care is a large part of the generalist's practice. Information technology (IT) is now an integral part of the generalist's office, often more so than in secondary care and therefore this chapter is a key starting point in the book. Initially there is an introduction of the role of IT in primary health and the many areas it may encompass. We then move onto organizing clinical information and the ways that this maybe represented electronically in the "cradle to grave" electronic health record. In addition to recording information, can IT help the primary care doctor? The area of IT in screening, prevention and alerts is discussed. The role of the computer in the clinician's office and the impact it has on the consultation is explored. Can computer help clinicians perform better? Areas of discussion include the role of computers in audit and systems using artificial intelligence to improve patient care. IT is increasingly important in scheduling both within the practice and at the local hospital. This can be done by the primary care doctor and in some instances by the patient his or herself. The ideal situation is the primary care doctor having a system which can "talk" to external systems (e.g. local hospital notes, with a secure portal). In some countries such as the United Kingdom, this is becoming a reality, though there are problems which are discussed.

INTRODUCTION INFORMATION TECHNOLOGY AND THE GENERALIST

The generalist medical function occupies an important role in most models of health service provision. The terminology may vary (Primary Care, Family Medicine General Medical Practice) however there are a number of consistent themes which characterise this role and impact on the information requirements.

1. Generalists have long term, relationships with patients covering the whole spectrum of medical, psychological and social functioning.
2. Successive generalists looking after a patient should inherit the entire existing record and its summary, add to it appropriately and pass it on in a coherent state to the succeeding clinician.
3. Generalists manage many of the day to day issues of patient care in house and refer and accept back patients from episodes of specialist or increasingly multidisciplinary care and need to record these events and their outcomes, both for the coherence of the record and to retain information pertinent to further requests for specialist advice or intervention

Hence clinicians, patients and administrators demand much of our medical record systems.

Different elements of the record (datasets) are required for different clinical situations, such as the recording of allergies, the past obstetric history, the most recent blood pressure measurement. Each element of the history assumes a different importance at different times.

- Some conditions may be recurrent; recording post natal depression in the past may alter and direct the care offered in a further

pregnancy and change the index of suspicion for the obstetrician.
- Some conditions change the subsequent risk profile. Gestational diabetes though resolved postnatally remains a risk factor for Type 2 diabetes in later life.
- Some elements of the record become highly relevant only in very specific situation – a difficult endotracheal intubation has little relevance to a generalists care but is critical information to an anaesthetist. This information may not transfer in a hospital to hospital situation an argument for patient held records in the form of an accessible alert.

Medical decisions are often dependent on observing trends in a specific test or measurement or recognising a constellation of features of the medical history which point to a recognised pathological process. Recording and presenting data to highlight these trends aids correct management of the clinical situation. The maintenance of accurate, comprehensive and up to date records supports this process

Communication with other health care professionals often requires specific datasets of information to be mutually agreed and easily transferred and integrated into the appropriate record. Standardisation of the method of recording, transferring and distribution data is central to the effectiveness of multidisciplinary medical care.

Organised proactive care of patient subgroups in the form of screening, vaccination and analysis of combined risk factors requires a recall or reminder system which has to be updated in real time. Missed recalls need to be recorded and acted on while the patient choice to cease or postpone recall need to be respected. Opportunities to remind patients opportunistically allows further explorations of the patient's choice and the presentation of personalised explanation and encouragement – backed up by specific literature explaining why engagement with the service is in the patient's interest.

Increasingly the quality and the outcomes of medical activity need to be fed back to the central authorities for payment, audit, public health (or sometimes disciplinary or medico-legal) reasons. The aggregated records of patients and those specific subgroups of interest have to be organised with this requirement in mind.

A further and very topical theme related to the recording of medical information relates to the contrasting pressure to share and combine information about patients for a number of very worthy administrative or policy making aims including the analysis of gaps in service provision and tailoring better quality services. This can be in conflict with an overriding need for confidentiality of the patient/clinician relationship and the records content.

There are also tensions between a patient viewing or even holding their records and the need for records to be secure and contemporary. Patients are encouraged to view their records as an aid to involving them in informed choices about their care. Patients can edit or contest them if they are inaccurate and may want part or all of what they consider to be contentious or sensitive deleted or made available in a specific restricted distribution. Experience shows that what a patient may consider sensitive is a highly individual issue and not easily predicable even by the clinician that knows them well.

For these reasons the long term health record (sometimes called the 'cradle to grave' record) is best placed in with the generalist. Increasingly in part or in full this is and electronic record. Generalists tend to be at the hub of the patient care and hence inevitably the electronic record.

Clinicians develop skills and experience in tacit areas of knowledge i.e. the ability to consult with patients in a caring and effective manner. As far as the generalist is concerned it is impossible to keep fully abreast of changes in medical knowledge, advances in pharmacology and specialist

practice. Computer systems can aid the reference and acquisition of what might be termed 'just in time knowledge' for the physician and increasingly by way of algorithms and other techniques advise on therapy for example the specific doses of anticoagulants.

Full clinical pathways can be modelled on computer systems; prompts can be set up to alert for opportunities for productive intervention and the agreed form and datasets for multidisciplinary interaction

Computerisation of the generalist medical record holds many advantages for the generalist but also involves some threat in terms of the new IT skills required and often a perceived loss of autonomy of behalf of the (perhaps senior) clinician. New computer systems and advances in functionality need to be handled sensitively, by consensus and allied to training.

Computers should do what they're good at and people should do what they're good at. Modern medical computer systems store and organise large volumes of patient data in an easily accessible and consistent format however this comes at a price of embracing and managing the change from paper records which has significant potential pitfalls.

ORGANISING CLINICAL INFORMATION ON COMPUTER

Data, information and knowledge (and arguably wisdom) are on a continuum of increasing complexity and uncertainty. Binary data stored on computer discs as areas stored and organised by the computers operating system and is the province of the computer engineer scientist and computer programmers. Major challenges relate to how the storage of increasing amounts of data can produce clinically useful information and enhance medical knowledge while avoiding information overload.

The discipline of health informatics sits between computer science and clinical medicine and attempts to understand the needs and language of both activities, in particular creating guiding principles by which effective clinical record systems are developed. The nature of medical information is complex, uncertain and ever-changing the task of modelling the convoluted processes of medicine falls to the system developer. Well-designed information systems will easily integrate new knowledge, will support the decision maker and also the choices and information available to the end user of the service the patient. It will in other words enhance the familiar medical process.

Interest in structuring the medical record going back over many decades and change related to the introduction of the problem orientated medical record in the late 1950s by Larry Weed. Thinking about records changed from simple maintenance of a list of past events to an orientation around problems. A problem could be anything of relevance to the patient and their care and evolves with time. Generalists who are dealing with patients over time have a specific need to be able to edit the record to reflect the way that the problems change with time.

Menorrhagia and pelvic pain was initially recorded as a problem in general practice, after investigation and referral, ultrasound scanning and laparoscopy the problem evolves to a diagnosis of endometriosis in secondary care then treated by a combination of hormonal and surgical intervention. Once treated and asymptomatic endometriosis is regarded a an inactive problem but may become reclassified as active in the future when subsequent complications of pelvic scarring become apparent.

The problem begins as a symptom then is overwritten as a diagnosis then a complication but the database maintains the underlying links with the data items that supports the progressive understanding of the evolution of this problem. A modern database system will also have the functionality to recreate the state of the database in the past for audit purposes.

This change modelled the real world medical process more closely and offered the possibility of enhancing ongoing clinical care by using the problem list as a predefined query for medical knowledge databases in real time as an aid to the clinician (Problem /Knowledge Couplers) resulting in Time magazine leading with the headline 'The computer will see you now'.

However implementing problem oriented medical records (POMR) in paper form suffered from significant limitations which hampered its universal adoption. In a Problem Oriented approach each observation may be relevant to more than one problem. This means that in POMR, an observation could be entered more than once. For all but the most avid advocates this was difficult to maintain. The underlying reason for this difficulty is that relationships between data can be more convoluted than is apparent at first glance and change over time.

One-to-one relationships between data exist for instance the patients date of birth. This is not going to change with time as long as it is correct, you don't need the ability to edit it once entered.

Some data relationships are more complex, for example patients requiring a cervical smear test on a regular basis both for screening and for follow-up following colposcopy. It is not predictable at the outset how many cervical smears will be needed during the course of a lifetime and each point we need to record data about the smear including the date of the test the cytological result and the name of the smear taker and the analyser. This is an example of a one to many relationship in information terms (One patient can have many smears) and in relational database system terms is represented by two tables, one which relates to the patient and one which relates to the smears linked by a column containing an identifier common to both tables.

Other complex and subtle data relationships exist. Consider for instance the patient has two problems. The patient is taking the oral contraceptive pill (Contraceptive Care-Problem1) and is also hypertensive (Hypertension-Problem2). Blood pressure measurements are relevant both problems. How does the clinician record one measurement with both problems without recording the same data under two headings?

This is an example of a many to many relationship. The blood pressure recording is relevant to more than one problem and the blood pressure needs to be recorded under more than one problem heading. This can be modelled by the system developer by creating a linking intermediate table of data which only contains records blood pressure values and the links to both problems. This can be achieved seamlessly in a modern relational computer database system from the enduser's point of view – the reading once entered appearing automatically under both problems.

Medicine it is a complex subject and many different concepts need to be represented in clinical records. Clinical concepts such as in Snomed CT are in general hierarchical and need to be linked in subtle ways.

To illustrate a hysterectomy (Concept: Hysterectomy) is an example of an operation (Concept: Operation). Since all operations can have complications (Concept: Post operative complication) such as infection (Concept: Post operative Infection) then following a logical path a hysterectomy can be coded as complicated by a post operative infection.

A clinical nomenclature or coding system models these relationships and is not just a list of concepts. Coding systems also has the advantage to the programmer that the concepts can be allocated a shorthand code which saves storage space and allows for combined concepts to be recorded in coded form as above. For more on coding see chapter 3.

A further issue is that different users have different requirements of the coding system if they each create their own system it will lead to multiple poorly compatible systems in healthcare.

Hence a method of translating between coding systems has to be developed and maintained.

The large overhead in maintaining and translating between coding systems has increased interest in producing a single extensive health nomenclature where different users will view and use relevant subsets of the same system. One of the most obvious benefits is to provide medical language translations so that the user enters data in their native language but other users can view the same data in their own tongue by use of their specific language subset and a table of synonyms connecting concepts.

MOVING TO ELECTRONIC INFORMATION SYSTEMS

Paper records whether handwritten or typed have major limitations of storage (they are bulky and degrade over time), access (only one copy exists able to be read in one place at one time) and safety (loss through physical damage or simply being misfiled). Radiological and other images such as histology, electrophysiological recordings such as CTGs, sound recordings and video streams can be incorporated by modern database systems filed by a single patient identifier and accessible to appropriate staff (sometimes remotely by access to the Internet).

However adoption of computer systems involves significant financial investment and management drive not least in running the legacy paper systems in parallel for a time and converting the historic paper based data to electronic form. Most large scale business now runs electronically and benefits from the resulting efficiencies and the clinical barriers and the assurances required both to clinicians and patients can be addressed.

The adoption of electronic records can be thought of as a stepwise process and the key to acceptance include an appropriate user interface for each type of user depending on their role and computer literacy, appropriate training in protected time and environment and an early gain for the users.

To illustrate this early primary care computer systems often concentrated on prescribing, which was often chaotic and poorly recorded on paper. By converting to electronic systems early adopters banished the drudgery of writing prescriptions by hand, the system became safer (introducing allergy checks and better legibility) and was now easily auditable. News of these early gains spread and encouraged take-up and supported development of more sophisticated systems.

The developing computer systems then look to solve more clinically contentious issues such as recording sensitive patient data and working with computers during consultations. There are real dangers in aggregating patient data in a searchable patient database format and issues such as confidentiality have become a significant barrier in the UK to take up of the national Summary patient record as well as the formidable technical challenge of a national database of some 60 million records.

Modern database systems have sophisticated user definable interfaces, can check data entry between specified parameters can issue warnings and advice triggered automatically and because of their structure allow complex queries involving multiple parameters to be developed. Practice defined options such as drug formularies can be enabled and every aspect of practice clinical activity can be monitored.

Do we really have a choice about using Electronic Medical Information Systems in the information age, is it reasonable to expect that patients were able to look at their bank balance on the Internet would not have access to their medical records?

In my opinion there is not really a choice about changing or about moving to electronic information systems in the information age however the principles of good practice in developing clinical systems have to be followed.

The introduction of information systems fail

- When they do not involve the users fully in development
- They don't work at an acceptable level of speed and reliability.
- They are not seen to be an improvement on the paper based system.
- Their specification and functionality is not determined correctly at the outset

If we are asking users to adapt the process by which they work than that must be to move to a more efficient system. The system doesn't have to be perfect but it has to be acknowledged to be better than what went before by a measure relevant to the user.

HEALTH INFORMATICS IN ACTION

Health informatics is essentially a practical discipline which allows a medical process to progress as effectively as possible, to illustrate this some case studies are presented. The reader is invited to consider what contribution informatics makes at each stage and how practical and effective it would be without computers.

Prevention Case Study Involving Osteoporosis

The aim is to detect the subtle, progressive age and gender related process of osteopenia/osteoporosis in order to prevent a negative outcome for the patient in the form of pathological fractures with their associated morbidity and mortality.

Initially requires a systematic process of inquiry requiring team input to establish a protocol which will involve defining characteristics of patients who should be screened (By DEXA scan) by reference to literature searching, previous policy, national policy or directives.

The implementation group then defines the risk factors to search for on computer and identify all the codes that would be relevant. Can we search free text? It is possible with some systems- it's likely however to be much slower and less precise.

Identify other risk factors such as prolonged steroid use by querying the patient database.

Identify within the potential screening group already established on treatment or unsuitable for screening in some other respect.

Be aware of the need to manage the process at all levels so that secondary care not overwhelmed and can establish what level of take-up is expected, consider doing a pilot study.

Make sure that there is sufficient capacity and finance for performing the Dexa scans, for assessing the results, and the pharmaceutical budget to treat patients once identified.

Establish a method of contacting these patients about the new facility for screening for osteoporosis and look into providing them with information required to make an informed choice whether to go ahead.

Contact patients by their preferred method. Look to raise the awareness in staff to bring the issue up opportunistically. Address confidentiality issues.

A number of audits of outcome measures will need to be in place looking at issues such as the uptake of the service, the number of positive results and the progress of those established on treatment. Formal cost/benefit and cost effectiveness studies could be performed.

Case Study. Early Detection of Disease - Cervical Cytology

Although many of the organisational issues are in common with osteoporosis cervical screening has been in place for many years and data is now available to suggests it reduces death and morbidity rates for cervical cancer

Cervical cytology and associated call/ recall systems did predate use of computers in general practice in the UK. This was a card based system whereby the patients recall status was determined by the position of their card - as they came to the front they were invited for screening, once screened satisfactorily the card was replaced at the back of the box. Woe betides anyone who inadvertently tipped the cards out of the box.

Some other Issues that Relate to Cervical Screening

Part of the population to be screened is young and mobile so it is critical that contact data is correct, and that the contact is in a form the patient prefers -software is now available to send smear and vaccination reminders by SMS message.(texting)

Further targeting the invitation for screening contact may be appropriate. Does for instance one age group require a tailored invitation letter to encourage compliance? A particularly difficult group is those that have declined smears in the past. It is ironic that this group has a higher rate of cervical cancer

Audits are in place to judge the quality of the sample takers as well as the cytology screeners and cytopathologists, new systems of image pattern recognition by may mean that the initial image analysis is done by computer in the future. See Chapter eleven for more information.

Screening can occur in several settings - GP surgery, hospital clinics, colposcopy clinics for follow up, family planning clinics and privately. All this has to be coordinated by exchange of information.

In the future identifying patients who have had or not had a prior course of HPV vaccination - these patients represent a different risk group from those that haven't had the vaccination. Hence should they be screened less often if at all? This illustrates the need for vaccine status to follow the patient in the generalist record over an extended period of time.

CAN COMPUTERS ENHANCE THE CONSULTATION?

Currently in the UK majority of general practitioners record consultations on a computer and the written records are not retrieved for each consultation (but are still usually available on site). This is in contrast to the position 10 years ago where so called paperless practices were in a small minority. This change has had a number of drivers not least since 2004 the contractual climate rewards information gathering in a systematic and predefined way in the Quality and Outcomes Framework (QOF) which determines a significant proportion of income. The QOF clinical points score is solely determined by computer audit.

Personal experience suggests the historical consultation data and its relevance to the current concentration relates mainly to its age, the most recent entries seems to the most relevant and so when a few years worth of consultation data and the important older historical data is held in the problem list the doctor rapidly sheds the need to refer back to paper to function effectively.

More generalist consultations are now structured evidence and observation gathering activities reviewing chronic or recurrent disease which sit well with systematic computer data entry but less so with the patient centred intuitive 'freestyle' that many GPs feel produce the best doctor patient interactions. Structured consultations are easier to model from an informatics perspective but all consultations have some information content and opportunistic intervention.

There remains hostility from clinicians who dislike 'button pushing', or seeming inexpert in front of the patient (by fumbling with a keyboard or mouse). Using a computer positively to enhance the consultation requires new skills on behalf of the clinician and informatics is involved directly in system design, functionality and user friendliness enhancing rather than hindering the medical process.

Moving further into the future will computers enable the doctors and patients to take better decisions? We have already noted support required in the repeat prescribing area is fairly clear so that a contemplated current prescription can be checked against allergies and previously recorded side-effects. Should not the computer suggest which alternative drugs or modalities of treatments are appropriate, and rank them according to established efficacy? Should decision support software and pharmaceutical database suggest in certain cases that the patient may be experiencing a side effect from an existing prescription as the reason for consultation and suggest modifications?

Increasingly scheduled care for chronic disease is being organised around predetermined pathways, clinical staff other than doctors are making therapeutic changes and initiating investigations according to agreed protocols. This situation seems primed for the introduction of increasingly sophisticated decision support systems which interact in real time according to the current and historical data entered on the computer.

In contrast there are political moves in the UK to remove the GPs hold on first contact care in the community setting and to open walk in centres open for extended hours of the day manned by a number of different team members where at present there can be no real time exchange of data until the Summary care record arrives in 2014 or there are some rapid advances in patient held data or data held on the internet such as healthspace. Only as a recent development and with a number of outstanding unsolved issues have GPs been able to transfer the majority of the electronic record to another GP directly.

Clinical Knowledge Summaries are a computerised tool, a development from Prodigy (http://www.prodigy.nhs.uk/home), which allows clinicians to use the computer to assimilate the evidence behind a clinical guideline rapidly and accurately and suggest the rationale for intervention in defined clinical scenarios.

Some referrals from primary care are principally around seeking advice. Can we upgrade the GP to be confident in managing conditions to a higher standard by using computer tools which may obviate the need for referral or at least target them in an improved fashion, saving both the patients time and the clinic's resources?

Modern aspects of artificial intelligence seek to model the medical process, medicine is an information rich activity and there are difficulties in disseminating and applying the sheer volume of new knowledge that is published. Knowledge management and Knowledge engineering are developing area of activity in many organisations; the reader is referred to the National Library for Health as an example of how different information sources can be brought together to smooth this process

CAN COMPUTERS HELP CLINICIANS PERFORM BETTER?

Modern health services need to demonstrate improving quality of service whether these are organisational or clinical matters. The concepts of clinical governance have now taken root in all aspects of medicine. Reviewing procedures and auditing clinical outcomes and the assessment of patient satisfaction has become part of everyday practice.

Using paper methods it's been difficult and time-consuming to audit even a simple aspect of a hospital service or general practice. Computerisation offers the opportunity of a continuous background process of audit taking away the emphasis on laborious data collection and analysis and focusing on changing clinical outcomes.

By structuring the input of clinical data in a way to facilitate subsequent audit we immediately realise a number of gains. The process of data entry can be standardised by means of input screens (called forms in database systems). During the process of data entry the system can

remind us of missing data, can alert to abnormal or possibly erroneous or rogue data, and can be programmed not to consider the data entry complete until obligatory items have been entered. The clinical system can also remind users about conditions that are due or overdue for review; these commonly take the form of messages or notes on the screen to perform certain actions or to check certain results.

The business process of a medical practice and medical communication can be facilitated by an electronic document management system. Modern systems scan and electronically file paper documents into the medical database, can identify and code pieces of information with user supervision and can conduct the distribution of the important issues identified for follow up. These can be an efficient and auditable way of communicating between different medical and paramedical personnel based at different sites and/or in different specialities.

By creating the correct output of the data (in database terms a report) we can customise a presentation of data in a usable and understandable format whether it by text, graphs or columns of figures. These can be compared with targets and by directing the output to a spreadsheet the remaining numeric targets to be achieved can easily be appreciated.

It is possible to drill down further into the data to compare the data to national or international norms not just local targets. By accumulating data automatically in particular in relation to activity we can pose quite tricky questions. Do we have enough appointments? Do we have enough access to pathology tests or imaging and how does this impact on the total waiting time and patient experience? Are there things we like doing or have traditionally done which are ineffective?

Beyond this in British general practice the audit is not only being used as a clinical tool but also as a contractual and financial tool rewarding practices which achieve the requisites quality of service and patient satisfaction over a range of activity. Payments relate to an external audit by way of questionnaire evaluating the patient experience and we can see the whole face of medicine changing from the traditional somewhat paternalistic approach where the doctor knows best to one where the system has to become flexible and responsive to the needs, and arguably wants, of its users to flourish.

This driver for change is potent comprising both the pressure of the personal relationship that the practice has with its patients to correct issues where it falls below par combined with the pressure from the quality, contractual and financial pressures that concern the Health Authority. There are some predictable difficulties resulting from this approach in terms of game playing by contractors and health authorities and creative presentation of data commonly known as spin.

Taking this one step further the results of these audits and assessments are being made public with the intention to influence the choice of the patients in terms of their choice of general practice or hospital.

League tables are considered a blunt instrument in terms of assessing quality however in a health service driven by government objectives and in a situation where information about public bodies is readily available through statute such tables are an inevitable development.

A NATIONAL ELECTRONIC PATIENT RECORD SYSTEM

Not only local healthcare systems are undergoing a revolution but systems at a national level also have to adapt and mature. Modern standards of data storage and transfer mean that multiple function specific legacy systems are redundant and in the UK a decision was made to start again from scratch. The model chosen in the UK was a central database with multiple functionality or services - those relevant to doctors include:-

- **Patient demographic service:** To maintain non clinical patient data.
- **Secondary user service:** Collect anoymized management information
- **Care records service:** A limited subset of exchangeable clinical data.
- **Choose and book:** Electronic referrals according to patient choice
- **GP2GP:** Transferring electronic records between GPs
- **ETP:** Electronic prescriptions direct to the pharmacy

Coalescing patient information to one database has obvious advantages to information accuracy and cascading changes for example patients address changes only have to be edited once at the point the patient interacts with any part of the health service, however recent experience in data security point up that the systems are highly vulnerable to unthinking or sloppy practices which may reduce public confidence in the system to the point it becomes less effective in meeting its goals.

However as with any bespoke IT solution these systems are expensive, prone to delay, difficult to project manage and roll out and vulnerable to continuing changes in specification and in the case of national projects to the political climate of the time.

Adopting a new IT infrastructure and national database gives potential clinical and organisational advantages to the generalist and these include:-

- The chance to retrieve at least a minimum dataset of information in the unscheduled care situation.
- Potential to aggregate information to inform the reorganisation of the service.
- Opportunities to support different ways of working including working at a distance e.g. telemedicine, to have advice on hand

from specialists remotely or for clinicians seeking support from experts.

- To standardise and audit referral systems into pathways while offering patient choice backed up with up to date patient relevant information concerning their choice.
- Information for patients and clinicians can be held centrally and be modified or adapted efficiently from a central distribution point.
- Becoming a more coherent service from a patient perspective.

ELECTRONIC PATIENT SERVICES

It is relevant to consider how patients may benefit from advances in health related IT systems since it is considered that the reintroduction of patient choice allied to better information about the performance of healthcare providers will create pressure to innovate and improve health services.

National patient oriented UK services online include

- NHS Direct, a telephone based advice and triage services accessible to patients. Also available online.
- NHS Choices website that brings together patient information on NHS services and their performance information as well as magazine style articles on healthy living and information on specific diseases and self help.
- National Library for health has some searchable patient oriented information.
- Map of Medicine UK mainly contains information for professionals about care pathways but links to patient information on NHS choices for specific diseases.
- Choose and Book allows a patient armed with a unique booking reference number (UBRN) and password supplied by their GP

to book their own outpatient appointment by negotiating directly with secondary care.

- Healthspace ('a secure online health organiser') it is envisaged will allow patients to view their summary care record as well as entering their own health notes online and will act as a patient portal for choose and book.
- Department of health website tells patients amongst other things how successful the government health reforms have been to date and will be in the future.
- Electronic Transfer of Prescriptions (ETP) will mean that electronically authorised prescriptions and in particular repeat prescriptions can be collected from a nominated pharmacy without requiring a paper based signed prescription form to be collected from the doctor's surgery.

GP clinical systems also give access to patient support information designed to be printed during the consultation, many GP practices have their own website to supply information to patients and many practices produce newsletters and annual reports for patients some distributed by e-mail.

With the emphasis now moving towards patient information on the web the plight of the information poor group i.e. without internet access is becoming increasingly problematic.

FUTURE RESEARCH DIRECTIONS

Clearly the area of health informatics in primary care is a fast moving field and is one of the leading areas for change. Much implementation is taking place across the world with an assumption that it will improve outcome. However, there is a not much research examining the real outcomes of importance: disease progression and illness, in parallel with these changes. Research in this area however is difficult as systems are often introduced across large groups in an ad hoc way. Data will emerge with time but will probably be retrospective based rather than randomised controlled trials.

The role of IT in supporting decision making is interesting and many workers are active in this area. Chapter X discussed the use in cardiotocograph interpretation and primary care doctors are already used to pharmaceutical drug alerts. It is likely that more complex systems will emerge in the future.

REFERENCES

Bolton, P., Douglas, K., Booth, B., & Miller, G. (1999). A relationship between computerisation and quality in general practice. *Australian Family Physician, 28*(9), 962-965.

Bomba, D. (1998). *A comparative study of computerised medical records usage among general practitioners in Australia and Sweden.* Paper presented at the Medinfo 9.

Department of Health UK. (1998). *Information for Health.* Retrieved. from.

Ho, L., McGhee, S., Hedley, A., & Leong, J. (1999). The application of a computerized problem-oriented medical record system and its impact on patient care. *International Journal of Medical Informatics, 55*(1), 47-59.

Llewelyn, H., & Hopkins, A. (1993). *Analysing how we reach clinical decisions.* London: Royal College of Physicians

Noone, J., Warren, J., & Brittain, M. (1998). *Information overload: opportunities and challenges for the GP's desktop.* Paper presented at the Medinfo 9.

Roger, F., De Plaen, J., Chatelain, A., Cooche, E., Joos, M., & Haxhe, J. (1978). Problem-oriented medical records according to the Weed model. *Medical Informatics, 3*(2), 113-129.

Tilyard, M., Munro, N., Walker, S., & Dovey, S. (1998). Creating a general practice national minimum data set: Present possibility or future plan? *New Zealand Medical Journal, 111*(1072), 317-318, 320.

Weed, L. (1971). The problem-oriented record as a basic tool in medical education, patient care and clinical research. . *Annals of Clinical Research, 3*, 131-134.

Weed, L. (1975). The problem-oriented record-its organizing principles and its structure. *League Exchange, 103*, 3-6.

Weed, L., & Zimny, N. (1989). The problem-oriented system, problem-knowledge coupling, and clinical decision making. *Physical Therapy, 69*(7), 565-568.

Zanstra, P., Rector, A., Ceusters, W., & de Vries Robbe, P. (1998). Coding systems and classifications in healthcare: the link to the record. *International Journal of Medical Informatics., 48*(1-3), 103-109.

Chapter V
The Electronic Health Record to Support Women's Health

Emma Parry
The University of Auckland, New Zealand

ABSTRACT

The seamless electronic health record is often hailed as the holy grail of health informatics. What is an electronic health record? This question is answered and consideration is given to the advantages and disadvantages of an electronic health record. The place of the electronic health record at the centre of a clinical information system is discussed. In expanding on the advantages several areas are covered including: analysis of data, accessibility and availability, and access control. Middleware technology and its place are discussed. Requirements for implementing a system and some of the issues that can arise in the field of women's health are elucidated. Finally, in this exciting and fast moving field, future research is discussed.

INTRODUCTION

Electronic health records (EHR) also known as Computerised Medical Records (CMR) and many other variations, have been an active area of research for more than 30 years. Many aspects of women's health lend themselves to computerised records, but the overarching aim of a computerised, holistic and appropriately accessible electronic record is still to be realised. A definition of the EHR from PubMed is "Computer-based systems for input, storage, display, retrieval, and printing of information contained in a patient's medical record." It is important to note that the existence of an EHR does not exclude the continuing existence of paper-based systems and that the EHR is just a part of a clinical information system. It is also common that information about individuals is held by multiple systems.

This chapter will give a brief history of the use of EHR, an introduction to what EHR systems are for, what they do, and how they can assist clinical care, research and administration. A review of the particular role EHR's hold in women's health and some speculation on future trends complete the chapter

History

Computers have developed with a speed that has surprised even those working in the industry. The well known "Moore's law" postulates a doubling of computer performance every year to 18 months (Schaller & Schaller, 1997). The medical profession have traditionally shunned computers in their practice as a just another time-wasting device, however in recent years computers have shown themselves to be useful and time-saving (Horwood & Richards, 1988). One of the most striking features of the development of EHR, has been the widespread adoption of administration, billing and laboratory systems ahead of the clinical record.

In 1968 the first attempt to use computers in obstetrics was initiated by Thatcher in Australia (Thatcher, 1968). A pilot system was introduced in Australia at the Royal Hospital for Women, Sydney in 1968. In 1971 a pilot study was set up at St Thomas's Hospital in London (South & Rhodes, 1971) and in Victoria Australia(Cope, Greenwell, & Mather, 1971) whilst in America, the Duke University Medical Centre also went on line in their obstetric department in 1971. All these systems were based around a mainframe computer, which were cumbersome and slow. These were the first 'microcomputers' which were within reach of smaller companies in terms of price.

In these early systems information was entered after the event (a retrospective system) by trained computer staff. The medical and midwifery staff had no role in data entry. It is well recognised data entered in this fashion is less accurate than data entered by a user (e.g. midwife) prospectively (at the time of the event).

As new faster microprocessors were developed, along with improved software and user interfaces, user based systems could be developed (Chard, 1987; Horwood & Richards, 1988; Lilford & Chard, 1981). The advent of the personal computer in the early 1980's made computers more accessible, smaller and cheaper (Shipton, 1979). The possibility of having computers in clinical areas began to be raised. Interest in computers in Obstetrics increased again. During the 1980's many hospitals developed systems, although most of these were retrospective in their method of data collection. One of the first hospitals to develop a prospective data collection system was King's College Hospital in London (Horwood & Richards, 1988). This system, EuroKing, relied on staff using a barcode reader and code book to take a booking history. This group found that with this system, the time to take a full booking history fell from one hour to ten minutes.

Systems in Current Use

Obstetrics lends itself to data collection. Each pregnancy is discrete with a final outcome. The options for most variables are limited. Most obstetric patients are well with no confounding illnesses. Over the last twenty years there has been a revolution in patient attitude and with it doctors have been called to account for their actions. This has resulted in all disciplines of medicine being required to keep records of the service they are offering. Audit has become an integral part of our training and clinical practice. Obstetrics as a speciality has responded relatively well to this challenge and most units will be able to quote numbers of deliveries, induction, caesarean section and forceps delivery rates. Increasingly through the necessity of data collection, computers are being introduced into obstetrics (Chard, 1987; Horwood & Richards, 1988; Kohlenberg, 1994; Lilford & Chard, 1981; South & Rhodes, 1971).

WHAT IS AN EHR?

An EHR is based around a person. The aim of the EHR is to support the clinical care of the patient, although other functions, such as data collection for secondary purposes or administration and billing may be included. It may form part of a larger clinical or health information system. Such systems are often very large and complex. Traditionally, computer systems are built as "proprietary" entities – that is the developing company owns the intellectual property associated with a system and may be reluctant to allow purchasers or users to modify or distribute it. Currently there is great interest in so-called "open source" software. The open source movement allows users of the software to copy it and modify it without payment. Often many users collaborate on the development and maintenance of open source products – such as the very popular "Apache" web server (McDonald et al., 2003).

Generally EHR systems are built around commercial Database management systems (DBMS), although open source solutions (Kantor, Wilson, & Midgley, 2003) which may be based on common standards such as the such as openEHR (openEHR Foundation, 2007) have been proposed. DBMS support the recording and search of structured and semi structured data. Many of the advantages that potentially accrue to the use of EHR depend on the degree to which the features of DBMS are exploited. The EHR records details of clinical findings, actions to be taken, and decisions made, including diagnosis and treatment.

The EHR sits at the centre of a clinical information system (Figure 1), and may communicate with other systems – such as a patient administration system, Laboratory systems, picture archiving and communication (PACS), and other electronic health records, that may exist for other clinical areas or care providers.

There are a wide range of approaches to the degree of coding included in an EHR. Although the coded representation of diagnoses and outcomes is often important (see Chapter III), some EHR systems simply record free text, along with some numerical data. Direct coding into the EHR can be difficult and there is a trade off between convenience and speed during the clinical encounter and accuracy of coding. Diagnostic codes cannot be assigned before a diagnosis is made. However, with the increasing use of clinical vocabularies

Figure 1. The electronic health record as a the centre of an information system

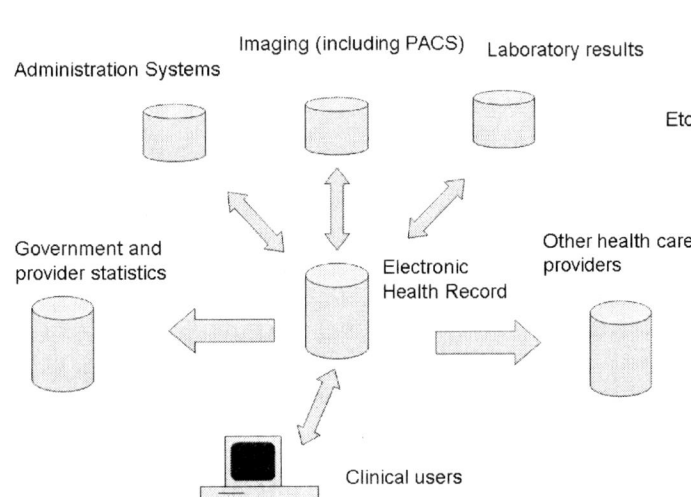

such as SNOMED CT (American College of Pathologists, 2000), coding of observations, symptoms and actions becomes easier. Indeed there is beginning to be some progress towards the goal of automatic coding of free text description using SNOMED(Patrick, Wang, & Budd, 2007).

Hybrid systems that track paper records or include scanned images of the paper record as part of a document management system have been used in a number of circumstances. In some cases these are used temporary solutions, but they may be useful when the implementation issues, including the wide diversity of requirements of different clinical areas prevent a fully digitised approach.

Disadvantages of Paper Records

Paper records have been used in medicine since at least the time of Hippocrates. One of the major aims of EHR has been to replace paper records, as these have a number of disadvantages.

Firstly, paper records can be lost or not available when needed (Bates et al., 2001). Some patient administration systems also record the location of the paper records in order to make them more easily available. Some maternity care providers have used patient-held notes to ensure higher availability, and increase patient involvement in the care process(Webster et al., 1996). Photocopies of paper records, or scanned copies of records can be made available, but these require strict procedures for version control – that is ensuring that the most up to date records are being used.

Secondly paper records are often difficult to organise. Although a lot of work has been done on problem-based records (Weed, 1968) this often requires duplication of effort by manually extracting a problem list, and keeping it up to date. Generally paper based records are organised in a temporal sequence, but linking relevant items together may be difficult.

Thirdly, paper based records may simply be difficult to read or understand – especially when

they are being used as a communication medium between clinical staff. It may not be obvious that a particular action has been performed, or where the results of a particular test will be recorded. The same issues arise when using records for research or audit purposes, where proving that a particular action has not been taken involves a huge amount of searching, and particular items of interest may be located in odd locations.

However, paper records are unaffected by power cuts, shortage of terminals or hardware or software failure. They are generally more accepted for legal purposes and generally do not require expensive conversion to be used in different health systems and are not rendered obsolete by hardware or software upgrades. Even electronic record systems produce vast quantities of paper in practice.

Advantages of the EHR

Apart from correcting the deficiencies of the paper records as described above, EHR have particular advantages.

Flexibility of Display and Data Entry

The use of a computer system means that there does not need to be a choice between temporally ordered and problem based records – both can be display as required. In addition, data trend lines can be produced for example to show response to therapy (see Figure 2).

This also extends to associated reports – for example letters to patients and referral destinations and communication with other systems. The vision of (Weed, 1968) can be realized with records that can change their display instantaneously. Not only can the record go from being a list of events, to a problem-based approach, but also time series of data, or events of particular interest can be identified. Modern interface technology can incorporate options to choose the "skin" that is the set of rules corresponding to appearance

Figure 2. Views of data from EHR

Temporal record

Time	Event
4/11/08 12:25 PM	Patient admitted, 36 weeks, ? Preeclampsia
4/11/08 1:51 PM	BP measured 160/110
4/11/08 3:44 PM	Proteinurea +++ on dipstick
4/11/08 3:58 PM	Antihypertensive given, Protein:Creatinine ratio elevated
4/11/08 5:18 PM	Diagnosis - Preeclampsia
4/11/08 6:44 PM	BP measured 150/95
4/11/08 8:01 PM	CTG - reassuring
4/11/08 9:27 PM	CTG - reassuring
4/11/08 9:59 PM	Admitted to HDU
4/11/08 10:49 PM	BP measured 140/90
4/11/08 11:35 PM	Consult with Perinatologist
4/12/08 12:29 AM	CTG - reassuring
4/12/08 1:06 AM	Normal obs HR 70, RR 15
4/12/08 2:00 AM	Perinatologist review
4/12/08 2:44 AM	BP measured 130/85
4/12/08 2:49 AM	CTG -Not reassuring
4/12/08 2:49 AM	BP measured 120/80
4/12/08 3:09 AM	OBGYN called
4/12/08 4:38 AM	Admitted to Theatre
4/12/08 5:41 AM	Cesarian section completed

Problem List

Diagnosis - Preeclampsia

Action - LSCS

Trend Lines

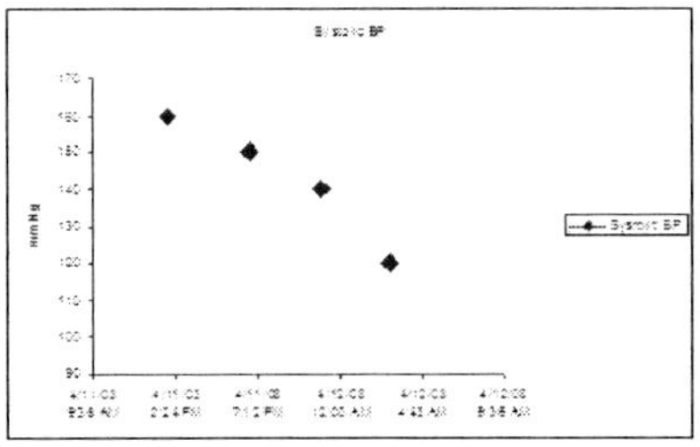

of the screen, and allow sorting of data lists and arrangement of windows on the screen according to personal preferences.

Analysis of Data

Analysis of data – and use for decision support – is simple and virtually instantaneous. Reminder and recall systems can be integrated into or communicate with e.g., the PRODIGY system (Wilson, Purves, & Smith, 2000). In this case, the EHR triggers warnings or reminders when certain criteria are met. This allows the encoding of clinical protocols, and treatment rules within a system. This approach is particularly useful for triggering recall messages eg when an abnormal PAP smear is discovered, or when the patient requires regular health checks for example after starting oral contraceptives. Other uses of data are covered later in the chapter. There is a wide literature concerning the importance and usefulness of electronic systems that can support decision making The NEONATE extension for the HELP system described in (Franco, Farr, King, Clark, & Haug, 1990) used an expert system to produce a problem list automatically.

Accessibility and Availability

Accessibility and availability of data is much higher. Compared to paper records, access to data can be controlled if there is private or sensitive information contained in a record. For example, past obstetric or sexual health history may not need to be accessible by all legitimate users of the record. At the same time, data can be simultaneously accessed and updated in different locations, by different users – as may be the case if ultrasound results are being produced while the patient is at the antenatal clinic.

Access Control

Audit of access and change to records is possible in a computerised system. By assigning each user a user ID, individual's use of the system can be monitored. Role-based access, where users are assigned rights to see and update data based on their function can assist in making such rules flexible but enforceable. For example administrative staff may require access to all patient's demographics, and clinic booking information, which may take some data from the EHR. However, only the patients own OBGYN, or their locum may be allowed access to sensitive data. In an emergency, most systems allow an override function which allows normally unauthorized access – for example in the case where a woman is admitted to hospital without their own physicians being available. However, a record of this access is maintained which may be helpful when reviewing this activity. Similarly, EHR systems should maintain a change log, so that when important data is changed, the previous values can be recovered if necessary. These approaches are vital if the EHR is to retain the status of a legal document held by the paper record. Users of the EHR must be confident that the record includes not only the correct data but that the source of that data is verifiable and traceable.

On a different note, access tracking can also be used as part of a reminder system so that clinical staff are prompted to review results, or note outcomes, if there has not been any viewing of the record.

DBMS Technology

As most EHR systems are based around DBMS, it should be noted that all these features noted above are common to many electronic record systems, such as those used by banks or law-enforcement agencies. Indeed modern DBMS include many tools to support multiple views of data and analysis tools, access and change logging, security and links to "triggers" – programs that run when particular combinations of parameter values are discovered. Modern DBMS are also designed to store multimedia information, which in clinical terms could include images or ultrasound cineloops. One of the greatest advances in DBMS technology in recent years has been the explosion in XML-based data transfer and Web interfaces to data. This allows data within databases to be reliably converted to and from transfer formats – such as HL7 CDA (see Chapter III). The use of standard Structured Query Language (SQL) to build and maintain databases also allows the structure and content of databases to be saved and transferred to other varieties of DBMS systems relatively easily. Native XML databases – that is where data is stored within the DBMS in XML format, and queried using XQUERY and other techniques are becoming more popular, although performance issues may restrict their growth.

This is not intended to be a tutorial on database design, but one important aspect of SQL-based DBMS is the need to link tables, often by means of an unique identifier, and maintaining these across systems is a major task in countries without national health index numbers.

The "middleware" approach to the EHR accepts that data will be stored in different systems, but needs to be drawn together for clinical decision making. For example screening systems such as cervical or osteoporosis testing may feed in information to a web or other portal that also includes feeds from lab results, discipline-based systems e.g., nursing and midwifery systems and specialised areas such as operating room or outpatient management. A modern approach to the use of DBMS in system design may use n-tier approach, where the data level is separate from the business rules level – which may include for example editing and audit processes, which is again separate from the presentation layer, which is seen by the user.

Figure 3. A middleware approach to the EHR

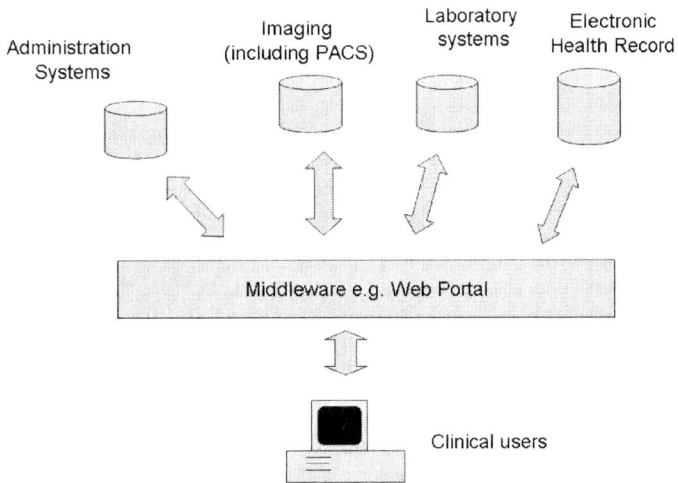

In classical database design, the normalisation process attempts to remove multiple storage locations for data to avoid conflicting information being held. Given the often heterogeneous nature of health records, with data being held by different providers in different places, this approach is often not yet practicable.

REQUIREMENTS

In order to act as a replacement or adjunct to a paper-based system the EHR must act as a legally useful record of the observations, results, diagnosis, plans and actions made as part of the clinical process. As different professionals are often involved in the care of women, each group should be assured that the EHR reflects their needs, and identifies where information came from, and presents it in a usable form.

User interface design is a vital aspect of electronic systems. Just as the views of the data held in the record may need personalisation, data entry and avoidance of error requires careful thought. In many cases for example, bench space is at a premium, so mouse-driven systems may be awkward. Recent work using tablet PC's

(Main, Quintela, Araya-Guerra, Holcomb, & Pace, 2004) and personal digital assistants (PDA) (Skov & Th. Hoegh, 2006) has indicated that these systems may be more usable in the clinical environment than traditional desktop machines. Such systems bring their own overheads in the form of the need for secure wireless networks, and means of securing expensive devices and keeping batteries charged.

The EHR acts a source of data for many purposes(Kenney & Macfarlane, 1999) and the concept of the 5 (or 6) uses of clinical data has been introduced.

Data collected should be available for:

- Supporting clinical intervention – in direct patient care and public health surveillance.
- Clinical Governance – including audit and performance management
- Administration (in all parts of Health) – both for funding, and logistic purposes
- Strategy and policy development – at all levels
- Research – including the identification of rare events and support for clinical trials.

A 6th use – patients self-management is becoming increasingly important – patients are getting more involved in the decision-making process and the "Smart patient" (R. L. Sribnick & W. B. Sribnick, 1994) is a partner rather than a consumer.

EXAMPLES IN WOMEN'S HEALTH

Supporting women's health offers a number of opportunities for EHR. Pregnancy care offers the opportunity for time-limited "stand-alone" databases, often known as Perinatal databases.

Perinatal systems have a number of differences from common episode-based EHR systems. Collaboration between care groups is common in pregnancy, and such systems need to support this. Uniquely, pregnancy episodes end with more patients involved than in the beginning, so that the offspring's data may need to be transferred to neonatal and infant information systems (see chapter 9). Perinatal systems often record information about previous gynecological and medical history, and in a integrated system, this can come from primary care or personal health information. Similarly, at the end of the pregnancy, appropriate information needs to be fed back to primary care.

In contrast to perinatal systems, screening programs require administrative support in terms of recall and results notification systems, for long-term care.

Systems to support "well woman" and screening programs are often use to support recall for PAP smears etc. and ensure that appropriate interventions are performed. Genetic and familial information may also be needed to assist with counseling before conception and uring early pregnancy. The extensive use of imaging in pregnancy will often require integration with an ultrasound reporting and assessment, including appropriate growth charts and risk calculated from Nuchal translucency.

ISSUES

Privacy issues change considerably when personal health information is stored electronically. Recent work has shown (Whiddett, Hunter, Engelbrecht, & Handy, 2006) that patients have strong views on who can view their data, and that many are unaware of the degree of data sharing that already occurs. Generally EHR systems are covered by data protection legislation, and usually patients would have the right to view information held about them and alter it if incorrect. There is a conflict here between the rights of the health provider, to record events, and the rights of the patient to adjust or delete those records. The chapter on ethics (Chapter II) deals with this in more depth. Because of the personal and sometimes sensitive nature of the data being stored woman's health informatics has particular issues in this regard.

However privacy rules are addressed – whether for example, different information is available to different users, a reliable method of identification of users is required. Currently most EHR systems use individual accounts with "role-based" access. That is a user will log in, be identified as a particular person, and then have rights to view and change data depending on rules relating to their role in relation to a patient. Thus an administration clerk may have unlimited rights to view and change demographic data relating to any patients, but no access to any clinical details, whereas a OBGYN may be able to access any clinical data relating to patient's identified as being under their care. Complexities arise when people change roles or locums are brought in and there are often fairly complex rules dealing with these cases. What is "sensitive" information can vary between cultures and situations and individuals, and many EHR systems provide a fairly crude method of identifying sensitive information during data entry.

Unauthorised access to data, either by using other peoples user identification or password, or by back-door access to the system e.g. by directly accessing the DBMS is a serious disciplinary offence in most organisations. However, unjustified data access that is, access to data which the system allows, but is not necessary for care, may be harder to detect. Some systems record all data access by users and can be audited to discover "suspicious" activity, for example apparently inappropriate access to data concerning famous people or staff members or their relatives. This can be followed up, but is time consuming and may be used in a limited number of cases.

Security of data is obviously vital to the success of EHR's. There is extensive guidance on protecting the security of information systems in the international standards such as IS0 17799, and these are particularly applicable to health systems. Security includes not only the prevention of unauthorised access but also this includes reliability and availability of the data on the system. There is therefore a need to backup the EHR data, in a suitable fashion, and ensure that the process for backup and restoration is reliable. Consideration also needs to be given to disaster recovery, and the use of paper records for example if there is a hardware or network failure.

Even in normal operation, EHR systems have a role as a contemporaneous record, so that data that is revised, should be noted as such. This often involves the retention of a revision log, as for example, if the estimated date of delivery (EDD) is changed, decisions that were made based on previous EDD may other wise seem incomprehensible. Generally, all data entered into an EHR should be recoverable, just as a paper system record that fact that writing may have been crossed out or marked as incorrect.

Although computerised systems are often thought to reduce the time taken to perform tasks, this may not be true in the case of EHR systems, and computerised order-entry systems that are used for ordering laboratory tests etc. A recent systematic review (Poissant, Pereira, Tamblyn, & Kawasumi, 2005) showed that although nurses appeared to take less time in documentation tasks, this was not true of physicians. There is still no

certainty in this area – it may be that time spent documenting via EHR's reduces the need for other means of communication, which is considerable (Coiera & Tombs, 1998), that EHR's do not fit into workflow patters so well, or that availability of terminals is an issue.

One of the most concerning gaps in research at the moment is the relative paucity of studies that actually show benefit to patient care by the use of EHR (Mitchell & Sullivan, 2001). This is a relatively difficult area to research, and impossible to blind. Cost benefit in some areas has been shown (Wang et al., 2003), but clinical benefit is more elusive, partly because of the fact that the introduction of EHR is often associated with other changes in practice and , for example the introduction of decision-support tools.

The process of implementation of EHR and clinical information systems seems particularly fraught, and failures are relatively common (Littlejohns, Wyatt, & Garvican, 2003). As with all information technology implementations, an understanding of the domain is vital. Comparisons between health systems, although controversial,(Feachem et al., 2002), seem to indicate that, on balance, increased spending on information technology does provide benefit.

FUTURE WORK

As with many other aspects of computerisation, the focus of much work appears to have moved to the web. Both Microsoft and Google have announced plans to develop personal health records, stored on the web. Issues arise in terms of security, privacy, accuracy and accessibility in the case of emergency. Who owns the data in the EHR is a matter of some debate, and it may be that women feel that they should choose the custodians of the data. Web-based systems offer the possibility of effectively free storage, integration with web-based health tools, and availability of the data in any context.

The rise of pervasive and ubiquitous computing (Weiser, 1993), has raised the expectation that information should be collected and used everywhere, though devices that quietly work in the background of our everyday life (Honey et al., 2007). Mobile phones have become the most common expression of this stream of development and some systems are already collecting clinical information via sensors attached to the phone, or giving health advice in this way.

Electronic health record systems have had a very diverse range of uptake, and there are major projects underway to increase their use in a number of countries, for example the UK, Canada and Australia and in particular organisations such as Kaiser Permanente. Success in these implementations requires more than just technical expertise, clinical staff and patients must all agree on the need to gain the benefits and the appropriate uses of the technology to improve care. Such agreement will require education, debate and acceptance of change.

REFERENCES

American College of Pathologists. (2000, 2000). About SNOMED. Retrieved January 11, 2002, from http://www.snomed.org/about_txt.html

Bates, D. W., Cohen, M., Leape, L. L., Overhage, J. M., Shabot, M. M., & Sheridan, T. (2001). Reducing the Frequency of Errors in Medicine Using Information Technology. *J Am Med Inform Assoc, 8*(4), 299-308.

Chard, T. (1987). Computerisation of Obstetric Records. In J. Studd (Ed.), *Progress in Obstetrics and Gynaecology: Volume Six* (1 ed., pp. 3-22). London: Chuchill Livingstone.

Coiera, E., & Tombs, V. (1998). Communication behaviours in a hospital setting: an observational study. *British Medical Journal, 316*(7132), 673-676.

Cope, I., Greenwell, J., & Mather, B. S. (1971). An Obstetric Data Project- General Description. *Med J Aust, 1*, 12-14.

Feachem, R. G. A., Sekhri, N. K., White, K. L., Dixon, J., Berwick, D. M., & Enthoven, A. C. (2002). Getting more for their dollar: A comparison of the NHS with California's Kaiser Permanente. *BMJ, 324*(7330), 135-143.

Franco, A., Farr, F. L., King, J. D., Clark, J. S., & Haug, P. J. (1990). "NEONATE"--An expert application for the "HELP" system: comparison of the computer's and the physician's problem list. *J.Med.Syst., 14*(5), 297-306.

Honey, M., Øyri, K., Newbold, S., Coenen, A., Park, H., Ensio, A., et al. (2007). *Effecting change by the use of emerging technologies in healthcare: A future vision for u-nursing in 2020.* Paper presented at the Health Informatics New Zealand (HINZ), 6th Annual Forum., Rotorua.

Horwood, A., & Richards, F. (1988). Implementing a Maternity Computer System. *Mid Chron Nurs Notes*(11), 356-357.

Kantor, G. S., Wilson, W. D., & Midgley, A. (2003). Open-source software and the primary care EMR. *Journal of the American Medical Informatics Association, 10*(6), 616.

Kenney, N., & Macfarlane, A. (1999). Identifying problems with data collection at a local level: survey of NHS maternity units in England. *BMJ, 319*(7210), 619-622.

Kohlenberg, C. F. (1994). Computerization of Obstetric Antenatal Histories. *Aust NZ J Obstet Gynaecol, 34*(5), 520-524.

Lilford, R. J., & Chard, T. (1981). Microcomputers in antenatal care: A feasibility study on the booking interview. *B Med J, 283*, 533-536.

Littlejohns, P., Wyatt, J. C., & Garvican, L. (2003). Evaluating computerised health information systems: Hard lessons still to be learnt. *British Medical Journal, 326*(7394), 860-863.

Main, D. S., Quintela, J., Araya-Guerra, R., Holcomb, S., & Pace, W. D. (2004). Exploring Patient Reactions to Pen-Tablet Computers: A Report from CaReNet. *Ann Fam Med, 2*(5), 421-424.

McDonald, C. J., Schadow, G., Barnes, M., Dexter, P., Overhage, J. M., Mamlin, B., et al. (2003). Open Source software in medical informatics--why, how and what. *International Journal of Medical Informatics, 69*(2-3), 175-184.

Mitchell, E., & Sullivan, F. (2001). A descriptive feast but an evaluative famine: systematic review of published articles on primary care computing during 1980-97. *BMJ, 322*(7281), 279-282.

openEHR Foundation. (2007). Welcome to openEHR. Retrieved 1st April 2008, from http://www.openehr.org/home.html

Patrick, J., Wang, Y., & Budd, P. (2007). *An automated system for conversion of clinical notes into SNOMED clinical terminology.* Paper presented at the Conference Name|. Retrieved Access Date|. from URL|.

Poissant, L., Pereira, J., Tamblyn, R., & Kawasumi, Y. (2005). The Impact of Electronic Health Records on Time Efficiency of Physicians and Nurses: A Systematic Review. *Journal of the American Medical Informatics Association, 12*(5), 505-516.

Schaller, R. R., & Schaller, R. R. (1997). Moore's law: past, present and future

Moore's law: past, present and future. *Spectrum, IEEE, 34*(6), 52-59.

Shipton, H. W. (1979). The microprocessor, a new tool for the biosciences. *Annual Review of Biophysics and Bioengineering, 8*, 269-286.

Skov, B., & Th. Hoegh. (2006). Supporting information access in a hospital ward by a context-aware mobile electronic patient record. *Personal Ubiquitous Comput., 10*(4), 205-214.

South, J., & Rhodes, P. (1971). Computer Service for Obstetric Records. *B Med J, 4*, 32-35.

Sribnick, R. L., & Sribnick, W. B. (1994). *Smart Patient, Good Medicine: Working With Your Doctor to Get the Best Medical Care.* New York: Walker and Company.

Thatcher, R. A. (1968). A package deal for computer processing in Obstetric records. *Med J Aust, 2*, 766-768.

Wang, S. J., Middleton, B., Prosser, L. A., Bardon, C. G., Spurr, C. D., Carchidi, P. J., et al. (2003). A cost-benefit analysis of electronic medical records in primary care. *The American Journal of Medicine, 114*(5), 397-403.

Webster, J., Forbes, K., Foster, S., Thomas, I., Griffin, A., & Timms, H. (1996). Sharing antenatal care: Client satisfaction and use of the 'patient-held record'. *Aust N Z J Obstet Gynaecol, 36*(1), 11-14.

Weed, L. L. (1968). Medical records that guide and teach. *New England Journal of Medicine, 278*(11+12), 593–600 + 652–597.

Weiser, M. (1993). Some computer science issues in ubiquitous computing. *Communications of the ACM, 36*(7), 75-84.

Whiddett, R., Hunter, I., Engelbrecht, J., & Handy, J. (2006). Patients' attitudes towards sharing their health information. *International Journal of Medical Informatics, 75*(7), 530-541.

Wilson, R. G., Purves, I. N., & Smith, D. (2000). Utilisation of computerised clinical guidance in general practice consultations. *Studies in health technology and informatics, 77*, 229-233.

ADDITIONAL READING

Implementing an Electronic Health Record System (Health Informatics) by James M. Walker, Eric J. Bieber, Frank Richards, and Sandra Buckley

Electronic Health Records: Understanding and Using Computerized Medical Records by Richard W. Gartee

Electronic Health Records: A Practical Guide for Professional and Organizations, 3rd Edition by MBA, RHIA, CHPS, CPHIT, CPEHR, FHIMSS Margret K. Amatayakul

Chapter VI
Imaging and Communication Systems in Obstetrics and Gynecology

Graham Parry
Middlemore Hospital, New Zealand

ABSTRACT

Information technology and communication systems have made imaging in women's health easier at many levels. There are now many commercial systems on the market, which improve the management of appointment systems, digital storage, and reporting of images, transmission of reports, teaching, and consultation particularly in large departments. This chapter discusses the use of communication technology for many aspects of imaging including transfer of images, data storage, teaching, and training as well as audit and accounting or budgeting, information sharing and research. Ultrasound imaging is used within the examples for this chapter, although many of the comments apply equally to other imaging modalities such as Xray, CT scanning, or MRI.

INTRODUCTION

Information technology and communication systems have made imaging in women's health easier at many levels. There are now many commercial systems on the market, which improve the management of appointment systems, digital storage and reporting of images, transmission of reports, teaching and consultation particularly in large departments.

Computer technology is also used as post processing to digitally manipulate the data acquired to look at the images in a different format.

I will use Ultrasound imaging as my examples for this chapter, although many of the comments apply equally to other imaging modalities such as Xray, CT scanning or MRI.

APPOINTMENT SYSTEMS

Computerisation of appointments allow:

- Appropriate allocation of time for different examinations. Many manual systems are rigid in time scheduling. Many computerised appointment systems can have an expected time for a particular examination customised into the software and therefore automatically generate the correct time allowance.
- Allocation of appointments from different clinics or receptionist sites. If different sites can access the computer program, rather than a manual system at one site, time can be saved by reducing the need for telephoning that site as well as reducing error from mishearing the time that is spoken.
- Generation of appointment letters
- Reappointments for patients who DNA (Do Not Attend)
- Generation of worklists on ultrasound equipment. When the worklist is on the ultrasound screen then patient data can be selected.

- Allocation of staff and equipment depending on the workload of the day.
- Integration with systems such as the electronic health record.

DATA STORAGE

Image Storage

In medical imaging, **picture archiving and communication systems** (PACS) are computers or networks dedicated to the storage, retrieval, distribution and presentation of images. The medical images are stored in an independent format. The most common format for image storage is DICOM (Digital Imaging and Communications on Medicine). For more information on DICOM refer to chapter 3.

PACS systems handle images from various medical imaging equipment, including ultrasound, MRI, CT and Xrays.

PACS replaces hard-copy based means of managing medical images, such as film archives.

Figure 1. A first trimester scan as stored on PACS

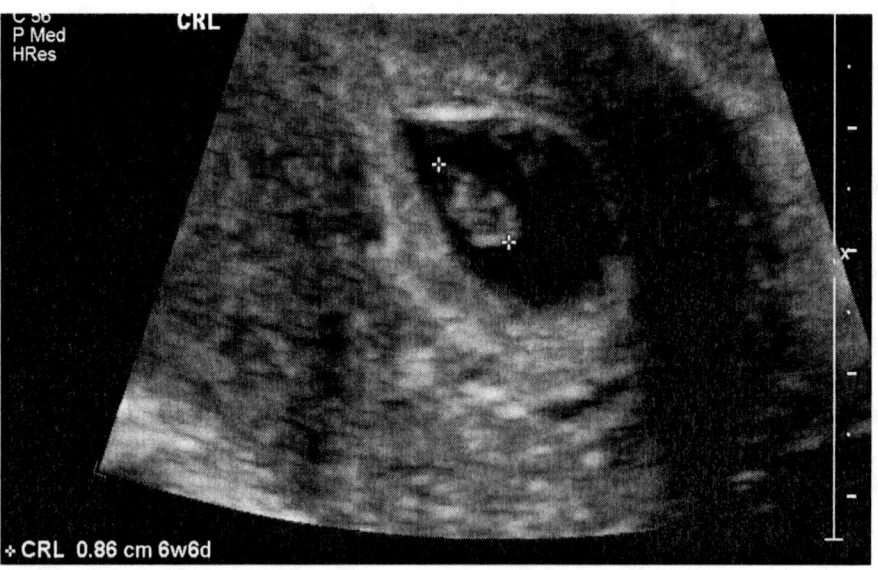

It expands on the possibilities of such conventional systems by providing capabilities of off-site viewing and reporting. Additionally, it enables practitioners at various physical locations to access the same information simultaneously. With the decreasing price of digital storage, PACS systems provide a growing cost and space advantage over film archives (as well as reducing the need for processing films with potentially toxic chemicals).

The most difficult area for PACS is interpreting the DICOM image format. DICOM has enough latitude to allow various vendors of medical imaging equipment to create DICOM compliant files that differ in the internal tags used to label the data.

A feature common to most PACS is to read the data from all the images into a central database. This allows the PACS user to retrieve all images with a common feature no matter the originating instrument.

Typically a PACS network consists of a central server that stores a database containing the images connected to one or more clients via a LAN (Local Area Network) or a WAN (Wide Area Network) which provide or utilize the images. Web-based PACS is becoming more and more common: these systems utilize the Internet as their means of communication, usually via VPN (Virtual Private Network) or SSL (Secure Sockets Layer). The software (thin or smart client) is loaded via ActiveX, Java, or NET Framework. Definitions vary, but most claim that for a system to be truly web based, each individual image should have its own URL. Client workstations can use local peripherals for scanning image films into the system, printing image films from the system and interactive display of digital images. PACS workstations offer means of manipulating the images (crop, rotate, zoom, brightness, contrast and others).

Modern radiology equipment feed patient images directly to the PACS in digital form.

A full PACS system should provide a single point of access for images and their associated data (i.e. it should support multiple modalities). It should also interface with existing hospital information systems: Hospital Information System (HIS) and Radiology Information System (RIS). For more information on interfacing see the following section on multi-equipment connection.

Report Storage

As well as digital storage of images, dictated reports can be stored. This can be as a preliminary report while waiting for the report to be verified by the author. There are a number of commercial software packages that do this, including Détente. Once the reports have been authorised they can be transferred electronically to a Medical Document storage system such as Concerto (Orion Health), thus creating a digital patient record. As the patients are entered into the system they can be coded as to the type of examination being performed. This allows the codes to be analysed and data produced for trends, planning and accounting.

Multi-Equipment Connection

Interfacing between multiple systems provides a more consistent and more reliable dataset:

- Less risk of entering an incorrect patient ID for a study – modalities that support DICOM worklists can retrieve identifying patient information (patient name, patient number, accession number) for upcoming cases and present that to the technologist, preventing data entry errors during acquisition. Once the acquisition is complete, the PACS can compare the embedded image data with a list of scheduled studies from RIS, and can flag a warning if the image data does not match a scheduled study.

• Data saved in the PACS can be tagged with unique patient identifiers (such as a social security number or NHS number) obtained from HIS. Providing a robust method of merging datasets from multiple hospitals, even where the different centers use different ID systems internally.

An interface can also improve workflow patterns:

• When a study has been reported the PACS can mark it as read. This avoids needless double-reading. The report can be attached to the images and be viewable via a single interface.
• Improved use of online storage and nearline storage in the image archive. The PACS can obtain lists of appointments and admissions in advance, allowing images to be prefetched from nearline storage (for example, tape libraries or DVD jukeboxes) onto online disk storage.

Recognition of the importance of integration has led a number of suppliers to develop fully integrated RIS/PACS systems. These may offer a number of advanced features:

• Dictation of reports can be integrated into a single system. The recording is automatically sent to a transcriptionist's workstation for typing, but it can also be made available for access by physicians, avoiding typing delays for urgent results, or retained in case of typing error.

It provides a single tool for quality control and audit purposes. Rejected images can be tagged, allowing later analysis. Workloads and turn-around time can be reported automatically for management purposes. Below is the flow diagram of one commercial system illustrating the above points

Figure 2. GE View point (www.gehealthcare.com)

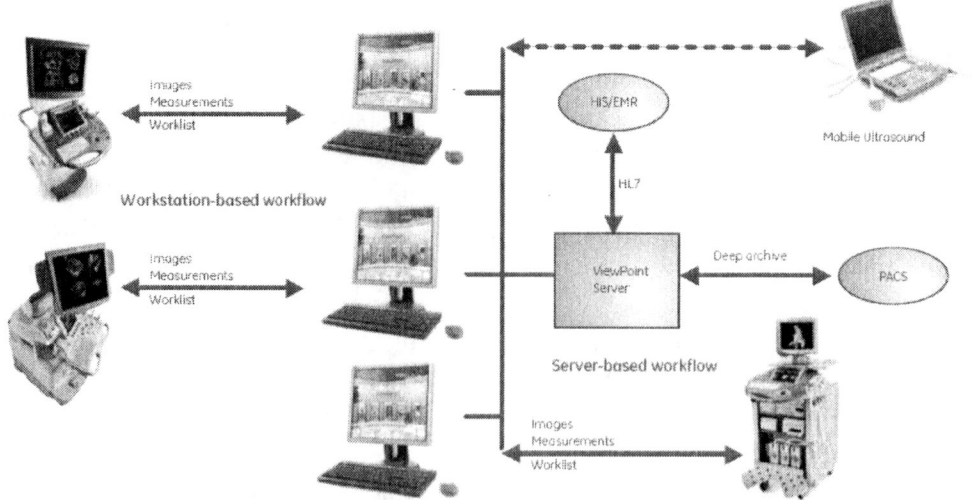

OTHER USES FOR STORAGE TOOLS

Audit

It is important to maintain good standards of measurement and of diagnosis, as these are the basis for making clinical decisions.

The collection of images allow for the ease of image review

- Correct diagnosis
- Measurement – film analysis

Audit can be performed by using the stored images by using a cumulative sum technique (CUSUM). A cusum chart is basically a graphical representation of the trend in the outcomes of a series of consecutive procedures performed over time. It is designed to quickly detect change in performance associated with an unacceptable rate of adverse outcome. At an acceptable level of performance, the cusum curve runs randomly at or above a horizontal line (no slope). However, when performance is at an unacceptable level, the cusum slopes upward and will eventually cross a decision interval. These are horizontal lines drawn across a cusum chart. Thus it provides an early warning of an adverse trend.

For a series of observations $X1, X2, \ldots\ldots\ldots X_n$, the cusum can be defined as

$$S_n = S (X0 - Xi)$$

Where $Xi = 1$ for a success and $Xi = 0$ for a failure. $X0$ is a reference or target value set for the level of performance. A success of nine out of ten is deemed acceptable than $X0$ would have a target value of 0.9 (ie equivalent to 90% success). In practice, this means that for every failed attempt the cusum increases by an increment of 0.9 and each success reduces the cusum by 0.1.

For example, in a series consisting of a success followed by a failure and four successes,

the cusum would take the values -0.1, 0.8, 0.7, 0.6, and 0.5.

CUSUM has been used in fetal measurement (biometry) both in training (Weerasinghe et al., 2006) and audit (Salomon et al., 2007).

Controlling for the distribution of biometrical measurements in comparison to reference measurements is a preliminary step for quality assessment. Z-scores have proven useful in such quality assessment processes. Cumulative sum (CUSUM) charts offer a simple way to detect changes in the mean of a quantity of interest. They focus on the cumulative sum of the deviations between the measurements and a target value.

Theoretically, Z-scores should follow a normal distribution with 0 and 1 for mean and standard deviation (SD) respectively.

In the study by Salomon et al a single sonographer prospectively measured biparietal diameter (BPD), head circumference (HC), abdominal circumference (HC), and femur length (FL) at 20-24 weeks gestation (Salomon, Poercher, Bernard, Rozenberg, & Ville, 2007). All measurements were transformed into Z-scores. CUSUM charts and tests were used to pick up any deviation greater than half an SD in the distribution of Z scores. 1266 examinations were included. Mean and SD were all statistically different from 0 and 1 respectively. CUSUM charts and test allow the authors to prospectively monitor sonographic measurements and to pick up trends towards deviant measurements for all four parameters.

The same technique has been used by the same authors in assessing the quality of Nuchal Translucency measurements (Salomon, Porcher, Bernard, Rozenberg, & Ville, 2007) as well as in quality control of images (Salomon, Nasr et al., 2007; Salomon, Winer, Bernard, & Ville, 2007).

For the quality control of images in the emergency room, five standard ultrasound planes illustrating key organs were defined (two for the uterus, one for each ovary and one to look for intraperitoneal fluid) (Salomon, Nasr et al., 2007).

Twenty examinations made of these 5 planes were selected from an ultrasound database. These 100 images were analysed by 2 experienced reviewers. Each image was scored by three to five criteria making a 23 point score for a complete examination. Inter- and intra-reviewers' differences for each criteria were analysed using adjusted Kappa. Reproducibility of scoring a complete examination was assessed by means of intra-class correlation (ICC) coefficients and Bland and Altman plots. Feedback and training were given to sonographers and another set of 20 examinations was scored to assess improvement in the quality of examinations.

The results of this study showed adjusted Kappa coefficients above 0.8 in 100% of the criteria. Before training, mean (±SD) examination score was 10.2 ± 2.8. ICC was 0.93 for examination scores. Bland and Altman plot analysis confirmed good reproducibility: mean difference and 95% limits of agreement were: -0.35 (-0.84; 1.4). Following feedback and training, there was a statistically significant increase in the mean score of 16.1±3.3 (p < 0.05). ICC remained high (0.96) and mean difference and 95% limits of agreement were: 0.3 (-0.1; 0.7).

The CUSUM technique has been used in training and in assessing trainee proficiency in fetal biometry measurement (Weerasinghe, Mirghani, Revel, & Abu-Zidan, 2006). In this study three primary healthcare doctors with no prior ultrasound training were recruited. Each trainee measured the fetal biparietal diameter (BPD), head circumference (HC), abdominal circumference (AC) and femur length (FL) on 100 consecutive pregnant women. The supervisor repeated the measurements. The CUSUM for each set of trainee measurements was calculated at a set failure rate of 10%. The point at which the graph fell below two consecutive boundary lines indicated the number of examinations required to achieve competence. The CUSUM graphs showed that the rate of learning measurement skills varied among the three trainees. The graph for the CUSUM series for BPD and HC measurement for all trainees fell below two consecutive boundary

Figure 3. CUSUM chart showing candidate proficiency (Weerasinghe et al., 2006)

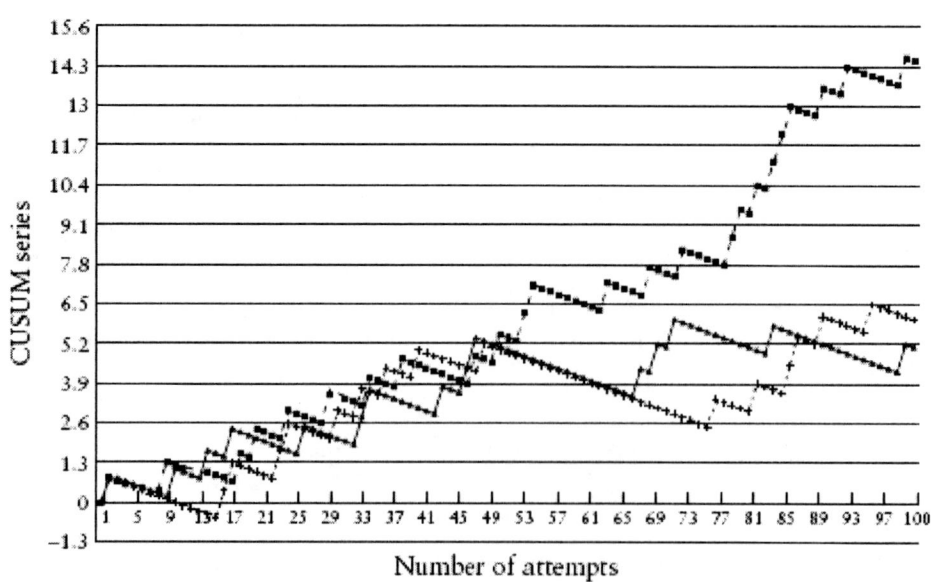

lines and remained there, indicating competence. The CUSUM series for AC measurement for two of the trainees indicated that competence was achieved; however, for the third trainee, while the graph fell below two consecutive boundary lines, indicating competence, it rose again, crossing two consecutive boundary lines. This indicated a loss of competence and the need for further training. FL measurements for the same trainee never fell below two consecutive boundary lines, indicating failure to achieve competence; the other two achieved competence, but failed to maintain it.

Figure 3 illustrates how one candidate never achieved competency as the graph continued to climb. The other two were initially competent, but failed to maintain that competency as the graph climbed above 2 consecutive boundary lines (Weerasinghe et al., 2006).

In conclusion, it can be seen that CUSUM is a useful tool for identifying points of competence and for quantifying the duration of ultrasound training required for each trainee. It provides an early indication of performance, and highlights difficulties in individual performance.

A website (http://www.sfape.com/) (Salomon, Bernard et al., 2007) is available using an automated tool that can help sonographers assess the quality of their examinations. Quality assessment is available for first, second and third trimester examinations.

This is a four step process:

1) Support is provided to help the sonographer choose the reference ranges that best fit their practice.
2) The sonographer can routinely check for the distribution of the biometrics
3) Biometrical images can undergo external qualitative audit based on a scoring system
4) Standard anatomical images can undergo external qualitative audit based on a scoring system

Accreditation

Images can be stored and selected for accreditation process. Accreditation can be streamlined with customisable data-mining.

Accounting/Budgeting

The integration of accounting systems with the appointments and image procedures allow these procedures to be accessed at the end of the month and compared to those that have been billed.

This allows:

- Bill payment for private/insurance schemes
- Generation of reports for accounting purposes
- IRD and tax audit
- Budget planning
- Reduction of billing errors.

Reporting

Reporting of imaging is pivotal in communication between all those caring for the patient as well as the patient herself.

- Image review via study list allows the selection of the studies to be reported. Some systems allow an archive module that can compare previous exams side by side on the screen with the current study.
- Exams can be read at a workstation that can be at a different site. This will improve workflow and enhance productivity. The use of the internet allows images to be read in a different timezone or country. This means that images can be read overnight and reports available first thing in the morning.
- Customisable reports and templates allow structured reports that ensure consistency of reporting of essential clinical information.

- Simultaneously review of images and reporting of data can be done with proforma templates on a computer workstation and the report immediately available. Dictation can be remote and need a typing pool or can be dictated using electronic voice recognition systems.

If a separate typing pool is used then reports need to be checked, corrected and then authorised before released to the referring clinician.

All reports are then stored in a central database and are integrated electronically.

Electronic reporting and storage of reports reduce the potential for human error by eliminating the tedious job of tracking charts, reports being missed or not signed off.

INFORMATION SHARING

Transfer of Images

Documents and images can be distributed using multiple options, including fax, email, PDF and DICOM formats. Images can be transferred between hospitals and community scanning sites for reporting as well as for consultation. This can be done in realtime using tele-ultrasound.

Integrated Systems

Integrated systems (Figure 4) allow the full use of IT and computers to streamline workloads by managing

- Appointments
- Records
- Image storage
- Reports
- Audits
- Data analysis
- Connection of multiple ultrasound machines to one server

- Connection of multiple sites to one network
- Exchange of patient data with ER, HIS/RIS and other IT system

The integration of all these tasks reduces the risk of loss, mistakes and decreases the work by reducing the repetition of tasks. Integration also allows improved communication between patient, referrer, technician and consultant as well as feedback to technician for quality control.

Consultation

Transmission of images allows consultation with experts. This can be done electronically or with large numbers of images they may need to be downloaded onto a DVD or video.

If these are rare cases they can then be posted on the internet for teaching purposes. The most well known website in the field of perinatology for interesting images is www.thefetus.net.

TEACHING AND TRAINING

Electronic storage of images is very useful for teaching pathology and demonstrating correct biometry and technique. The pathology will be stored as standard 2D images.

3D images are stored as volumes that can be manipulated with equipment specific software after they have been stored on DVD. This enables the volumes to be studied in a classroom situation with interactive practice using individual computers.

Two particular examples are outlined below: biometry and anatomy teaching.

Biometry

Biometry is the accurate measurement of fetal growth parameters. It requires accurate images and accurate caliper positioning.

Figure 4. An integrated system as installed by Millenium Technology (MillTech)

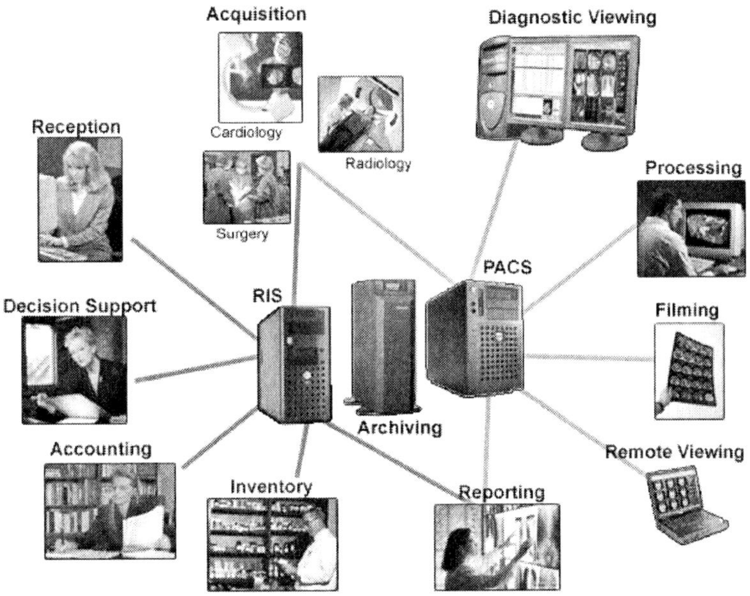

Acquisition

Diagnostic Viewing

Cardiology

Radiology

Reception

Surgery

Processing

PACS

RIS

Filming

Decision Support

Archiving

Remote Viewing

Accounting

Inventory

Reporting

Figure 5. A 3D fetal head dataset

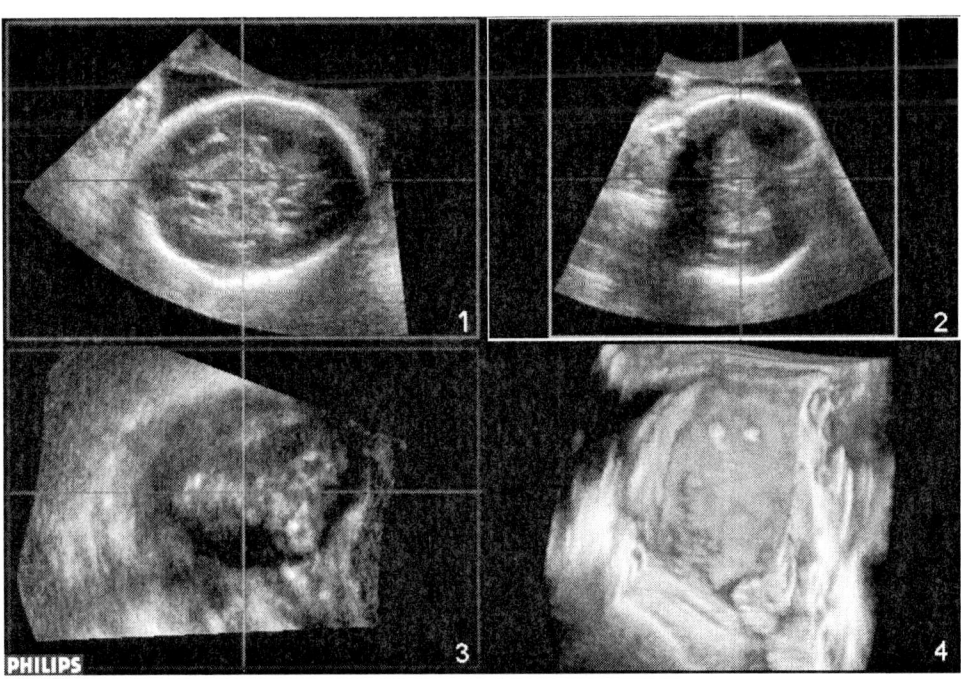

3D data sets allow image manipulation at the computer screen to select the correct image plane and assess correct positioning of calipers (Figures 5 & 6). This can be done by deliberately having an incorrect biometry plane and the trainee has to use the computer to obtain the correct plane and then position the calipers correctly.

This can be done as a group setting with multiple laptops, rather than each individual attempting to find the correct planes in a patient.

A small study (Lau, 2007) has demonstrated the use of this technique shortens the time taken to acquire the skills to be competent at doing biometry measurements.

Teaching Library

Electronic storage of images makes the development of a teaching library much easier than with a film library. Images can be copied and used for teaching at multiple sites when teaching:

- Standard pathology
- Normal anatomy
- Unusual cases
- The library can be used to collect cases to be used in an examination situation.

Anatomy

The images below can be manipulated to demonstrate fetal anatomy relationships. These were captured and demonstrated using a commercial system Philips Qlab ™.

I slice (Figure 7) is the Philips Qlab™ system which can divide the image into slices of variable thickness similar to a CT scan. This is also useful to teach anatomical relationships.

Figure 6. Fetal 3D volume

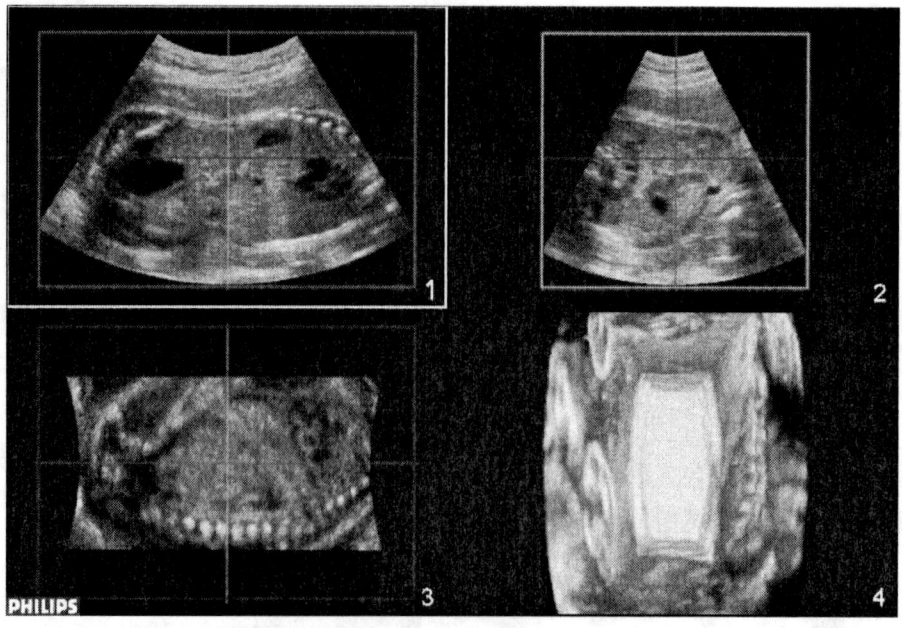

Figure 7. I-slice representation of 3D fetal volume

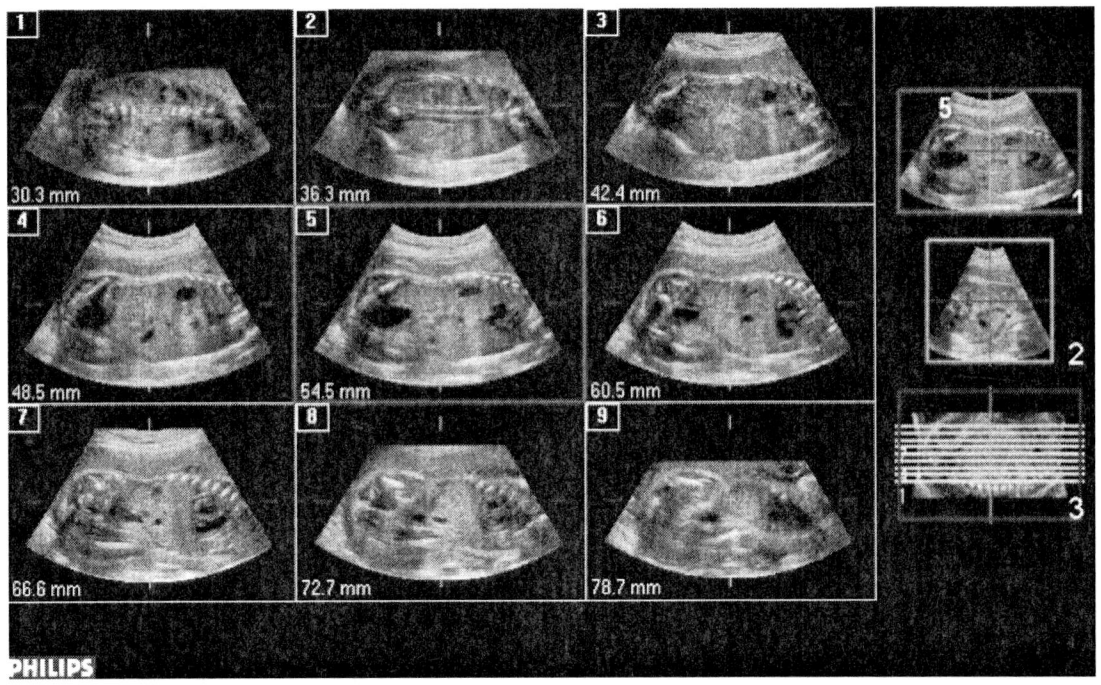

IMAGE ANALYSIS

2D On Cart Analysis

Analysis on the ultrasound equipment (on cart) is most useful in the ability to measure a fetus and determine its size and/or the rate of growth as well as the size of any organ within the body.

All ultrasound machines have software incorporated to allow the conversion of measurements to a gestational age.

There are a number of different software packages available and it is important that the one chosen is appropriate for the local population.

Many machines will allow these to be graphically presented. These include:

- Biometry (Measurement of fetal anatomical size)
- Estimation of Fetal Weight
- Doppler measurement and calculation of systolic and diastolic indices to give resistance indices.

3D Offline Analysis

Obstetrics

This includes the ability to measure volumes from 3D datasets as well as do a full anatomy survey. A recent study by Benacerraf showed that 3D volumes had a speed advantage over traditional 2D scanning (Benacerraf, Shipp, & Bromley, 2006).

In the study fifty consecutive women undergoing fetal anatomic survey at 17-21 weeks of gestation formed a study cohort. After standard 2D US was performed by one of eight sonographers, the same sonographer also obtained five 3D volumes to encompass the entire fetal anatomy. Three physicians interpreting the scans independently evaluated the completeness of the examination and time needed to read the scans, comparing the standard 2D method with the 3D volume reconstruction technique. The paired t test was used to compare biparietal diameter (BPD), femur length, and performance times between the 3D measurements and the 2D measurement. The t test was used to compare fetal anatomy according to volume angle.

The results showed that the mean time to perform 2D US was 19.6 minutes per examination, whereas mean time to perform complete 3D volume acquisition was 1.8 minutes. Mean times needed to interpret 3D images and measure the BPD and femur were 5.53, 4.79, and 5.34 minutes for the three interpreting physicians. Compared with complete fetal surveys performed with 2D US, individual fetal anatomic landmarks (except for fetal arms and cavum septum pellucidum) were identified more than 94% of the time by using 3D US. Grouping anatomic views by region, the heart, head, extremities, and abdominal views were completely seen in 88%, 90%, 90%, and 95% of patients, respectively. No significant difference was seen between the three physicians regarding completeness of the 3D examinations (P = .7).

The authors found that overall, the standard fetal anatomic survey could be performed in less than 2 minutes with 3D volume US, and the volumes can be interpreted in 6-7 minutes, compared with a mean of 19.6 minutes to perform standard 2D US.

Thus 3D reduced the time for a scan by 12 minutes, including image review.

Other advantages of 3D volumes for routine scanning include reduced fetal exposure to ultrasound, increased number of patients per room, especially with no waiting for the sonographer to find the sonologist to check the findings.

The down side to this is a reduction in patient satisfaction. A pregnancy scan is almost a social event with patients wanting to be shown each part of baby and to have an interaction with the person performing the scan (Benacerraf et al., 2006).

3D analysis can also be used to identify structures which are difficult to see on 2D scanning e.g. the corpus callosum.

Gynecology

Using advanced post-processing (examining and manipulating the images after they have been stored) applications for volume review in

Figure 8. 3D volume of the non-pregnant uterus

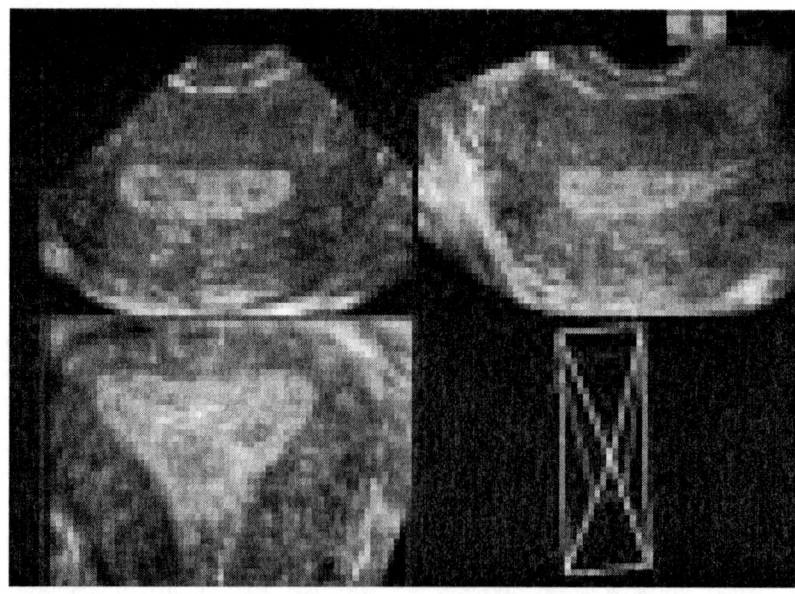

gynaecology allows the imaging of planes that are otherwise not possible to image.

In the 3D volume shown in figure 8, the top two images are the transverse and longitudinal planes. The bottom left image is a digitally manufactured image of the coronal plane. It is not possible to get this image on a transvaginal scan any other way.

Spatio-Temporal Image Correlation (STIC) Analysis

Post processing is useful to look at fetal hearts by using a 3D/4D process called STIC (Spatio-Temporal Image Correlation).

Figure 9 shows this technique combined with I slice. In this format it is possible to show all the essential components of a fetal heart study on one set of images (Espinoza et al., 2008)

DATA ANALYSIS

USS studies produce data in terms of fetal measurements. These have been traditionally biometry, which compares the fetal size to expected norms and alerts the physician to deviations.

More recently nuchal translucency has been evaluated and is now measured routinely also. The nuchal translucency is a measurement of a fluid filled space at the back of the fetal neck. An increased measurement is associated with an increased risk of Down syndrome, as well as other abnormalities.

There is an increasing risk of Down syndrome with increasing maternal age.

The Fetal Medicine Foundation has produced a computer program based on Baysian techniques (see chapter 15 for more information re Bayes theorem). This will calculate the risk of Down syndrome in that fetus after the maternal age, the size of the fetus and the measurement of the nuchal translucency are entered onto the computer.

Figure 9. STIC data volume represented using I-slice

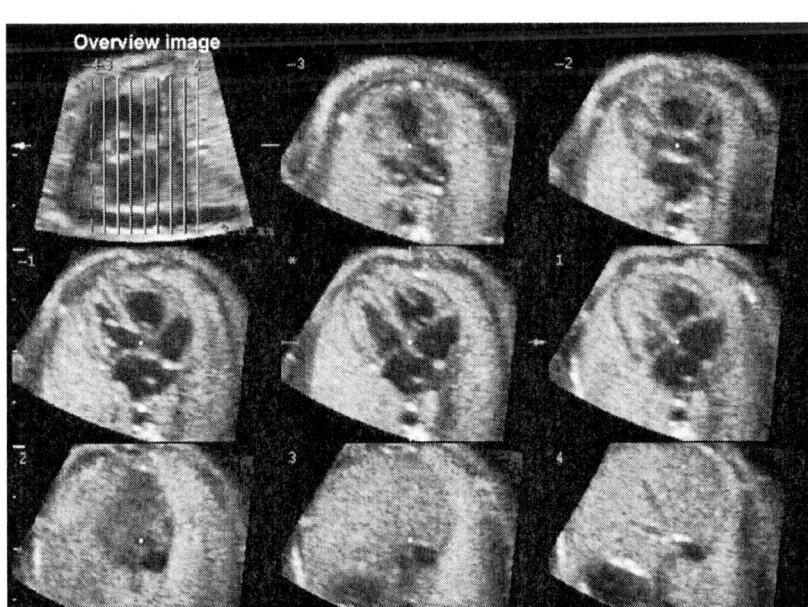

This is also a very good example of the ability to audit practice because to be able to access the program the scanner must submit images to the Fetal Medicine Foundation to ensure ongoing quality.

The data from the program is also collected to allow continued updating of the risk assessment. This would have to be the largest database with the collection of worldwide data.

RESEARCH

The new 3D imaging systems have produced a number of research projects in Women's Health, including Estimation of Fetal Weight.

One of the major problems in obstetric medicine is the estimation of fetal weight. There is a margin of error in any fetal weight estimations, which is increased in the larger fetuses, especially for pregnancies of diabetic women.

Figure 10. Fractional Thigh Volume

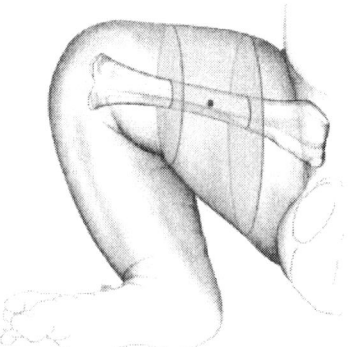

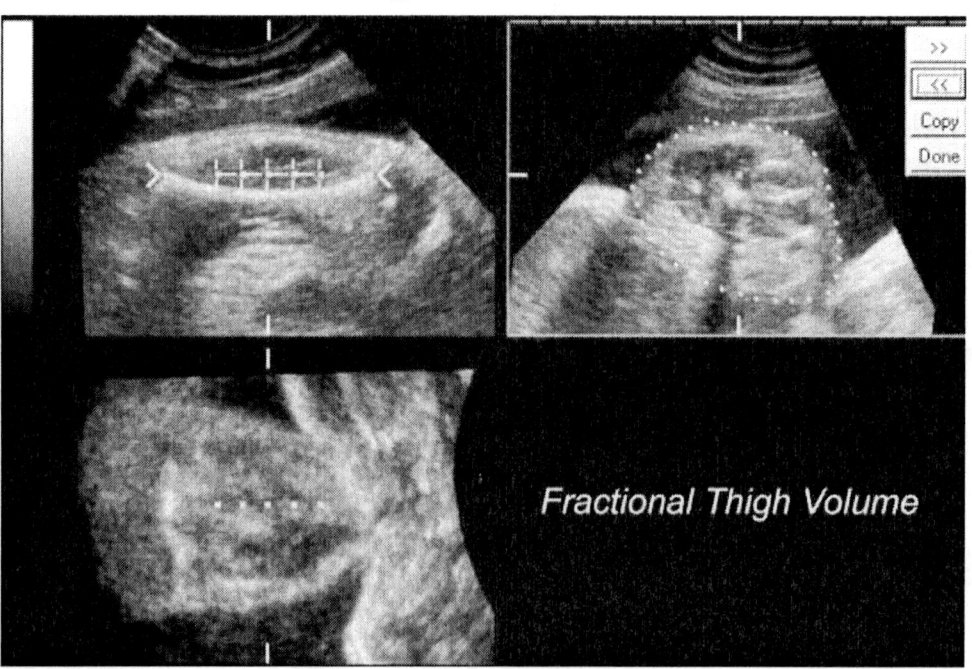

Lee (Lee et al., 2004) has introduced the concept of Fractional Thigh Volume to estimate fetal weight by incorporating soft tissue assessment in the equation.

The rationale for this can be seen from figure 10.

The centre of the femoral diaphyseal length is found and 50% of the diaphyseal length measured around this centre point. The volume of the soft tissue is then measured as is shown below.

Research continues into the accuracy of this estimation in diabetic fetuses as well as growth restricted fetuses.

FUTURE DIRECTION

I think the future is in the distribution of teaching by luminaries and in the audit and assessment of standards as well as pooling of knowledge and accumulation of data on rare cases.

SUMMARY

Informatics has revolutionised imaging and communication in Women's Health.

The future for sharing of information and pooling of data looks very bright. This will allow a greater understanding of disease processes, especially in rare conditions.

REFERENCES

Benacerraf, B. R., Shipp, T. D., & Bromley, B. (2006). Three-dimensional US of the fetus: volume imaging. *Radiology, 238*(3), 988-996.

Espinoza, J., Romero, R., Kusanovic, J. P., Gotsch, F., Lee, W., Goncalves, L. F., et al. (2008). Standardised views of the fetal heart using four-dimensional sonographic and tomographic imaging. *Ultrasound in Obstetrics and Gynecology, 31*, 233-242.

Lau, T. K. (2007). *3D Aids Biometry Skills.* Paper presented at the ISUOG.

Lee, W., Deter, R. L., McNie, B., Goncalves, L. F., Espinoza, J., Chaiworapongsa, T., et al. (2004). Individualized growth assessment of fetal soft tissue using fractional thigh volume. *Ultrasound in Obstetrics and Gynecology, 24*(7), 766-774.

Salomon, L. J., Bernard, J. P., Perl, B., Hamon, H., Calla, M., Auger, M., et al. (2007). An internet based tool for quality assessment of fetal ultrasound examination. *Ultrasound in Obstetrics and Gynecology, 30*(4), pp. 532-532(531).

Salomon, L. J., Nasr, B., Beoist, G., Bouhanna, P., Bernard, J. P., & Ville, Y. (2007). Implementation of quality control for standard gynaecological examination. Feasibility and reproducibility of an image scoring method for gynaecological ultrasound examination in the emergency room. *Ultrasound in Obstetrics and Gynecology, 30*(4), 512.

Salomon, L. J., Poercher, R., Bernard, J. P., Rozenberg, P., & Ville, Y. (2007). Cumulative sum (CUSUM) charts and tests: A simple method to assess the quality of fetal biometry. *Ultrasound in Obstetrics and Gynecology, 30*(4), 480-481.

Salomon, L. J., Porcher, R., Bernard, J. P., Rozenberg, P., & Ville, Y. (2007). Quantitative quality assessment of nuchal translucency measurements at 11-14 weeks: A role for cumulative sum (CUSUM) charts and tests. *Ultrasound in Obstetrics and Gynecology, 30*(4), 391.

Salomon, L. J., Winer, N., Bernard, J. P., & Ville, Y. (2007). Feasibility and reproducibility of an image scoring method for quality assessment of standard ultrasound planes at second trimester examination. *Ultrasound in Obstetrics and Gynecology, 30*(4), 370.

Weerasinghe, S., Mirghani, H., Revel, A., & Abu-Zidan, F. M. (2006). Cumulative sum (CUSUM) analysis in the assessment of trainee competence in fetal biometry measurement. *Ultrasound in Obstetrics and Gynecology, 28*(2), 199-203.

ADDITIONAL READING

PACS and Imaging Informatics: Basic Principles and Applications by H. K. Huang - 2004

Picture Archiving and Communications System (PACS) - NHS www.connectingforhealth.nhs. uk/systemsandservices/pacs

Section III
Obstetrics and Neonatology

Chapter VII
Statistical Measures in Maternity Care

Emma Parry
The University of Auckland, New Zealand

ABSTRACT

Pregnancy is unique in medicine in providing a discrete event with a fixed end. It is well suited to data collection and statistical assessment. This chapter systematically reviews the antenatal, intrapartum, and postnatal (both maternal and neonatal) aspects of care. The range of events that can occur and their classification is discussed. In many cases there is variation in classification around the world and between different organizations. These complexities are discussed. Once data is collected there are a number of ways to analyze it depending on what is wanted. Issues of appropriate numerator and denominator are discussed and the pitfalls which can occur. Use of data, both original and derived, is discussed in terms of type of use: planning, benchmarking, process review and research, and by whom: individual, local unit, country level, or internationally.

INTRODUCTION

Obstetrics lends itself to data collection. Each pregnancy is discrete with a final outcome. The options for most variables are limited. Most obstetric patients are well with no confounding illnesses.

Over the last twenty years there has been a revolution in patient attitude and with it doctors have been called to account for their actions. This has resulted in all disciplines of medicine being required to keep records of the service they are offering. Audit has become an integral part of our training and clinical practice.

Obstetrics as a specialty has responded relatively well to this challenge and most maternity units will be able to quote numbers of deliveries, induction of labor, caesarean section and forceps delivery rates. Increasingly through the necessity of data collection, computers are being introduced into obstetrics (South and Rhodes 1971; Lilford and Chard 1981; Chard 1987; Horwood and Richards 1988; Kohlenberg 1994).

The data collected can be a small collection of discrete variables or a large number of both discrete and continuous variables. There are many ways to examine and present the data and many ways to effectively use the data. It must always be borne in mind though that the quality of outputs depends on the quality of the data entered and the best outputs have checks of data validity.

In this chapter I will describe the variables of data that can be collected, commonly used definitions within maternity care and an introduction to the range of uses of this data. Other chapters within this book will examine more closely perinatal databases and data use.

MATERNITY VARIABLES

Antenatal

At the time of booking a number of demographic variables will be recorded. These will usually include data on the woman's age, ethnicity, contact details and primary health care physician. Previous pregnancies, their progress and outcome will be recorded. In many 'booking forms' there will be a series of general health questions for the woman and her family eg 'do you have diabetes or is there any history of diabetes in your family?' 'Have you had any surgery?'

There will be a large section of questions devoted to the current pregnancy. These will include information on last menstrual period (LMP), estimated date of delivery (EDD), confirmation of pregnancy method (urine test, scan). Was the pregnancy planned and if so was folic acid or vitamins taken periconceptually in countries where this is recommended? Where there has been a scan is the pregnancy confirmed to be singleton or multiple? Any problems so far?

Information on factors which may affect pregnancy and where modification is advised will usually be included. This includes smoking, alcohol intake and recreational drug use. Adherence to primary health strategies such as pap smears and sexually transmitted diseases (STD) swabs will often be included.

Most booking regimes will include some basic assessment of socio-economic status such as highest level of qualification or postcode/zipcode assessment.

As pregnancy progresses a series of visits will take place and investigations and screening options offered. The visits will usually include regular checks of blood pressure, urinalysis and abdominal palpation (to check the fetal growth and position). The woman's height and weight will often also be recorded. Routine blood tests will usually include a complete blood count (CBC), screening for hepatitis B, syphilis, HIV and checks for blood group and rubella immunity. In many countries women are offered scans and/or blood tests to assess the risk of Trisomy 21 (Down syndrome) and general fetal anatomy. Some countries also offer additional blood tests for screening. Some women may have invasive diagnostic tests such as amniocentesis.

All this information gathering and testing has evolved as part of the management of pregnancy over the last 100 years. For an individual woman it allows detection of problems in a timely fashion to allow appropriate intervention. However, with the advent of computerization, this information gathering has become a powerful tool to provide statistical measurement of many areas of maternity care delivery. Clearly though, the accuracy of the data depends on the care with which it is entered.

Commonly generated data include: pregnancy rate, average age of mothers and range, parity and gravidity, distribution of ethnicity and/or socio-economic group, smoking, drugs and alcohol use rates. Analyses of uptake of screening and diagnostic interventions may be evaluated. In addition there maybe an analysis of fetal abnormality and termination of pregnancy rates.

Delivery

At delivery there is usually high ratios of health care professionals to women. This is with good reason as it is a time of highest risk for the mother and fetus. This also means that there is usually a health care professional available to 'fill in forms'. A significant amount of paperwork is involved with delivery, but this is usually filled in by the person conducting the delivery which in turn generally ensures a high level of accuracy. In many maternity units, much of the necessary government paperwork is generated from the perinatal database after entering all the delivery details. This creates an incentive for the person conducting the delivery to enter information into an electronic form.

Details regarding type of labor onset (spontaneous or induced), drugs used, length of labor, type of delivery and indication and delivery of the placenta. If there was an induction the indication will usually be included. If there is a caesarean section whether it was planned before labor (elective) or required in labor (emergency) will be recorded along with the indication for caesarean section. The gestation at delivery will be recorded. There will usually be details about the mother's blood loss and the neonates first minutes of life.

Postnatal

Most women who deliver in hospital will have a short postnatal stay on a hospital ward. There are a number of events during the postnatal stay which will generate outcome measures. Complications such as wound infections, urinary tract infections and thromboembolic disease will generally be recorded, along with the requirement for medications and extra treatments. Method of infant feeding will be recorded and maybe important

for accreditation schemes eg Baby friendly hospital initiative (BHFI). Measures of bed stay and complexity eg high dependency unit admission are generally noted.

Neonatal

For babies who are unwell, there will usually be admission to a neonatal unit. A large proportion of these admissions will be due to prematurity and less often infection and poor condition at birth.

In the developed world nearly all-neonatal units will have a database of varying complexity. For more information on these read chapter nine which follows this one.

Data recorded will include sex, weight at birth, gestation at birth and delivery details. Details regarding feeding, interventions and treatments may be recorded. Length of stay and discharge treatments will usually be detailed. In many units follow-up care as an outpatient will get recorded in a database so that long term outcome statistics become available with time.

MATERNITY DEFINITIONS

Maternal

1st Trimester

Even before a woman has reached the end of the first trimester useful statistical measures can be measured and reported. Many countries will report pregnancy rates. These are usually presented as a rate per 1000 women of fertile age (e.g. age 15 to 50). Teenage pregnancy rates are often quoted as an independent subset.

Abortion rate and miscarriage rate will usually be expressed as numbers per thousand pregnancies.

In early pregnancy many women will be offered screening blood tests which vary from country to country. The percentage of the maternity population who are rubella immune, have syphilis and hepatitis B are useful data. In many countries HIV testing is routinely offered (opt-off screening) and rates of HIV in pregnant women maybe expressed as a percentage or per thousand depending on the prevalence.

Multiple pregnancies place an extra strain on healthcare services and most maternity units will report the numbers of these and outcomes. They create potential confusion within perinatal databases as there are two or more separate fetal/neonatal outcomes to report for each mother. In some systems the fetus has an assigned health number prior to birth, but this is unusual. Great care must be taken in assessing statistics including multiples. Measurements often quoted are multiple pregnancy rates as a percentage of total pregnancies, average gestation at delivery in weeks, induction of labor rates and mode of delivery. All but the last pertain to the pregnancy and therefore are straightforward.

Most developed countries have screening programs in place to detect Trisomy 21 (aka Down Syndrome). These programs cost a great deal to implement and run, but reduce costs in care of handicapped children and adults as many parents opt for termination. For screening programs to be effective uptake must reach a certain level. Maternity data can be produced in some centers which gives a percentage of women offered screening and those which accept the offer.

2nd and 3rd Trimester

In most developed countries a woman is offered a routine anomaly screening ultrasound scan at 18-20 weeks gestation. Rates of anomalies such as neural tube defects and cardiac defects can be collected (see fetal/neonatal section).

During the rest of the antenatal period there are many routine activities, which are repeated on a regular basis to detect particular pregnancy complications.

Pre-eclampsia is one of the most common causes of maternal mortality in the world and it's detection is important. Unfortunately there are a number of definitions and therefore comparison of data maybe difficult. In many databases the label of pre-eclampsia is assigned by an individual clinician rather than being assessed within the database by blood pressure measurements and presence of proteinuria. Rates are generally presented as percentages.

Fetal growth restriction is also important and suffers the same vagaries as pre-eclampsia. Many units will actually report small for gestational age (SGA) which is a post-natal definition based on a neonatal weight below a certain weight cut-off (eg 10th percentile) on population based centile charts.

Bleeding in pregnancy can have a number of causes. Placenta previa is a concern as it is associated with significant maternal morbidity and even mortality. Placenta previa may be reported, though the rates are generally low and will need to be expressed as a rate per 1000 or 10,000 pregnancies.

Preterm birth is the leading cause of perinatal mortality amongst normally formed infants. A number of factors influence preterm labor (eg smoking) and rates are usually expressed as percentages. Preterm labor is defined as birth less than 37 weeks. In developed countries this includes many neonates who will do well and dilute out the effect of very preterm babies. As an alternative, many units will also report rates of preterm labor/ birth less than 32 weeks to define a high risk group.

Delivery

Delivery as previously stated generates a great deal of maternity statistics. These include several routinely used statistics: induction of labor rate, caesarean section rate, operative vaginal delivery rate, episiotomy/tear rate, third degree tear rate, PPH rate and neonatal sex and weight.

Induction of labor, like multiple pregnancy, can result in varying statistics that mean apples are being compared to pears. Although the numerator may clearly be induction of labor, the denominator may change. It could be all pregnancies or all women where it is planned to deliver vaginally (ie excluding elective caesarean section). Obviously the percentage for the former will be lower than the latter.

Mode of delivery is usually expressed as a percentage, but like induction of labor care needs to be taken in assessing statistics. Usual practice is to express the mode of delivery as a percentage of all pregnancies. Caesarean sections can then be further divided into emergency and elective. Further analysis of data may allow VBAC (vaginal birth after caesarean section) rate and spontaneous and iatrogenic preterm delivery rate.

When comparing units or practitioners, one concern is that the population expressed in the denominator maybe higher or lower risk, thus skewing results. One approach to this has been to examine numerators as a proportion of a pre-specified group. In the 'low risk primipara', rates of induction, caesarean and other important numerators can be examined within a group of women in their first pregnancy with no risk factors (eg non-smokers, singletons) (Cleary 1996). Alternatively for particular outcome the background risk of women with the outcome can be examined. In the case of caesarean section the 'Robson groups' have been developed (Robson, Scudamore et al. 1996). These provide a category for all women having a caesarean section so that unit/individual can see what proportion of their caesarean cases are secondary to a particular set of circumstances (eg elective caesarean as breech).

As previously mentioned multiple pregnancy has its own problems. Mode of delivery will have more than one baby per mother and there maybe two or more different modes of delivery. Probably one of the best ways to express this outcome is to have an elective caesarean section rate as a percentage of all multiple pregnancies. For women who enter labour the mode of delivery can be expressed as percentage rates of various combinations eg Pregnancy A: twin 1-forceps, twin 2-normal vaginal, Pregnancy B: twin 1-forceps, twin 2-caesarean section, etc.

The rate of post partum haemorrhage (PPH) is expressed as a percentage of all births. It is generally considered to be primary (within 24 hours of birth) or secondary (after 24 hours until 42 days post partum).

Postnatal

During the postnatal period infections are usually expressed as a percentage of total births. Thrombo-embolic disease is an important cause of maternal mortality and although it can occur at any time in the pregnancy it is more frequent in the postnatal period. It is usually reported as a rate per 10,000 pregnancies.

Maternal Mortality

Maternal mortality is usually rare in the developed world, but is sadly common in resource-constrained countries. It is seen as key indicator of improving maternity services when it reduces in resource-constrained countries.

The Tenth Revision of the International Classification of Diseases (ICD-10) defines a maternal death as *'the death of a woman while pregnant or within 42 days of termination of pregnancy, irrespective of the duration and site of the pregnancy, from any cause related to or aggravated by the pregnancy or its management but not from accidental or incidental causes'*.

The 42-day limit is somewhat arbitrary, and in recognition of the fact that modern life-sustaining procedures and technologies can prolong dying and delay death, ICD-10 introduced a new category, namely the late maternal death, which is defined as the *death of a woman from direct or indirect obstetric causes more than 42 days but less than one year after termination of pregnancy.*

According to ICD-10, maternal deaths should be divided into two groups:

• *Direct obstetric deaths* are those resulting from obstetric complications of the pregnant state (pregnancy, labour and the puerperium), from interventions, omissions, incorrect treatment, or from a chain of events resulting from any of the above.

• *Indirect obstetric deaths* are those resulting from previous existing disease or disease that developed during pregnancy and which was not due to direct obstetric causes, but was aggravated by physiologic effects of pregnancy.

Accidental or incidental causes would include such events as death during an earthquake or road traffic accident (RTA). Some care should be taken with RTA in particular though, as cases of suicide maybe hidden amongst these (Oates 2003).

The Maternal Mortality Ratio (MMR) is the maternal death rate per 100,000 live births. Given they are a rarity in developed countries they are usual collated from a region or whole country and maybe collated over several years to be able to provide meaningful data. An example is the UK Triennial reports. The Seventh Report of the Confidential Enquiries into Maternal Deaths in the United Kingdom is published by the RCOG press.

Fetal/Neonatal

At its most basic the outcome for the fetus/neonate will be survival. The death of a fetus in-utero (before birth) is defined as a stillbirth or intra-uterine fetal death. Prior to a cut-off gestation the term miscarriage should be used. In the past the cut-off used was 28 weeks gestation, but with the limits of viability being ever pushed to earlier gestations, this cut-off has fallen. In England in Scotland it is 24 weeks (http://www.rcog.org.uk/resources/public/pdf/goodpractice4.pdf) and in New Zealand it is 20 weeks or >400gms (http://www.legislation.govt.nz/libraries/contents/om_isapi.dll?clientID=1342601627&infobase=pal_statutes.nfo&jump=a1995-016&softpage=DOC). The WHO define a stillbirth as one after 24 weeks or >500gms.

Where a neonate is born with signs of life, but dies within 28 days it is termed a neonatal death. From 28 days to age one year is termed a post-neonatal death or infant mortality. These definitions tend to be universal unlike stillbirth. Neonatal mortality is divided into early: less than 7 days and late: 8 days to 28 days. This separation is to try to reflect the different reasons for neonatal death, with early neonatal deaths being more likely to be due to factors surrounding birth and later deaths more due to the environment the neonate is living in eg neonate in country where infectious diarrhoeal diseases are endemic.

The perinatal mortality rate is a further attempt to use the fetal/neonatal death to reflect the effect of obstetric and early neonatal care on outcomes. The definition of a perinatal mortality is usually all stillbirths (however they are defined) plus all early neonatal deaths in the first week of life per thousand births, although the WHO defines it as all stillbirths plus all early neonatal deaths up to 28 days as a per thousand births.

Rates of stillbirth and perinatal mortality are generally represented as per thousand of all pregnancies proceeding to a gestation where the lower limit of stillbirth is defined. Neonatal death rates are usually represented as a per thousand live births (http://www.who.int/healthinfo/statistics/indneonatalmortality/en/)

Congenital abnormality rates are often collected. These may include rates of chromosomal aberrations eg trisomy 21 or structural abnormalities eg neural tube defects. Depending on the rate of these they maybe expressed as per 1000 or less commonly 10,000 pregnancies. The numerator should include terminations for abnormality if all pregnancies are included denominator. If live-births only are included as the denominator then the live birth abnormalities are usually given as the numerator. These rates maybe very different due to terminations and natural fetal wastage amongst the abnormal group of fetuses.

For neonates admitted to the neonatal unit many other outcomes can be recorded. This is covered in the chapter on health informatics in neonatology.

STATISTICAL MEASURES IN ACTION

From the preceding sections it can be seen that a vast array and amount of data can be collected which is related to pregnancy. This data can be used by governments, regional administration, non-governmental organizations (NGOs), researchers and individual health care providers. The data can be used for many different activities. An overview of the areas covered in this section with examples are shown in Table 1.

International Planning

Maternity measures are important both in the developed and resource-constrained setting. Measures of teenage pregnancy rate, unplanned pregnancy and termination of pregnancy are useful indicators of healthcare provision and in some cases women's standing in the community.

Within the resource constrained setting, the Millenium Development Goals were set by the United Nations in 2000. They aimed to improve eight outcomes in all resource constrained countries by the year 2015. The fourth and fifth goals pertain to child and maternal health. There are specific outcomes for these goals and they form part of the tools used to decide on funding. Statistical data allows progress towards the goals to be tracked e.g. maternal mortality.

These datasets are used by many international organizations. They can be used for planning where funds should be distributed and to what degree. The World Health Organisation (WHO) uses data such as maternal mortality to assign funding programmes such as EmOC (Emergency Obstetric Care). The funding is used to provide centres which have the ability to perform common obstetric procedures such as caesarean section.

Table 1. An overview of potential areas for use of maternity data with examples

	Planning	Benchmarking	Process Review	Research
International	NGO funding streams	Program planning	Introduction of family planning initiatives	Effect of EMOC program introduction
National	Midwifery training	Identifying 'gaps' in service delivery	Maternal Mortality	Folic acid fortification
Local	Equipment purchase	Ensuring quality	Adherence to guidelines/protocols	Post dates management and outcomes
Individual	Patient volumes and clinics	Amniocentesis miscarriage rate	Checking referrals	N=1 studies

Maternity statistics form the basis of international reports such as Reproductive Health Response in Conflict Consortium 2004 report of EmOC http://www.womenscommission.org/pdf/EmOC.pdf.

Private organizations such as the Bill and Melinda Gates Foundation, also use maternity statistics to decide on where and how to support maternity in the resource constrained environment.

In the developed world statistics are used to plan services. For example, there are a number of new fetal therapies which are rarely performed and require a high level of expertise. In the case of fetoscopic intervention for congenital diagphragmatic hernia, in Europe the fetal medicine team in Belgium take referrals from surrounding countries as statistics have shown that it would not be worth setting up centers in each European country.

International Benchmarking

Crude maternity statistics are collected by WHO in resource constrained countries. The accuracy will vary considerably. Due to political events, it is sometimes difficult to collect data and if available may not be accurate. However, despite these limitations, international maternity datasets are a valuable tool for benchmarking. This allows serious deficiencies in a particular region of the world or country to be recognized (Bell and Oakley 2006).

In the 1990s in Afghanistan, the maternal mortality rates were reported as increasing out of proportion to their near neighbours (6000+ per 100,000 women). This was in part due to issues of access to maternity care at the time and a strong patriarchal society where women are considered less important. In the last six years significant funds have been directed into the country and it is hoped that maternal mortality will fall http://www.unicef.org/media/media_27853.html.

International Process Review

Process review of implementation of international initiatives allows interventions to be evaluated. For example Emergency Obstetric Care (EmOC) is a scheme which aims to improve access to poorer communities to emergency obstetric care. It involves training local nurses/ midwives and doctors to be able to provide basic and more advanced emergency obstetric care depending on the facilities available. The package is similar in different countries, but may not be so effective if not implemented correctly or appropriately to the environment. In Rwanda a review of the EmOC services highlighted improved outcomes (Kayongo, Rubardt et al. 2006) consistent with appropriate implementation.

International Research

Many interventions are introduced without proper evaluation. This sin appears to be worst in the resource constrained world. International level research such as evaluating different types of antenatal care has been carried out across country boundaries. Different customs of care allow different approaches to be examined by directly comparing different countries outcomes where data collection is comparable. Sweden introduced pap smear screening prior to Norway and showed a significant reduction in cervical cancer (Mählck, Jonsson et al., 1994).

National Planning

From the booking data, information on numbers of women entering pregnancy, the age, socio-economic distribution and parity can be evaluated. Booking statistics can be used to give an indication of the level of risk of a population eg socioeconomic group and smoking. This can be important at a national and regional level when planning services and implementing prevention programs.

National planning also includes calculations of bed space requirements. This can be very important in the case of neonatal cots as changes in birthrate and level of risk of the population can result in large changes in requirements. In addition as services improve the gestation at which neonates are expected to survive and require intensive care lowers. This is most often seen in the resource constrained setting as the healthcare expenditure increases and expectations increase.

If birthrate and complexity of cases increases, then there is an increased need for qualified doctors and midwives to care for the population. There is a significant lead time involved in training these individuals and good quality data is essential to try and predict the requirements in the next ten years.

The introduction of new procedures at a National or Local level can also be important. The uptake of Trisomy 21 (Down syndrome) screening has meant that most women will have an extra ultrasound scan. This may translate into a requirement for more ultrasound machines.

National Benchmarking

Maternity statistics can be used for benchmarking at a national level. Comparisons can be made between countries for standardized outcomes such as fertility rate, termination rate, perinatal mortality rate and maternal mortality. For countries who are increasing expenditure on health they can use these benchmarks to help identify gaps in their sevices or to identify areas that are performing well. For developed countries comparisons to neighbour countries can ensure that services continue to be at a high standard.

A major potential pitfall is that data may not be collected in the same way, as accurately or use different definitions. There is the possibility of comparing apples and pears rather than the same things! For national benchmarking to be useful the dataset used must be clearly defined, of good quality and comparable.

National Process Review

Maternity statistics can be used to assess processes at a national level. Many developed countries have introduced screening for Trisomy 21 using ultrasound scanning, biochemical tests on serum or both. The cost of introducing such a system is thought to be offset by an increase in terminations for Trisomy 21 and therefore reduced costs of caring for these children.

Maternal mortality is a rarity in developed countries and cases are reviewed on an individual basis to examine closely system faults and try to improve outcomes. There is an assumption that for each maternal death there are numerous 'near misses' and that by focusing on system failures deaths and morbidity can be avoided. Within the resource constrained setting maternal mortality is sadly a common occurrence. As a country's gross domestic product (GDP) increases and interventions are put in place to improve maternal outcome, maternal mortality rates are generally seen to reduce and become a useful long-term barometer of the quality of maternity care and access to services.

National Research

Folic acid supplementation prior to pregnancy and in the first 12 weeks of pregnancy reduces the development of neural tube defects by 80%. As only half of pregnancies are generally planned many women so not have the appropriate level of folic acid in their diet. In many countries fortification of food (usually flour) with folic acid has been introduced (De Wals, Tairou et al. 2007). Longitudinal maternity databases in countries where this has occurred are now showing a reduction in neural tube defects.

Local Planning

Data is generally collected on a year-by-year basis to show trends occurring. It is important that indicators are presented in the same way as change in definition or denominator can mean that trends cannot be accurately interpreted.

Local areas or individual hospitals may use data to plan new buildings (eg beds available), order equipment, staffing levels or referral patterns.

Local Benchmarking

It is important to note the denominator in all comparisons between data/ units. Caesarean section rates for example can quoted as a percentage of total births or as a percentage of women who enter labor- ie elective caesarean sections can be excluded. These two statistical measures are looking at different areas. One unit may have a low caesarean section rate for women who enter labor, but a high elective caesarean section rate overall as many women have an elective caesarean section. One way to level the playing field is to examine a known dataset, such as using Robson groups (Robson, Scudamore et al. 1996). With this tool caesarean sections are grouped depending on whether the woman is primiparous, has had a previous vaginal delivery or caesarean section and whether this caesarean section is elective or emergency. Induction of labor is also included as this is known to increase caesarean sections. Caesarean section rates are fraught with concerns of over-medicalisation of birth or the current popular concept of 'to posh to push' and woman's choice. The 'correct' caesarean section rate is a matter of opinion!

Operative vaginal delivery (OVD) rates are also fraught with pitfalls. The OVD rate may reflect a percentage of all pregnant women, those who enter labor and as a percentage of those who have a vaginal delivery. Clearly the rate will be much higher if as a percentage of women delivering vaginally compared to all women! It is also important to examine how cases are coded if data from different units are being compared.

Local Benchmarking is often concerned with ensuring that the care offered is of an appropriate standard for the setting. Institutions where standards are below that expected can be identified quickly and the situation rectified.

Local Process Review

Many countries have introduced smoking cessation programs in pregnancy (de Vries, Bakker et al., 2006). These can be evaluated over time by using the booking data to ascertain the number of women referred to these services (if included in the database) and over a longer period of time examining trends in conditions known to be related to smoking in pregnancy eg fetal growth restriction and abruption.

Another example of local process review is the audit of HIV testing where the test is opt-on and opt-off. Often process review highlights that when the test becomes an opt-off test (automatically done unless the women decides she doesn't want it) the testing rate is much higher as the process of testing is more routine.

Local Research

Statistical measures which are collected routinely can be used for research projects in an institution. Parry et al examined outcomes of post-dates induction of labour on method of delivery (Parry, Parry et al. 1998).

Individual Planning

For the individual clinician, maternity statistics can be invaluable in planning. For example a clinician maybe examining whether to advertise for a colleague in his/ her department. Patient volumes and complexity can be gleaned from computerized maternity data.

Individual Benchmarking

Most clinicians need to show evidence of continuing medical education. Many colleges are moving to part of this being compulsory review of practice which could include audit of practice or peer review. This allows a clinician to compare themselves to an accepted standard or their peers. Using standard datasets such as the standard primipara for example (a low risk, young primipara), caesarean section rates, third degree tear rates and others can be fairly compared.

In the field of fetal medicine amniocentesis can be audited against expected standards for bloody taps, > one needle insertion and miscarriage rate after the procedure.

Individual Process Review

Individuals can examine their personal processes eg how many women are referred for Glucose Tolerance Test who meet institution criteria.

Individual Research

Maternity statistics can be used to search for outcomes of women where different types of care have been undertaken, either in a randomized or non-randomized way.

FUTURE RESEARCH DIRECTIONS

In the future it is likely that more commercial perinatal databases will enter the marketplace, increasing competition and reducing costs. Hopefully this will translate into increased data storage allowing more accurate analysis, particularly in resource constrained settings. In the developed world more complex systems are being developed which will result in the perinatal database and electronic health record becoming seamless. Many perinatal databases produce an array of reports, but it maybe more in the future that databases use alerts to produce ad hoc reports highlighting concerns identified on routine internal checks e.g. increasing operative vaginal delivery rates after a certain time of day.

SUMMARY

Obstetrics encompasses a discrete event in a woman's life which is uniquely able to be documented to a high degree of accuracy. Many of the potential variables that can be documented can be clearly defined and recorded. However many errors occur. These are as a result of a number of issues: lack of capture of all women, lack of capture of all data on a particular woman, inaccuracy of data. Ultimately these can be identified and completed from written notes of the electronic health record where there is resource to do this. It is important when using this raw data to be aware of potential limitations of the data.

Once data is entered further errors can occur in analysis if numerator and denominators are not well defined and uniform.

If there is accurate complete data then there is enormous potential to use that data for planning, benchmarking, process review and research.

REFERENCES

Bell, K. N., & Oakley, G. P. (2006). Tracking the prevention of folic acid-preventable spina bifida and anencephaly. *Birth Defects Research. Part A, Clinical and Molecular Teratology, 76*(9), 654-7.

Chard, T. (1987). Computerisation of Obstetric Records. *Progress in Obstetrics and Gynaecology: Volume Six*. J. Studd (Ed.), London: Chuchill Livingstone (pp. 3-22).

Cleary, R. (1996). The standard primipara as a basis for inter-unit comparison of maternity care. *British Journal of Obstetrics & Gynaecology, 103*, 223-229.

de Vries, H., Bakker, M. et al. (2006). The effects of smoking cessation counseling by midwives on Dutch pregnant women and their partners. *Patient Education and Counseling, 63*, 177-87.

De Wals, P., Tairou, F. et al. (2007). Reduction in neural-tube defects after folic acid fortification in Canada. *New England Journal of Medicine, 357*(2), 135-42.

Horwood, A., & Richards, F. (1988). Implementing a Maternity Computer System. *Mid Chron Nurs Notes*, (11), 356-357.

Kayongo, M., Rubardt, M. et al. (2006). Making EmOC a reality--CARE's experiences in areas of high maternal mortality in Africa. *International Journal of Gynaecology and Obstetrics, 92*(3), 308-19.

Kohlenberg, C. F. (1994). Computerization of Obstetric Antenatal Histories. *Aust NZ J Obstet Gynaecol, 34*(5), 520-524.

Lilford, R. J., & Chard, T. (1981). Microcomputers in antenatal care: a feasibility study on the booking interview. *B Med J, 283*, 533-536.

Mählck, C. G., Jonsson, H. et al. (1994). Pap smear screening and changes in cervical cancer mortality in Sweden. *International Journal of Gynaecology and Obstetrics, 44*(3), 267-72.

Oates, M. (2003). Suicide: the leading cause of maternal death. *British Journal of Psychiatry, 183*, 279-81.

Parry, E. C., Parry, D. T. et al. (1998). Induction of Labour for post term pregnancy: An observational study. *Aust NZ J Obstet Gynaecol, 38*(3), 275-279.

Robson, M. S., Scudamore, I. W. et al. (1996). Using the medical audit cycle to reduce cesarean section rates. *American Journal of Obstetrics and Gynecology, 174*(1 Pt 1), 199-205.

South, J., & Rhodes, P. (1971). Computer Service for Obstetric Records. *B Med J, 4*, 32-35.

ADDITIONAL READING

WHO reproductive health data http://www.who.int/reproductive-health/

WHO – Making pregnancy safer initiative: http://www.who.int/making_pregnancy_safer/en/index.html

Chapter VIII
Building Knowledge in Maternal and Infant Care

Kiran Massey
University of British Columbia and BC Women's Hospital and Health Centre, Canada

Tara Morris
University of British Columbia and BC Women's Hospital and Health Centre, Canada

Robert M. Liston
University of British Columbia, BC Women's Hospital and Health Centre, and British Columbia Perinatal Health Programme, Canada

Peter von Dadelszen
University of British Columbia and British Columbia Perinatal Health Programme, Canada

Mark Ansermino
University of British Columbia, Canada

Laura Magee
University of British Columbia and British Columbia Perinatal Health Programme, Canada

ABSTRACT

Our ultimate goal as obstetric and neonatal care providers is to optimize care for mothers and their babies. As such, we need to identify practices that are associated with good outcomes. Although the randomized controlled trial is the gold standard for establishing the benefits of interventions, trials are very expensive and must be reserved for the most important of clinical questions. As an alternative, continuous quality improvement involves iterative cycles of practice change and audit of ongoing clinical care. An obvious prerequisite to this is ongoing data collection about interventions and outcomes, as well as demographics, pregnancy characteristics, and neonatal care that may affect the intervention-outcome relationship. In Canada (as in some other developed countries), much of the country is covered by regional reproductive care databases. These collect information on maternal demographics, pregnancy characteristics, labour and delivery, and basic information on maternal and perinatal outcomes. The primary objective of these databases is to monitor geographical trends and disparities in health outcomes. As such, there is little information about interventions, especially outside the period of labour and delivery. Also, there is no standardization of definitions, and efforts to produce a "minimal dataset" have not yet yielded agreement, even after many years of work. A more comprehensive system is required. Moving in this direction would serve many purposes: efficiency, economy in the setting of shrinking budgets, standardization of definitions, collaboration, and creation of stable background data collection onto which researchers could "clip" extra data required for specific studies. These activities would lay the foundation for the electronic health record, which cannot build its foundation on the "Tower of Babel" that is our current definitional structure in women's health and obstetrics, in particular. Continuous quality improvement efforts and interaction with regional reproductive care programmes will facilitate translation and transfer of knowledge to care-givers and patients. These efforts raise concerns about privacy and security which remain major barriers to the EHR. However, security must be balanced with the need for health information.

OBSTETRICS: AN HISTORICAL LEADER IN KNOWLEDGE BROKERING

Over the past few decades, obstetrics has been a leader in medicine in the dissemination of medical knowledge. In 1979, when Archie Cochrane proposed, "a critical summary, adapted periodically, of all relevant randomized controlled trials"(1), it was obstetrics that first seized the call. A registry was developed of controlled trials of interventions during pregnancy and early infancy(2). Thus was born the Oxford Database of Perinatal Trials, otherwise known as the "Odd Pot" (ODPT). This served as a resource for reviews of interventions in maternal and neonatal care, and an important tool used by those involved in quality of care promotion(3). In 1993, with the influence of the worldwide web and advanced software, the ODPT became an electronic publication known as the Cochrane Collaboration Pregnancy and Childbirth Database (CCPC). Archie Cochrane urged specialty fields to arrange significant summaries of such data in the 1972 publication *Effectiveness and Efficiency: Random Reflections on Health Series* (1). Over the years it was obstetrics that again answered the call by publishing the first

edition of *A Guide to Effective Care in Pregnancy and Childbirth* (1989) (4) which summarizes randomized controlled trials regarding maternal and infant care in order to better understand health practices and set policies(5). *A Guide to Effective Care in Pregnancy and Childbirth* (6) is still used today as an effective resource among health care providers and their patients.

This type of RCT analysis, systematic reviews, extended into many other health and medical fields to later form the Cochrane Database of Systematic Reviews (CDSR) in 1994. The rest is, as they say, history as this accomplishment proved to be an enormous step forward not just for obstetrics but for the future of medicine. Having the CDSR available on delivery suites is considered to be an important quality of care criterion when assessments are made of academic obstetrics and gynaecology services and programmes. Today, no application for research funding can be made without reference to the relevant Cochrane review. Book was the first evidence based book, now onto third edition.

The CDSR is predicated on the idea that the randomized controlled trial is the least biased form of information about interventions that improve maternal and perinatal outcomes. However, the many limitations of relying solely on randomized trials have become more obvious over time. First, for many of the questions posed in maternal/infant care, there are insufficient trials to guide clinical practice. Second, trials are onerous to mount and very expensive to conduct. As such, they must be reserved for the most important of research questions. Finally, there are other questions that are simply unethical to study by using a randomized trial design.

THE CANADIAN PERINATAL NETWORK (CPN)

The CPN is made up of Canadian researchers from 22 tertiary perinatal units across Canada who collaborate on research issues relating to perinatal health. The CPN was born of a desire to generate new knowledge in the area of obstetric care, by using a continuous quality improvement approach to study clinical practice. This approach is based on the desire to identify those practices that are associated with good outcomes for mothers and babies, correcting for potential confounders of that relationship. The approach is predicated on the PDSA cycle and is designed to improve the quality of care (7).

CONTINUOUS QUALITY IMPROVEMENT: THE "PSDA" APPROACH

The actual approach involves the following steps: 'Plan', 'Do', 'Study', and then 'Act'.

The 'Plan' tests an hypothesis or a theory for healthcare improvement, implements the plan with a study protocol and data collection ('Do'), examines and summarizes the data collected ('Study'), and lastly, determines the change and iteration for further steps ('Act')(8). Thereafter, possibilities include: a new iterative cycle, testing of an intervention in a randomized controlled

Figure 1. PDSA Cycle ('Plan', 'Do', 'Study', 'Act')

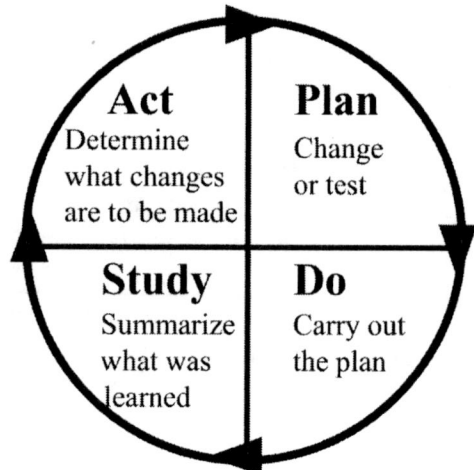

Source: Langley *et al.* (1996)

trial, or *translation* of new knowledge into clinical practice in order to reduce unwanted variability and produce organization-wide knowledge on carefully considered approaches.

Most readers will be familiar with the 'Plan' and 'Do' components. For example, readers are familiar with a knowledge audit, in which all potential sources of information are explored. However, there is often 'starvation in the face of plenty', because data are everywhere but they are not accessible. For example, a questionnaire was recently sent to all site investigators in the CPN. We inquired about basic information and characteristics about their tertiary perinatal unit. The findings showed that some of the largest centres in the country were having trouble finding basic information such as number of antepartum beds, or the percent of deliveries at a given gestational age. This was even true for some investigators who tried, in vain, to obtain the information from Department Heads. Clearly, these data are collected by the facility, but they are not readily accessible. In contrast, preparation of a recent grant application required knowledge about neonatal intensive care unit admissions among babies of hypertensive mothers; the Canadian

Neonatal Network database (discussed below) was contacted, and the co-ordinator was able to provide the data in 48hr by electronic analysis. In terms of the 'Do' component, readers will be very familiar with hospital guidelines for investigation and/or management of patients.

Unfortunately, readers will also be familiar with the lack of data collection that follows the 'Plan' and 'Do' steps. We do not know if most guidelines are being implemented, and if so, whether or not the outcomes of interest are being changed. Ultimately, what future steps should be taken. In contrast, the formal PDSA cycle ensures objectives are set and alternative solutions are considered, and forces *measurement* to take place(9). When used, the PDSA cycle encourages evidence-based solutions to develop knowledge and achieve the highest quality of care.

PDSA research builds knowledge(10). For example, at Birmingham Children's Hospital, it was observed that incoming emergency and elective patients were waiting for assessment until outgoing patients had vacated their beds. A proposed solution to decrease the waiting time was to create a discharge lounge where patients who were being discharged could wait for their prescriptions or paperwork(9). The 'Plan' was a written proposal for the discharge lounge with an operation protocol, followed by the 'Do' step, providing a facility for the testing of the idea to occur in. The actual 'Study' part included measuring the waiting times of the patients. The results showed that beds were freed up earlier, children were less upset about being in the hospital and that there was general improvement in patient and family satisfaction(9). As a result, a longer test was scheduled which produced similar results as the initial test. With multiple PDSA testing of the same concept at different facilities, it was found that the lounge was mainly used by patients waiting for their take-home drugs. This created a new piece of knowledge to be addressed by more PDSA cycles. This would not normally have been

highlighted if it were not for multiple cycles and fine adjustments to the PDSA cycle. Issues need to be assessed but more importantly, changes need to be monitored and re-evaluated.

It is of note that the PDSA cycle approach requires a focus in terms of content. CPN has chosen to focus on the major causes of spontaneous and iatrogenic threatened very preterm birth in Canada. Also, the PDSA cycle approach is predicated on the ability to collect data. As such, CPN needed to have a foundation for data collection. In exploring our options, we examined existing data collection, in the area of maternal and newborn health, in Canada.

EXISTING DATA COLLECTION IN CANADA

How to construct the CPN database, so as to honour the goals of sustainability, collaboration, and convergence with other models of data collection, has not been an easy process.

Research Projects (Opportunistic Databases)

With advancements in database technology, we are accumulating vast quantities of data at a record pace from a variety of sources. Many researchers have developed databases for local as well as multicentre, collaborative studies with the goal of collecting information for a special purpose or specific project. Each is designed and built to fulfill specific goals and objectives within the cost constraints of the project. Each is usually active only for the duration of the study. A wide variety of programmes and digital formats may be used even by the same researchers, depending on the expertise and longevity of employment of other team members, particularly trainees. For the few that are digitally compatible and employ the same software, the definitions of the data fields become the ultimate barrier, as they too have a great deal of discrepancy.

As local funding sources come to an end and researchers move on to other projects, the maintenance of these databases does not usually continue, and potentially valuable data are effectively lost. Also, stewardship is often delegated to residents or fellows who worked on a project, so that even when the principal investigator is subsequently contacted, data cannot be found or retrieved in a timely manner (if at all). The ineffectiveness of contacting authors for missing information is a well known issue that many reviewers encounter(11). This is a problem that could be potentially avoided if the lifespan of the database were dependent on an organization(s) or network(s), rather than on an individual(s).

In obstetrics, such special purpose databases gather much of the general information that is already collected by reproductive care programmes (see below), in addition to the very detailed information about the intervention(s) of interest, and the potential confounders of the relationship between the intervention and the outcomes. It follows that there is much duplication of effort and data collection, particularly for patient demographics, diagnosis and basic procedures. By working in isolation as researchers do, inefficiency and expense result.

Reproductive Care Programmes in Canada

In Canada, there are many regional reproductive care databases that collect data on maternal and initial maternal and newborn outcomes, for all deliveries. The purpose of regional databases is to monitor trends and disparities in perinatal health, with the intention of regional reporting to government and policy makers. Health outcomes may be improved for the entire population by decreasing health disparities(12), be they cultural, geographic, monetary (in terms of income), educational, ethnic, or medical (e.g., differences

in admission or access to procedures). These are knowledge transfer activities, but they do not generate new knowledge.

Reproductive care databases are located in Nova Scotia [Atlee Perinatal Database], British Columbia [BCPHP (BC Perinatal Health Programme)], Alberta [APHP (Alberta Provincial Perinatal Programme)], Ontario (NIDAY Perinatal Database), Prince Edward Island and Newfoundland and Labrador [N&L PPP (Newfoundland and Labrador Provincial Perinatal Programme)]. Data are collected on maternal demographics, pregnancy characteristics, details of labour and delivery, and initial evaluation of the newborn. For the BC Perinatal Health Programme (BCPHP), data may entered directly into the electronic database and periodically sent back to the provincial database, be collected using paper data collection forms that are returned to the BCPHP, or collected by a data abstractor from the central site who goes on-site to participating institutions periodically. Data on maternal mortality and morbidity are obtained by linkage with national discharge abstract databases (DAD); this forms our national data collection system. However, there is insufficient information collected about interventions to allow for identification of those practices associated with the best outcomes for mothers and babies. For example, no reproductive care programme has information about maternal transport, outpatient surveillance, uterine artery Doppler velocimetry, $MgSO_4$ use, or use of specific tocolytics, antibiotics, or antihypertensive agents. No more than half of the programmes include information about maternal blood transfusion

The Canadian Perinatal Programs Coalition Database Committee (CPPC), an organization composed of perinatal and reproductive care programmes, has recognized both the lack of standardization of definitions, and the variability in the information collected. For a number of years, work has been ongoing on a 'minimal dataset', which has not yet been finalized. Many of the currently proposed variables are not currently collected.

NATIONAL NETWORKS IN MATERNAL AND NEWBORN CARE

Canadian Neonatal Network (CNN)

We have used the Canadian Neonatal Network (CNN, 1995) as the model for CPN. (The successful Canadian Paediatric Surgical Network (CAPSNet, 2005) has also done so.)

The CNN was established by Dr. SK Lee in 1995 in response to the critical need for new knowledge in maternal and newborn care. Data are collected across Canada in the context of routine clinical care, and are entered into a computerized database. This Network provides an established infrastructure for collection of high quality standardized data for research and reduces the cost of research.

The CNN database has been a vehicle for the generation of new knowledge (as well as for the translation of existing knowledge into clinical practice and policy.) For example, using CNN data, Lee *et al* (13) reported large variations in neonatal outcomes and related them to variations in practice in Canadian neonatal intensive care units. Synnes *et al* found that following adjustment for baseline risk factors and neonatal illness severity on admission to NICU, treatment of acidosis and vasopressor use on the day of admission to NICU were associated with intraventricular haemorrhage(14). Data from the CNN database has been used to show that obstetric practice [beyond corticosteroid use(15;16)] may influence neonatal outcomes. For example, Synnes *et al* showed that mode of delivery was associated with the risk of intraventricular haemorrhage among babies admitted to NICU(17). More recently, Hayter *et al* showed that for pregnancy hypertension specifically, between-centre variations in obstetric practice are associated with variations in neonatal physiology and survival after correction for NICU practice and antenatal corticosteroid use(18). Lee *et al* determined that the most cost-effective strategy for screening for retinopathy of

prematurity is routine screening only of infants with birthweight <1200g(19).

CNN has also taken the PDSA cycle beyond a single turn, into an iterative approach. Lee, Synnes, and others in the CNN are currently using these data, in addition to other 'change ideas' from systematic review of the NICU literature, to conduct a national CIHR-funded Evidence-based Practice Identification and Change (EPIC) study to improve quality of care in NICUs ('03-'08, submitted to NEJM).

In summary, having established our method as the PDSA cycle, with an iterative future, and identified the need for additional data collection in Canada, we sought to develop a CPN database.

CHALLENGES OF BUILDING A DATABASE WITH CONVERGENCE & COLLABORATION IN MIND

We were acutely aware that the CPN database must not reinvent 'the wheel', but capitalize on existing infrastructure and definitions. Here, we review the issues that needed to be addressed in trying to build the CPN database and meet these goals.

Geography

We used the CNN as our model. However, the NICU is very geographically defined. Babies reside there until discharge home or to another unit. However, in obstetrics, patients may be managed as outpatients, inpatients (and then admitted to various wards), go to a wide variety of laboratories and ultrasound departments, and be seen by a wide variety of consultants, each of whom may keep their own patient record. This highlighted for us the many places from where information must be gathered.

In response to these concerns, as a first step, we chose to limit the geographical scope of CPN and focus on inpatients, admitted to one of Canada's tertiary perinatal units.

Standardization of Semantics

Before systems can connect to each other and before we can even begin to think about hardware, software, and programming, we need to be speaking the same language. In essence, databases and the future electronic health record are about concepts and their definitions first and foremost, and not about computers, cables, and internet connections.

Standardization of terminology is perhaps the least obvious but most important challenge for data sharing. Data terms must be universally understood (i.e., the definitions must be the same). In creating CPN, it was clear very early on that there is no standardization in the published literature for most obstetric or neonatal terms in common use. For example, perinatal mortality is defined differently by different reproductive care programmes between Canadian provinces (e.g., WHO definition by birth at ≥28 weeks vs. birth at ≥20 weeks or ≥500g). What constitutes reduced biological growth potential is variably defined, ranging from birth weight <2500g, to birth weight <3rd centile for gestational age and gender (20), which is further complicated by the skewness of birthweight data remote from term (i.e., as these babies were not normal, or they would not have been born).

The CPN terminology has relied on a strict classification system. The CPN terms have been drawn from the proposed CPPC 'Minimal Dataset', and the CNN database manual. However, many of terms (variables) were chosen from among a variety of definitions in the published literature.

In Canada and internationally, the most common health care coding system used by hospitals is another strict classification system called the International Classification of Diseases (ICD). The ICD codes were defined by the World Health Organization (WHO), and ICD-10-CA is an enhanced version of ICD-10 which was recently developed by Canadian Institute for Health Infor-

mation (CIHI) in 2006 to include classification of morbidity. ICD-10-CA includes codes for disease and related health problems as well as a number of conditions and situations that represent other risk factors to health, such as occupational and environmental factors, lifestyle and psycho-social circumstances. The terms, gestational hypertension, placenta previa and maternal blood transfusions can be coded and grouped into categories, which allows for aggregation and retrieval of information.

There are problems with a system of strict classification.

- First, the details of novel significance can be lost. For example, in pregnancy, women with pre-existing hypertension due to one of a number of endocrine causes (such as thyrotoxicosis or hyperaldosteronism) receive the same code, 'Pre-existing hypertension, unspecified (code O10.9).

- Second, healthcare is a dynamic environment. As researchers and clinicians learn new and better procedures and interventions, categories of coding systems change and evolve. For example, in 1993, ICD-9 795.8 was 'positive serological or viral culture findings for human immunodeficiency virus (HIV)'. By 1994, the same code had been deleted, and then re-introduced in 2006 but as 'abnormal tumour markers'. You can see that it would be difficult at best to compare data between versions of a classification system!

- Third, at present, data abstraction and coding is usually done by a trained clerk (with limited content knowledge) from information that can be deciphered from the medical record. This may be improved by electronic health records that will allow for coding of information at the bedside by the clinician. His/her content ('domain') knowledge and better understanding of the specific situation will facilitate a higher level of data reliability.

- Finally, perhaps the most interesting limitation that current coding systems encounter is the inability for codes to form 'relationships' with other codes. For example, a code for gestational hypertension is actually a form of hypertension, and women with gestational hypertension are at increased risk of long-term hypertension, but in ICD-10, these are completely different codes. Using the example of the secondary causes of hypertension (above), the thyrotoxicosis might be coded in addition to the pre-existing hypertension, unspecified, but there is nothing that links them together, so one doesn't know if they are related. Although these relationships may not seem critical to coding terms for easier retrieval, they are absolutely necessary in order for us to use this systems to ask and answer questions and generate knowledge.

Coding has been used by industry for many years, most commonly evident as the ubiquitous 'barcode' however, in building the CPN database, we have recognized that there is an alternative to our use of this strict classification system.

The Systematized Nomenclature of Medicine (SNOMED) Clinical Terms (CT®)

The future of universal health care is the semantic harmonization promised by SNOMED®. The International Health Terminology Standards Development Organization (IHTSDO) supports the effort to produce standardized global clinical terminology and governs and owns SNOMED-CT® intellectual property(21). Currently, the IHTSDO has nine countries as charter members: Australia, Canada, Denmark, Lithuania, New Zealand, Sweden, The Netherlands, United Kingdom, and the United States. Access to SNOMED-CT® is provided to clinicians, researchers, and administrators in these countries.

In SNOMED-CT®, human-readable terms are assigned computer-readable codes. This clinical terminology is not only a way of coding that preserves specific medical information, but it allows for different systems to easily and accurately exchange information. In essence, SNOMED-CT® is our new universal 'language'.

The basic elements of SNOMED-CT® include concepts, descriptions, hierarchies and relationships. A **concept** is a single clinical meaning which has its own concept code and a human readable name attached to it [e.g., pre-eclampsia (SNOMED concept ID)]. As illustrated by Figure 3, all concepts are organized into **hierarchies** (e.g., clinical findings and disorders, procedures, or observable entities), each of which contains sub-hierarchies (not shown in Figure 3). Each concept falls under one or more hierarchies. In Figure 3, pre-eclampsia falls under the clinical findings and disorders hierarchy; however, pre-eclampsia could be linked to other hierarchies such as 'laboratory' with low platelets being the linking concept. Each concept also has a number of human readable **descriptions**, such as pregnancy induced hypertension, pre eclampsia, and high blood pressure which would be associated with the gestational hypertension concept. Lastly, but most importantly, SNOMED CT® allows concepts to be linked through **relationships**. Relationships are a powerful and innovative feature that will allow for clinicians and researches to build complex concepts with multiple terms to describe a specific situation. Figure 3 illustrates SNOMED-CT® using 'pre-eclampsia' as an example.

Essentially, SNOMED-CT® has the ability to take a human written or spoken sentence, such as "a fetus has a gestational age of 24 weeks, is a male, and has a mother with eclampsia", and convert it into a series of codes which represent the description, the specific concept and the relationships. Whether this sentence is dictated in Spanish or Russian, it would be coded exactly the same in SNOMED-CT®, enabling someone in Japan to understand the diagnosis, procedure

Figure 2. SNOMED-CT® and the example of pre-eclampsia (Massey, Magee, & von Dadelszen, 2008)

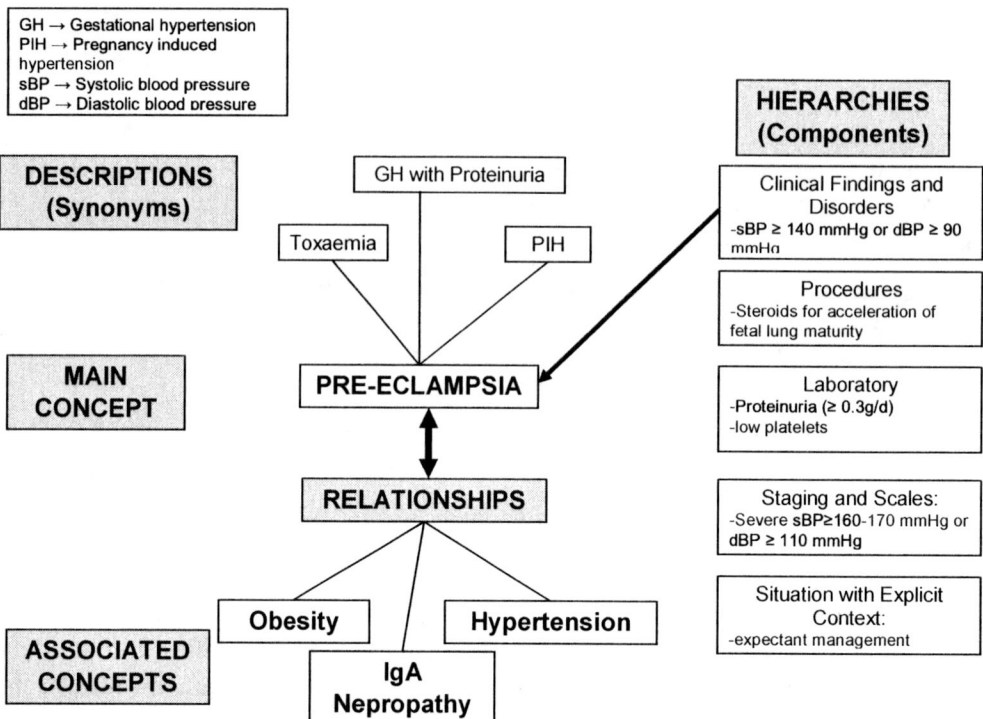

and clinical findings. As such, SNOMED-CT® has international capability and will become the universal language of medical care. In fact, any health informatics system that is marketed in Canada will soon have to be based on SNOMED-CT® terminology because it provides a consistent way to index, store, retrieve, and aggregate clinical data across specialties and sites of care and will form the backbone of the electronic health record, for quality of patient care and research.

Standardization of Digital Exchange of Information

Databases can be created using many different platforms, applications, interfaces and communication protocols. Interoperability is commonly limited to expensive, specifically designed interfaces that are limited in the amount of data

exchange and are not adaptive to changes in individual systems. Digital exchange of information between and among networks can be expensive, inaccurate (e.g., if probabilistic), and sometimes, impossible. However, with the future wave of electronic health records, it is absolutely crucial that existing systems be made digitally compatible. Clinical information should not only be accessible for care of the individual patient, but should provide knowledge for outcome improvements.

The CPN database shares the same digital technology as the CNN database. These are, in essence, the same database. CPN patients whose babies are admitted to neonatal intensive care, have the CNN number of the baby recorded in the database; thereafter, all neonatal outcome information can be obtained from CNN without any addition data collection by CPN. This digital integration has been a logical extension of other work within our unit in which all of our projects must have databases built with the same digital technology.

Ownership of the Data

As the Government of Canada Task Force for the National Consultation on Access to Scientific Research Data (NCASRD) points out(22), historically, research has been driven by individual researchers motivated by peer recognition and institutional reward, with collaborative team efforts aimed at improving the public good often coming second. It is not surprising then that there is little motivation for researchers to contribute to data-sharing initiatives once data are no longer linked to the individual. In addition, researchers involved in collaborative projects may also feel personally responsible for data that they individually collect at their centres, or may have concerns that their own research endeavours will be slowed down if they join larger multi-centre research efforts(23).

Local sites 'own' their data; they have free access to it and there is also a reporting function. However, access to national CPN data will require application to the CPN Steering Committee.

Changing the current mind set of well established organizations ultimately requires a paradigm shift away from competitive research. At the core of this issue is the idea of data ownership, which includes everything from intellectual ownership (for example, who can perform secondary data analysis, or who is entitled to authorship on publications), to where the data files will physically be stored(23). It is necessary to attend to these issues by creating inter-institutional committees so that specific guidelines can address, on a practical level, how data will be shared. (At present, a motivator for participation in the CPN is the fact that local data are owned and housed with the local site.) In the future, committees may choose to do away with the term "ownership" all-together, choosing instead the less emotionally-charged

term "stewardship"(23). Although this may seem like nothing more than semantics, it may be one small step toward a less individualistic research culture, driven by leaders and owners rather than collaborators. Universities could certainly facilitate this by recognizing collaborative research activities in performance reviews of faculty and Departments. Funding agencies are moving in the right direction. The Canadian Institutes of Health Research (CIHR) recognize the importance of collaborative research, and now offer team grants aimed at recognizing the achievements of groups of researchers, not just individuals. In the future, negotiation, open communication, and compromise will all be key elements in successfully dealing with the issues of data ownership, proprietary concerns, and authorship(24).

Privacy and Ethics

The sensitivity of personal health information is perhaps second only to financial information(25). Since 1988, COACH (Canada's Health Informatics Association) has been providing Healthcare Professionals and Healthcare Organizations with the guidance necessary to ensure that the security, privacy, and confidentiality of Personal Health Information (PHI) are upheld. The COACH Guidelines for the Protection of Health Information and are based on the Canadian Standards Association ten guiding principles for the protection of personal information, with the newly-released 2006 edition reflecting our increased use of information technology in the healthcare industry, in particular the risk that is introduced by the remote capabilities and access speed that are offered by electronic records(26).

Privacy and Confidentiality

Privacy is the fundamental right of every individual to dictate how their personal information is used and exchanged. Confidentiality is the organizational obligation to protect the personal information that is entrusted to it.

Canada made a commitment (as did other countries) to uphold an individual's right to privacy when we joined the global community in signing the OECD (Organization for Economic Co-operation and Development) Guidelines on the Protection of Privacy and Transborder Flow of Personal Data. These guidelines form the foundation for Canadian privacy legislation, and were used by the Canadian Standards Association as the basis for the Model Code for the Protection of Personal Information (CAN/CSA Q830-96), a set of ten guiding principles describing the minimum requirements that must be met in order to protect all forms of personal information (see Appendix 1). The CSA guidelines balance the individual right to privacy with the information requirements of private organizations, and are intended to assist organizations in developing appropriate policies and practices specific to their circumstances(27).

Security

Security is the process by which the information is protected(28). The mechanisms by which we prevent the unauthorized access, use and disclosure of PHI are known as security safeguards(29). Healthcare organizations should have security policies in place that are based on a national or international standard such as those developed by the International Organization for Standardization: ISO 17799 (The International Security Standard), or the soon-to-be-complete ISO 27799 (Health Informatics – Information Security Management in Health). The issues to address involve not only technology and policies, but the people who use them.

As electronic storage of PHI becomes increasingly straightforward, so does access to this information. As such, access control is becoming a fundamental component of data security. Preventing the unauthorized access to PHI has its challenges, not only from a technical standpoint (the implementation of user authentication systems, to password management systems, to securing remote or mobile access connections), but also from a management standpoint (deciding who should have access rights). As is so often the case, the latter may be the most complex part to tackle. Take for example the common situation where one individual performs multiple roles within a healthcare organization, each with different associated levels of access privilege, as might be true for a physician who is both a clinician and a researcher. In this situation, a role-based access control model needs to be implemented(30). Or the case where temporary access may be required for transient workers such as volunteers or students, which would necessitate regular and timely removal of access privileges when they leave. Finally, as information systems become increasingly complex, organizations often find that it is necessary to bring in third party specialists for system maintenance, and these individuals must still meet all the same privacy requirements as in-house users, complete with a contractual agreement that reflects this(31).

Advances in electronic databases bring with them not only data access challenges, but also those relating how to safely and efficiently store and archive data. We have moved well beyond the secure cabinet in a locked room. To enhance security, data should be stored on centralized servers, not on local workstations. In addition, to avoid increased security risk, servers should only be accessed using equipment maintained by specialized organizations. This can result in additional financial and time requirements, especially for data collection initiatives that span more than one health region, province/state/county/country, each jurisdiction having its own policies, procedures and legislation. When electronic data are archived, special considerations must also be made to account for the risk of data corruption, and the possibility of the eventual inaccessibility of data due to outdated storage technology(32).

E-health applications, mobile electronic devices, and Internet communications also introduce new security risks that require appropriate safeguards. If mobile electronic devices such as PDAs, laptops and removable media (such as memory sticks, DVDs and flash cards) are being used to access PHI, special security measures such as frequent data backups and special encryption procedures must be in place to mitigate the increased risk of loss of, physical damage to, or theft of these devices. Many e-health applications are also becoming increasingly dependent on Internet communications, as outlined in detail elsewhere(33). The general principles to keep in mind when considering Internet data transfers is that appropriate encryption methods are used to ensure that confidentiality is maintained, the information is not altered during the transfer, and that the sender of the information is always traceable(34).

Information system security measures need to be taken at every phase, from the inception of the system, to its development, administration and use(35). When the information system will be administered across healthcare organizations, the added challenge of having to meet the highly-variable policies and legal requirements of each organization is introduced. Not only is the security of PHI dependent on technology and policies, but more importantly it is dependent on users who employ the technology to abide by the policies in a security-conscious manner(36). While outside hackers are a concern, internal security breaches are probably more of a threat to the security of PHI, due more often to a lack of education and understanding than the express intent to breach security. It is the user who must not share their password or smart card with others, not log on to a computer and then leave it unattended, not remove computer equipment from secured areas, and not let security incidents go unreported.

The CPN relies on data access measures (i.e., username and password protected access), with storage of the database on a secure hospital network.

The implementation of any new information technology introduces new risk. It is important to identify and classify these risks based on their likelihood of occurring and the impact it would have if they did. By doing this, we are able to balance the benefit the technology provides with the risk that it introduces. It is becoming more common for jurisdictions to legislate risk assessment in the form of Privacy Impact Assessments and Threat and Risk Assessments to identify threats to privacy and security respectively, as well as safeguards against these risks. As technology is constantly being updated, so must we update these assessments(37).

Research Ethics Boards

Not only must healthcare and research institutions adhere to whatever regional and/or national privacy legislation exists, but they must also have an ethics committee in place to review how PHI is accounted for within the organization. Research Ethics Boards (REBs) in particular review all proposed research projects that involve the secondary use of data (i.e., data not used for direct clinical care administration). During the review process, REBs consider the purpose for the data collection, what type of patient consent process is necessary, and what limits should be placed on the collection, use, disclosure, and retention of the data. There are numerous challenges that we as health care professionals face, from the REB application process to following board recommendations and privacy laws.

In Canada, there is wide jurisdictional variability in how privacy legislation is interpreted(38), making national multi-centre research initiatives difficult to conduct. In the case of multi-centre collaborative projects, the same project must be reviewed by a separate REB in each institution where data will be collected. Some of the inefficiencies of this system could be avoided if Canada had a centralized REB application process similar to the UK. Not only is the application process itself a challenge, but so is the variation in each board's interpretation of existing privacy legislation. Perhaps this is best demonstrated by the variability in patient consent requirements for the secondary use of personal health information. For example, whether or not (or in what format) patient consent will be required for the same multi-centre project may vary, with one centre requiring no patient consent in any form, another requiring that the patient has the option of opting out, and yet another stipulating that express (written or oral) consent must be obtained(39). These decisions may have a direct impact on outcomes. For example, in the international PIERS project which is building a model of predictors for adverse maternal and perinatal outcomes in pre-eclampsia, the incidence of adverse outcomes fell in association with 'Standing Orders' for investigation of these women(40); however, the incidence did not appear to fall in centres where the REB required that patient consent must be obtained for the same 'Standing Order' investigations.

In summary, balancing the need to protect patient privacy with the need to share information is not a simple task. As a community of healthcare providers, we have a responsibility to circulate information to ensure the best possible treatments for patients, while at the same time protecting the patient's legal right to privacy. It can take significant time and resources to translate ethical and legal guidelines into concrete organizational policies and procedures, especially in light of the wide jurisdictional variations in legislative requirements in areas such as patient consent, safeguards, and risk assessment.

Stable Funding

This challenge reflects the reluctance of funding agencies to fund databases, as ongoing endeavours. As such, the national neonatal and paediatric networks (i.e., CNN and CAPSNet) as well as CPN, have chosen to focus on specific research projects to obtain initial funding. CPN has chosen

to focus on threatened very preterm birth (i.e., threatened birth before 29 weeks' gestation). This is both a major public health concern worldwide, and recognized to hold the greatest potential for improvement of outcomes for mothers and babies. Initially, CPN is focussing on the management of the major spontaneous and iatrogenic causes of threatened very preterm birth at 22^{+0}-28^{+6} weeks: spontaneous preterm labour, preterm pre-labour rupture of membranes (PPROM), gestational hypertension, intrauterine fetal growth restriction, and antepartum haemorrhage.

In order to demonstrate the need for, and justify, stable funding, we must be able to demonstrate that we have a core dataset onto which can be clipped additional data collection for specific research studies. We must also work with regional surveillance databases funded by government or health authorities; these regional databases also afford us the opportunity for knowledge interaction.

KNOWLEDGE INTERACTION

PDSA cycles should be not only *iterative* (in that knowledge learned from one cycle informs another), but these cycles should be *interactive*. Quality improvement involves sharing knowledge within *and* between organizations whether they be hospitals, networks, or regions, be they national or international.

There have been attempts to build organizations committed to building knowledge and sharing it. In 2003, The National Health Service (NHS), the United Kingdom's publicly funded health care system, introduced the "National Knowledge Service" (NKS) as a step towards the knowledge management program. There are three types of knowledge that the NKS concentrates on; knowledge from research (evidence), knowledge from collected and audited data (statistics) and knowledge from the experience of patients and clinicians(41). The basic idea of the National Knowledge Service is to use the leading and latest medical knowledge to educate health care professionals and patients in decision making (7). This is made possible by ensuring that quality information is not only available but by focusing on the technology needed to deliver it. By promoting the concept of coding the NKS also recognizes the importance of standardization in order to endorse knowledge growth in the health care system. The benefits to the quality of health care derived from already existing recourses, research, data and experience has a much larger and global impact when organized and combined with each other, reducing the most common problems in our current system including; unknown variables in clinical practises, errors and waste of data, inappropriate care, unsatisfactory patient experiences, and failure to implement new knowledge and technology(41).

It is this concept of knowledge interaction that has led us to look at a model of interaction between CPN, our national academic database, and the British Columbia Perinatal Health Programme (BCPHP), our provincial (regional) reproductive care programme (Figure 3). In this way, PDSA

cycles occur (and interact) in both tertiary perinatal units with high risk women (CPN), and community hospitals that serve the low risk, general obstetric population (BCPHP).

Knowledge Audit for National (Academic) Network Informing Regional Network (Figure 4)

A literature search for questions that the CPN wished to ask and answer for gestational hypertension yielded two pieces of high quality evidence that represented best practice: antenatal corticosteroids for acceleration of fetal pulmonary maturity (42), and magnesium sulphate ($MgSO_4$) for eclampsia treatment and prevention in women with severe pre-eclampsia (43). As such, use of steroids and $MgSO_4$ should be monitored in BC, with a goal of them being used in ≥80% of eligible women. However, we learned that $MgSO_4$ is not a term field collected by the BCPHP, and a revision to this database has been proposed.

Figure 3. Model of knowledge interaction (Massey, Magee, & von Dadelszen, 2008)

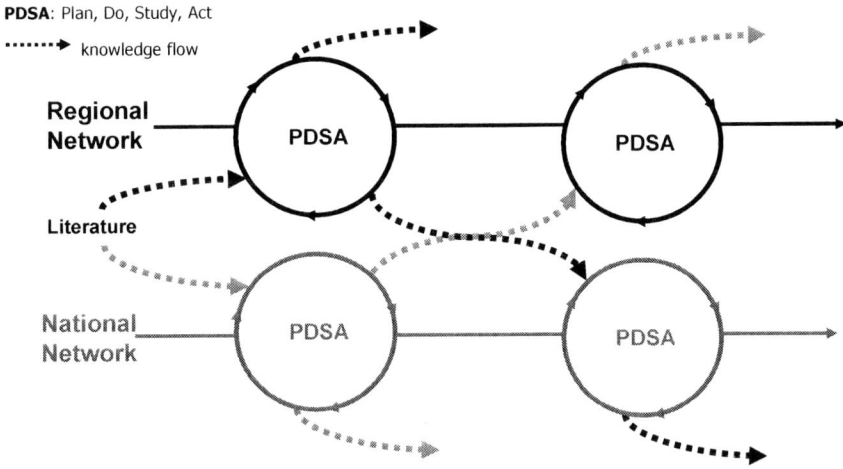

Figure 4. Knowledge audit for National (academic) network informing Regional network (Massey, Magee, & von Dadelszen, 2008)

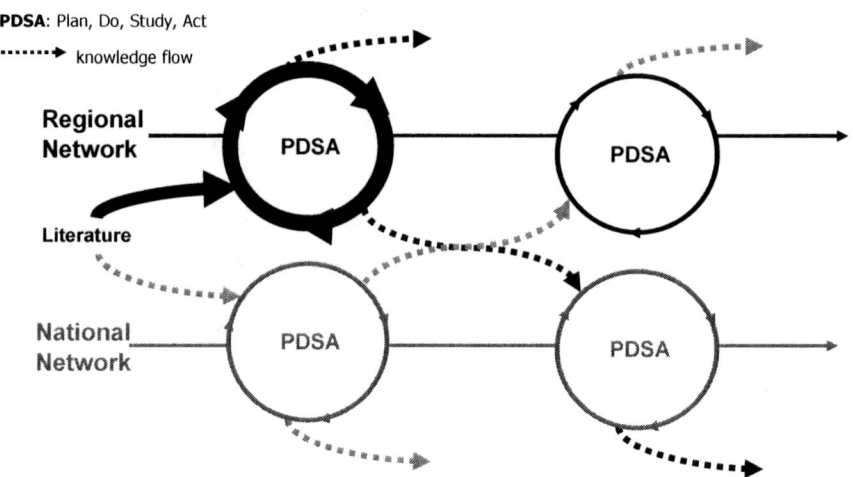

Iterative BCPHP PDSA Cycles (Figure 5)

Recently, provincial guidelines were implemented for the hypertensive disorders of pregnancy (44). A focus of these guidelines was judicious fluid administration for women with pre-eclampsia, given that an initial audit of the BCPHP database (in general and for BC Women's in particular) revealed a high incidence of pulmonary edema compared with a comparable unit in Australia(45). The BCPHP database will be audited two years after implementation of the guidelines, for performance indicators including pulmonary edema. If the incidence of pulmonary edema does not decrease, as anticipated, then a PDSA cycle devoted to this will begin anew, perhaps with pre-printed orders with high concentrations of oxytocin and $MgSO_4$ (IV drugs used in the setting of severe pre-eclampsia) in order to minimize fluid administration to 80mL/hour.

Iterative CPN PDSA Cycles (Figure 6)

Nifedipine is an excellent antihypertensive for treatment of acute, severe hypertension in pregnancy. Despite good arguments for its safety in hypertensive pregnant women (as opposed to older patients with coronary heart disease)(46), and its ease of administration, concerns linger about use of nifedipine on delivery suite. One question that CPN is asking is whether emergency Caesarean section and/or maternal intubation are more common with use of hydralazine, labetalol, or nifedipine. If nifedipine is no different, then plans will be made to have it re-introduced into perinatal pharmacies throughout BC.

BCPHP PDSA Cycle Informing a CPN Cycle (Figure 7)

Weights in pregnancy have been increasing over time, and so have relevant pregnancy complications (e.g., Caesarean section, and post-operative wound infections). The BCPHP monitors such

Figure 5. Iterative BCPHP PDSA cycles (Massey, Magee, & von Dadelszen, 2008)

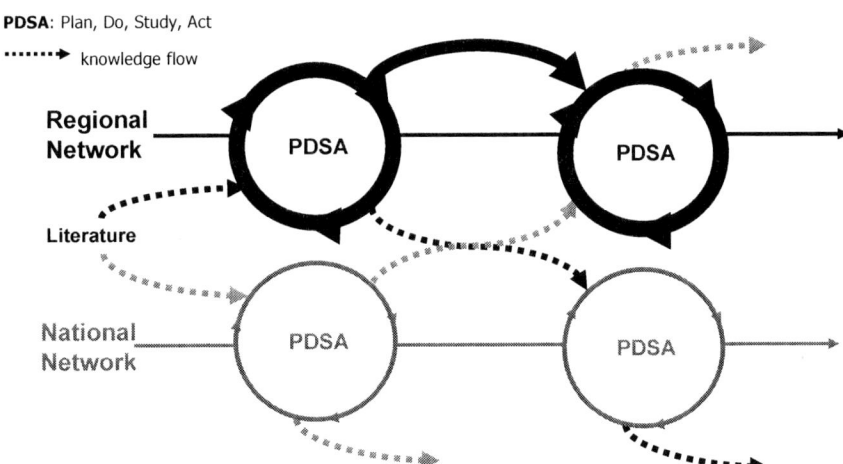

Figure 6. Iterative CPN PDSA cycles(Massey, Magee, & von Dadelszen, 2008)

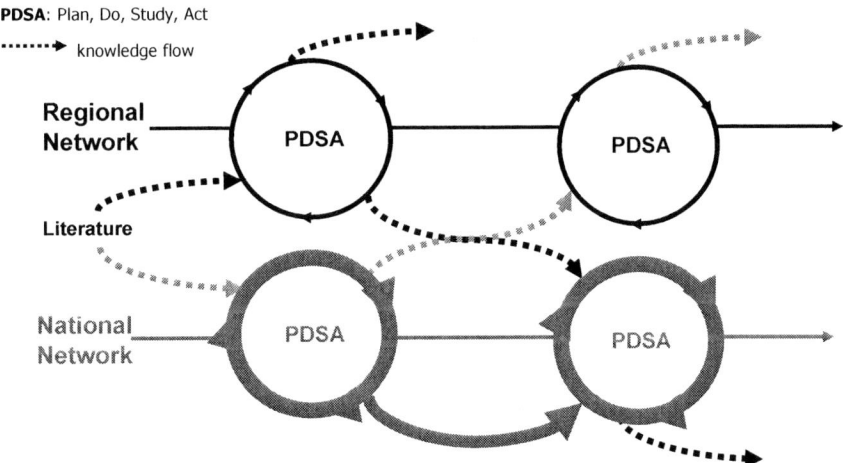

parameters, and they could, for example, take an idea about intervention to CPN. This initiative might target obese women following complicated pregnancy, and attempt to alter diet and lifestyle. If successful in effecting weight loss, and in improving pregnancy outcome, this initiative could be fed back to BCPHP for wider implementation.

CPN PDSA Cycle Informing a BHPHP Cycle (Figure 8)

One question that CPN is asking of the data is whether beta-lactam antibiotics are associated with more necrotizing enterocolitis, a serious bowel problem in preterm babies, than are mac-

Figure 7. BCPHP PDSA cycle informing a CPN cycle (Massey, Magee, & von Dadelszen, 2008)

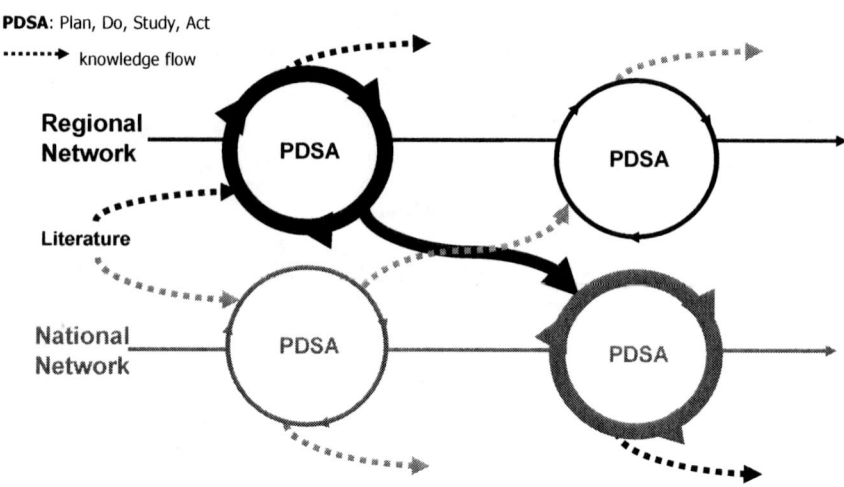

Figure 8. CPN PDSA cycle informing a BHPHP cycle (Massey, Magee, & von Dadelszen, 2008)

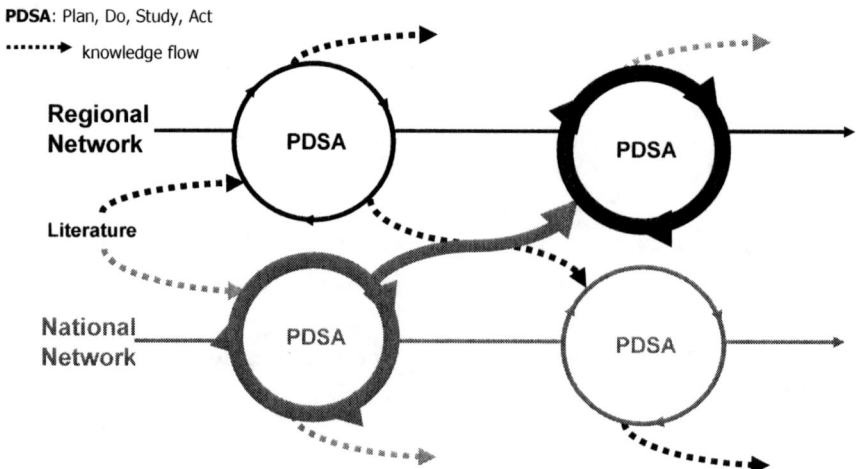

rolide antibiotics, when these antibiotics are given for PPROM. If CPN finds that one is superior, then a policy of that antibiotic's administration can be implemented provincially, with ongoing audit of the neonatal outcomes of interest.

CONCLUSION

The Future: The Electronic Health Record

At present, in the course of clinical care, data are collected, but not in a way that facilitates knowledge generation and improves care. Patients are treated in a variety of settings, by a variety of healthcare professionals and according to various hospital policies. The first goal of an EHR will be to provide for retrieval and storage; this has been achieved in many settings. However, with standardization of terminology, we can move beyond this to interpretation of the data and generation of knowledge. SNOMED-CT® will be an integral part of the new language that healthcare providers learn during their early training and that form the basis of EHR data screens.

Use of the electronic patient/medical records has been minimal. However, interest in use is growing exponentially. In the United Kingdom, the National Health Services (NHS) aims to have 60,000,000 patients with a centralized EHR by 2010, while in Canada the goal is to provide EHR to fifty percent of the population by the same year. This goal was set by Canada Health Infoway, a "not-for-profit corporation mandated to accelerate the modern systems of information technology" (47) after receiving $500 million from the Canadian government in 2001 followed by an additional $600 million in 2003. Vast amounts of money are being spent.

Canada Health Infoway and its partners aim to deliver the electronic heath record (EHR) and as a result, provide timely access to accurate information, enhance disease management, and

enable long term sustainability. Built on patient and provider registries, the EHR will facilitate sharing of clinical information allowing for easier identification of patient problems, laboratory test results, clinical reports, immunization history, and medication profiles, while avoiding duplicate history taking, investigations, treatments, and data collection(47). The systems likely to be the most valuable will be adaptable to changing needs within the organization, and will be able to be linked to other systems.

The United Kingdom is currently a leader in the switch to the electronic health record and has already encountered difficulties with safeguarding electronic data. One instance of mishandling identifiable data occurred in October 2007 when two computer discs were lost that contained the personal details of 25 million parents and families in the UK receiving child benefits (48). During this 'child benefit scandal' the discs, owned by Her Majesty's Revenue and Customs, were sent by junior staff from HM Revenue and Customs (HMRC) to the National Audit Office (NAO). The data were sent as unrecorded internal mail on October 18 and by October 24 the NAO complained to the HMRC that the data had not yet been received (49). It was not until early November that senior officials at the HMRC were informed of the loss. The lost data, which was believed to affect approximately 25 million people in the UK, included names, addresses and dates of birth of children, as well as the National Insurance numbers and bank details of their parents(50). The blame was initially placed on junior officials from the government; however, upon closer review, many believe that the problem lay with senior management and the flow of identifiable data between centres. This is based on the fact that the NAO had actually requested that identifiable bank information and details be stripped from the data they were to receive. Unfortunately, this did not occur since the HMRC claimed the removal of such data would be "too costly and complicated"(51).

Figure 9. EHR data access and exchange (Massey & Magee, 2008)

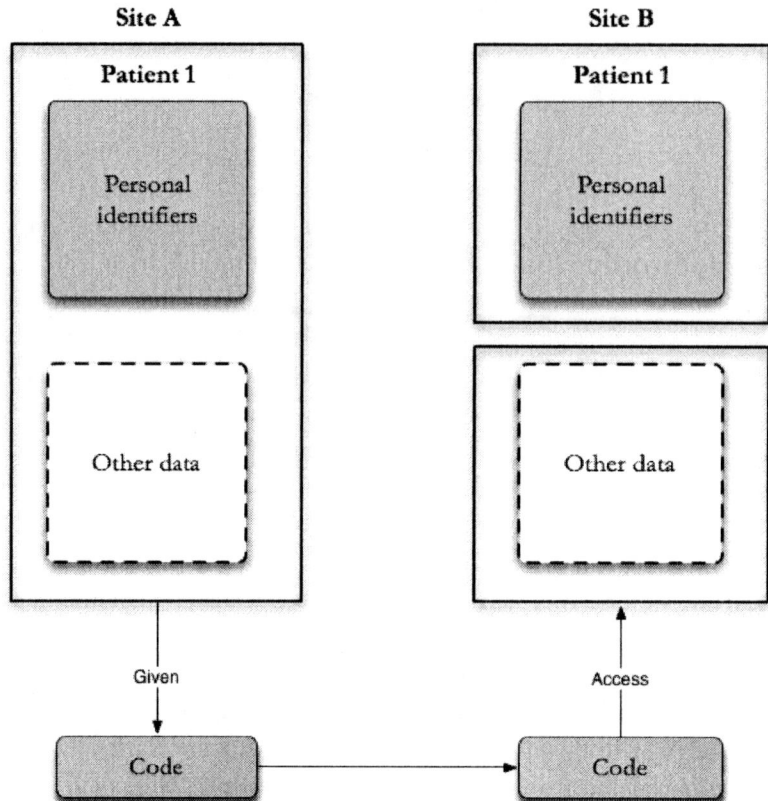

Episodes like this have caused concern among local centres sharing detailed identifiable data with the NHS. Potential breaches of security and privacy failures that could potentially arise increase greatly when sharing large amounts of data from multiple sources and locations. In an editorial by McGilchrist *et al.*(52) he identifies the concept of pseudonymisation. This concept allows the combination of anonymised data such as laboratory reports and diagnosis, but excludes linkages to any other personal identifiers such as personal health number, date of birth and postal code (Figure 9). The anonymised data could be accessed via a new common identifier, such as a study or research code, that links different records to the same patient whose personal information may otherwise only be accessed with a personal

health number. For example if a pregnant woman with diabetes arrives at Site A and her doctor at that site wishes to get her results from her eye appointment at the ophthalmologist (site B), he may send Site B her "code". The main concept is that any data within the site is secure and may include personal identifiers; however any data accessed from outside the site requires a code and does not include personal identifiers.

Many measures have been taken to avoid security breaches. This includes the reconfiguration of all personal and company computers to prevent downloading of data on to removable media which could only be reactivated with the approval of a senior manager for a specific purpose(53). At it stands now authorized system users and management are the only ones with access privileges.

While Standard Operating Procedures (SOP) are valued, they can only be effective if staff are trained to use them correctly and consistently. Likewise there needs to be no malicious intent, incompetence or mistakes in the SOP(54). Instead of having closed systems of SOP's, it has been suggested that crosschecking and supervision may be needed. This however, requires a great deal of trust from the patients and if their private personal information is displaced or mishandled, then the confidence and trust in such agencies is diminished.

Ultimately the challenge that prevails is balancing the need for health information with the need for security. As it stands, there is an imperative need to proceed with the EHR as many believe that the benefits greatly outweigh the security risks. As Flegel suggests in his editorial, an electronic patient record could inform a physician about a patient's history in a timely matter so they do not prescribe a drug that is harmful to the patient (55). It seems as though the situation has become counterproductive by allowing the potential risks to impede progression. At some point we must recognize that our concerns with privacy and security may actually do more harm than good.

FINAL THOUGHTS

Continuous quality improvement involves iterative cycles of practice, change, and audit, of ongoing clinical care. An obvious prerequisite to this is ongoing data collection about interventions and outcomes, as well as demographics, pregnancy characteristics, and neonatal care that may affect the intervention-outcome relationship.

In Canada (as in some other developed countries), much of the country is covered by regional reproductive care databases that monitor geographical trends and disparities in health outcomes. As such, there is little information about interventions, especially outside the period of labour and delivery. Also, there is no standard-

ization of definitions, and efforts to produce a 'minimal dataset' have not yet yielded agreement, even after many years of work.

A more comprehensive system is required. The rate-limiting steps in this process of data acquisition and knowledge generation/translation will be semantics/definitions, not computers and cables. Moving in this direction, particularly with respect to standardization of definitions, would lay the foundation for the electronic health record, which cannot build its foundation on the 'Tower of Babel' that is our current definitional structure in women's health and obstetrics. Efficiency and economy aside, the EHR is needed *for* patient safety, however concerns about privacy and access remains major barriers.

FUTURE DIRECTION

The next critical step is standardization of our scientific database language. SNOMED CT® will underpin these efforts. Research groups and sub specialty clinicians are encouraged to contact the IHTSDO for information about who to contact in their own country in order to access the SNOMED CT ® database. By doing so, one can get a better understanding of what currently exists in the database, and what remains to be described clinically. The step in standardizing our medical terminology is the responsibility of the clinical experts in the field, not solely the onus of informaticians and system administrators.

REFERENCES

"Brown apologises for records loss." BBC 21 Nov. 2007.

"E-mails reveal data check warning." BBC 23 Nov. 2007.

SNOMED. www.update-software.com/history/clibhist.htm . 2007.

British Columbia Reproductive Care Program. BCRCP Obstetric Guideline 11 Hypertension in Pregnancy. 2006. Vancouver BC.

Canada Health Infoway. 2015: Advancing the Next Generation of Health Care in Canada. 2006.

Canadian Standards Association. Canadian Standards Association: Privacy Code. http://www.csa.ca/standards/privacy/code/Default.asp?language=english . 2007.

Carey, T. S. et al. (2005). Developing Effective Interuniversity Partnerships and Community-Based Research to Address Health Disparities. *Academic Medicine, 80.11,* 1039-45.

Chien, L. Y. et al. (2002). Variations in antenatal corticosteroid therapy: A persistent problem despite 30 years of evidence. *Obstet Gynecol, 99.3,* 401-08.

Childbirth Connection. (2006). *About This Book: A Guide to Effective Care in Pregnancy and Childbirth.* http://childbirthconnection.org/article.asp?ck=10014 .

COACH: Canada's Health Informatics Association. Guidelines for the Protection of Health Information. 16-12-0007. Toronto, Canada.

Cochrane, A. L. *(1972). Effectiveness and Efficiency: Random Reflections on Health Services.* London: Nuffield Provincial Hospitals Trust.

Croll, P. R., & Croll, J. (2007). Investigating risk exposure in e-health systems. *International Journal of Medical Informatics, 76,* 460-65.

Crowther, C. A., Hiller, J. E., & Doyle, L. W. (2002). Magnesium sulphate for preventing preterm birth in threatened preterm labour. *Cochrane. Database.Syst.Rev., 4,* CD001060.

De Lusignan, S. et al. (2005). A knowledge audit of the managers of primary care organizations: Top priority is how to use routinely collected clinical data for quality improvement. *Medical Informatics & the Internet in Medicine, 30.1,* 69-80.

Enkin, M., Keirse, M., & Chalmers, I. (1989). *A Guide to Effective Care in Pregnancy and Childbirth.* 1 ed. London: Oxford Medical Publications.

Enkin, M. et al. (2000). *A Guide to Effective Care in Pregnancy and Childbirth.* 3 ed. London: Oxford University Press.

Flegel, K. et al. (2008). Getting to the electronic medical record. *CMAJ, 178.5,* 531, 533.

Grant, A. & Chalmers, I. (1981). Register of randomised controlled trials in perinatal medicine. *Lancet, 1.100.*

Hayter, M. A. et al. Variations in early and intermediate neonatal outcomes for inborn infants admitted to a Canadian NICU and born of hypertensive pregnancies. *JOGC* submitted July 2004; MS# pending (2004).

Khoshdel, A., Attia, J., & Carnery, S. L. (2006). Basic concepts in meta-analysis: a primer for clinicians. *International Journal of Clinical Practice, 60.10,* 1287-94.

Kramer, M. S. et al. (2001). A new and improved population-based Canadian reference for birth weight for gestational age. *Pediatrics, 108.2,* E35.

Lee, S. K. et al. (2000). Variations in practice and outcomes in the Canadian NICU network: 1996-1997. *Pediatrics, 106.5,* 1070-79.

Lee, S. K. et al. (2001). Evidence for changing guidelines for routine screening for retinopathy of prematurity. *Arch.Pediatr.Adolesc.Med., 155.3,* 387-95.

Love, D. et al. Data Sharing and Dissemination Strategies for Fostering Competition in Health Care. *Health Services Research, 36.1,* 277-90.

Magee, L. A., Cote, A. M., & von Dadelszen, P. (2005). Nifedipine for severe hypertension in pregnancy: Emotion or evidence? *J. Obstet. Gynaecol. Can., 27.3,* 260-62.

Mcgilchrist, M., Sullivan, F., & Kalra, D. Assuring the confidentiality of shared electronic health records. *British Medical Journal, 335,* 1223-24.

Menzies, J. et al. Instituting surveillance guidelines and adverse outcomes in preeclampsia. *Obstet.Gynecol., 110.1,*121-27.

Muir Gray, J. A. (2006). Best Current Evidence: Concepts and Plans (pp. 5-28). National Health Services.

Parliamentary reporter. (2007). Three million records lost in another government data scandal. *Computing, 18,* Dec. 2007.

Roberts, D., & Dalziel, S. (2006). Antenatal corticosteroids for accelerating fetal lung maturation for women at risk of preterm birth. *Cochrane. Database. Syst. Rev., 3,* CD004454.

Shoultz, J. et al. Reducing health disparities by improving quality of care: Lessons learned from culturally diverse women. *Journal of Nursing Care Quality, 21.1,* 86-92.

Speroff, T., & O'Connor, G. T. (2004). Study designs for PDSA quality improvement research. *Qual. Manag. Healthcare, 13.1,* 17-32.

Starr, M., & Chalmers, I. (2003). *The evolution of The Cochrane Library,* 1988-2003. www.update-software.com/history/clibhist.htm . 2003.

Strong, D. F., & Leach, P. B. (2005). *National Concultation on Access to Scientific Research Data: Final Report.* 31-1-2005. Ottawa, Canada, Canada Institure for Scientific and Technical Information.

Synnes, A. R. et al. (2001). Variations in intraventricular hemorrhage incidence rates among Canadian neonatal intensive care units.*J Pediatr., 138.4,* 525-31.

Thornton, C., Hennessy, A., von Dadelszen, P., Nishi, C., Makris, A., & Ogle, R. An international benchmarking collaboration: measuring outcomes for the hypertensive disorders of pregnancy. *J Obstet Gynaecol Can.,* 29.10 (7 A.D.), 794-800.

Walley, P., & Gowland, B. (2004). Completing the circle: from PD to PDSA. *Int. J. Health Care Qual. Assur. Inc. Leadersh. Health Serv., 17.6,* 349-58.

Wikipedia contributors. 2007 UK child benefit data scandal. Wikipedia, The Free Encyclopedia . 29-2-2008.

ADDITIONAL READING

SNOMED_Clinical_Terms_Fundamentals.pdf (http://www.ihtsdo.org/fileadmin/user_upload/ Docs_01/SNOMED_Clinical_Terms_Fundamentals.pdf)

This presentation gives an introduction to SNOMED CT: What is SNOMED CT, what is it for, how is it organized, etc.

APPENDIX: CPN COLLABORATIVE GROUP

		Principal Investigator (CIHR)	Co-Investigators (CIHR)	Steering Committee Member	Collaborator (Site Investigators)
Victoria Allen	IWK Health Centre, Halifax NS		✓	✓	✓
Mark Ansermino	BC Children's Hospital, Vancouver BC		✓	✓	
François Audibert	Hôpital Sainte-Justine, Montréal QC			✓	✓
Jon Barrett	Women's College Hospital, Toronto ON		✓		✓
Emmanuel Bujold	Centre Hospitalier de l'Université Laval (CHUL), Québec QC			✓	✓
Craig Burym	St. Boniface General Hospital, Winnipeg MB Winnipeg Health Science Centre, Winnipeg MB				✓
George Carson	Regina General Hospital, Regina SK				✓
Joan Crane	Women's Health Program, Eastern Health, St. John's NF			✓	✓
Jerome Dansereau	Victoria General Hospital, Victoria BC				✓
Nestor Demianczuk	Royal Alexandra Hospital, Edmonton AB			✓	✓
Duncan Farquharson	Royal Columbian Hospital, New Westminster BC				✓
Rob Gratton (*pending*)	Saint Joseph's Health Centre, London ON				✓
Shoo Lee	iCARE, University of Alberta, Edmonton AB		✓	✓	
Robert Liston	BC Women's Hospital, Vancouver BC	✓		✓	✓
Laura Magee	BC Women's Hospital, Vancouver BC	✓		✓	✓
Angela Mallozzi (*pending*)	Royal Victoria Hospital, Montréal QC				✓
Sarah McDonald (*pending*)	McMaster University Medical Centre, Hamilton ON				✓
Jean-Marie Moutquin	Centre Hôspitalier Universitairé de Sherbrooke, Sherbrooke QC			✓	
Femi Olatunbosun	Royal University Hospital, Saskatoon SK				✓
Jean-Charles Pasquier	Centre Hôspitalier Universitairé de Sherbrooke, Sherbrooke QC				✓
Bruno Piedboeuf	Centre Hospitalier de l'Université Laval, Québec QC		✓	✓	
Frank Sanderson (*pending*)	Saint John Regional Hospital, Saint John NB				✓
Graeme Smith	Kingston General Hospital, Kingston ON		✓	✓	✓
Peter von Dadelszen	BC Women's Hospital, Vancouver BC		✓	✓	✓
Mark Walker	The Ottawa Hospital, Ottawa ON		✓	✓	✓

continued on following page

Appendix. continued

Wendy Whittle	Mount Sinai Hospital, Toronto ON			✓	✓
Liz Whynot	BC Women's Hospital & Health Centre, Vancouver BC			✓	
Stephen Wood	Foothills Medical Centre, Calgary AB				✓

Chapter IX
Informatics Applications in Neonatology

Malcolm Battin
National Women's Health, Auckland City Hospital, New Zealand

David Knight
Mater Mother's Hospital, Brisbane, Australia

Carl Kuschel
The Royal Women's Hospital, Melbourne, Australia

ABSTRACT

Neonatal care is an extremely data-intensive activity. Physiological monitoring equipment is used extensively along with web-based information tools and knowledge sources. Merging data from multiple sources adds value to this data collection. Neonatal databases assist with collecting, displaying, and analyzing data from a number of sources. Although the construction of such databases can be difficult, it can provide helpful support to clinical practice including surveillance of infectious diseases and even medical error. Along with recording outcomes, such systems are extremely useful for the support of audit and quality improvement as well as research. Electronic information sources are often helpful in education and communication with parents and others, both within the unit and at a distance. Systems are beginning to be used to help with decision making – for example in the case of weaning neonates from ventilators, and this work is likely to become more important in the future.

INTRODUCTION

This chapter will outline the potential value of and barriers to the use of an informatics approach in neonatology. The term neonatology refers to the branch of medicine concerned with the care, development, and diseases of newborn infants [1]. Although the term neonatal strictly defines the newborn period from birth to four weeks of age, we will refer to neonatology in a broader sense.

This may include everything from routine care of the normal newborn infant with the mother, on the postnatal ward or at home, through to provision of intensive care for the smallest and sickest of infants. In many cases this will involve premature infants who are often older than four weeks of chronological age but less than 44 weeks corrected gestational age. This type of care is complex and generates large amounts of clinical, monitoring and laboratory or imaging data. However, it also has some information requirements that are in common with that of an uncomplicated term infant on the postnatal wards. Specifically, there is a need to link infant details with the antenatal history, maternal demographic data and clinical coding.

The five main areas where neonatology and informatics relate well are the provision of clinical care, including physiological monitoring and computer based clinical guidelines; data collection and management incorporating quality or benchmarking issues; education and training of staff; support of parents, including providing clear accessible information; and research.

CLINICAL CARE

An informatics approach has much to offer in terms of both efficiency and clinical safety. Firstly, it may serve as a web-based resource or repository for information. Secondly, it can

Figure 1. Clinical workstation interface in our institution

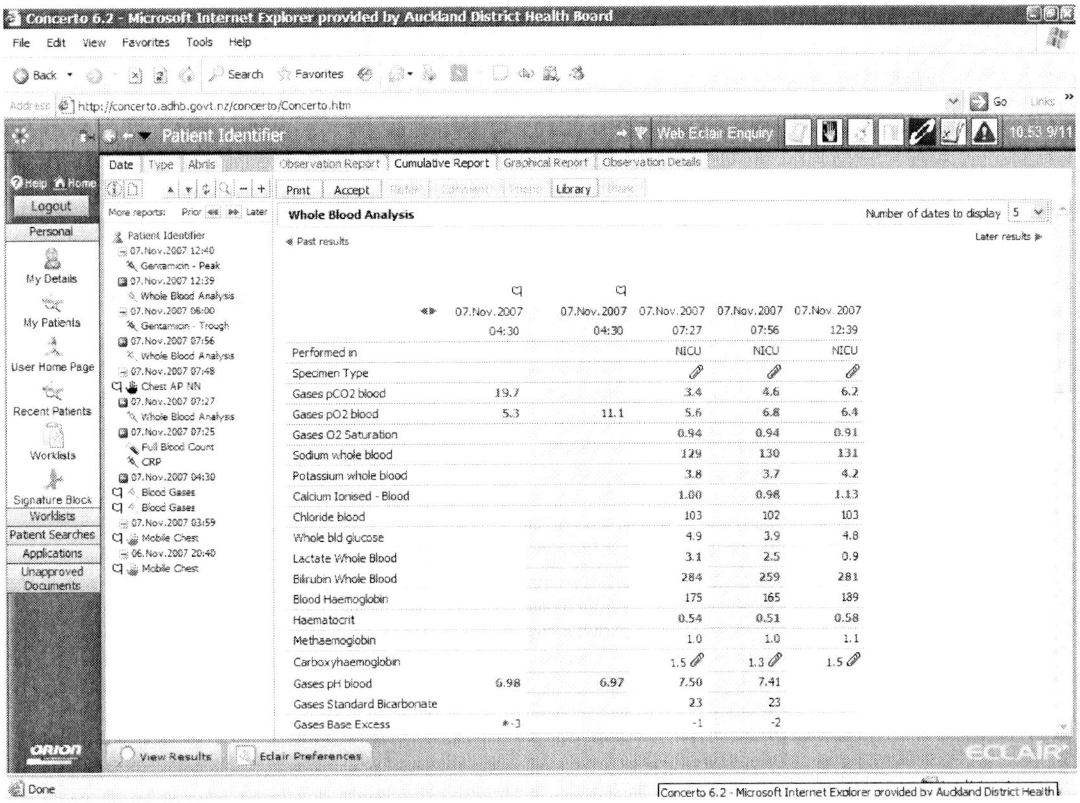

provide web-based tools, such as drug calculators or nomograms, which aid the clinician with procedures such as estimation of length of insertion of catheters or endotracheal tubes [2, 3]. Thirdly, informatics may include the provision of a portal or web-based interface with other applications giving up-to-date access to clinical information stored elsewhere such as radiology, lab results, and clinical documents. Fourthly, data from physiological monitoring can be analyzed, albeit largely after a clinical event requiring review. Finally once data has been collected it can then be used to generate an automated discharge summary that includes physiological parameters, radiology and laboratory results, as well as clinical information.

In the screenshot above, an example is given of the clinical workstation interface in place in our institution. The menu to the left provides the user with access to clinical information for specific patients (Figure 1). Electronic results can be "signed off" by the clinician once the results have

been acknowledged or acted on. Other results, such as radiology reports, can also be viewed. Radiology images can be viewed directly for this patient by choosing the logo resembling an x-ray of the hand. Similarly, the electronic clinical record used within our institution can be accessed directly through this interface. The triangle logo with an exclamation mark alerts the user to the presence of important specific information such as a drug reaction, child protection issues, or infection with an organism that may have infection control implications.

In its simplest form, physiological review may take the form of a perusal of data stored within a monitor, evaluating trends in parameters such as heart rate, respiratory rate, oxygen saturation, and blood pressure over time. This may be helpful when evaluating the effect of an intervention or interventions over time as demonstrated in the two examples given below. In the first trend graph saturation data are displayed before and after intervention with prostaglandins then

Figure 2. Trend graph of pulse oximeter saturation in a newborn infant with congenital cyanotic cardiac disease

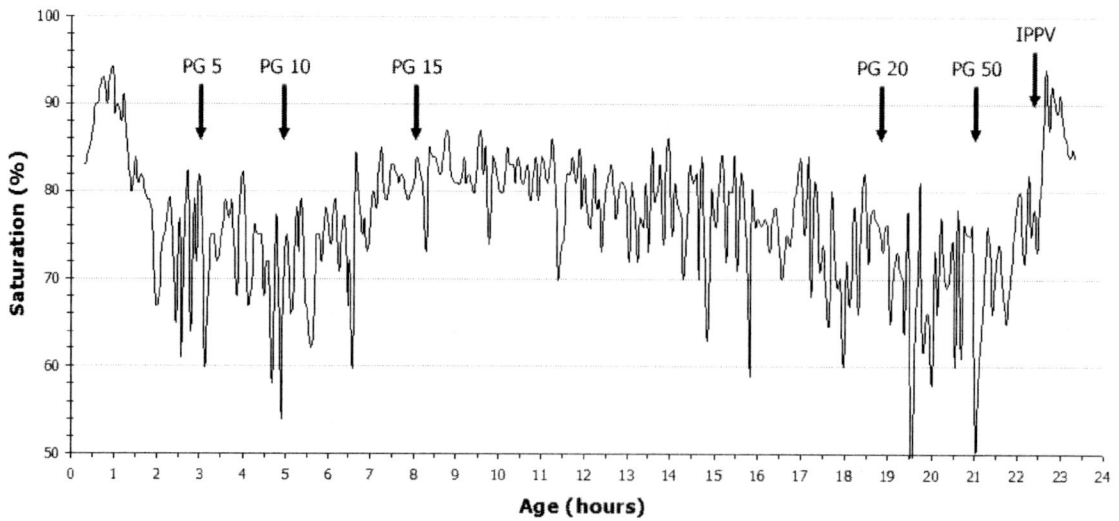

ventilation. In the second graph output from a bedside amplitude-integrated EEG (aEEG) monitor demonstrate the value of both real-time and trend analysis in diagnosis and determining the response to a treatment. Another typical use for trend analysis would include ventilator parameters and lung compliance data following administration of surfactant.

Data have been downloaded from the cardio respiratory monitor, via a network server where data are stored every 60 seconds. The graph shows an initial period of acceptable oxygenation for the first 90 minutes, followed by a decline. At 3 hours of age, prostaglandin E1 is commenced at a dose of 5 nanograms(ng)/kg/min (PG 5) to maintain patency of the ductus arteriosus to assist with oxygenation. However, the baby does not improve and the dose is increased further to 10 (PG 10) and then 15 ng/kg/min (PG 15). The saturations are maintained largely between 70 and 85%, but there are increasing periods of desaturation. The prostaglandin dose is increased further

Figure 3. Output from a bedside EEG monitor demonstrating both real time raw EEG data (upper two boxes) and trend amplitude integrated summary data (bottom two boxes) to assess response to treatment

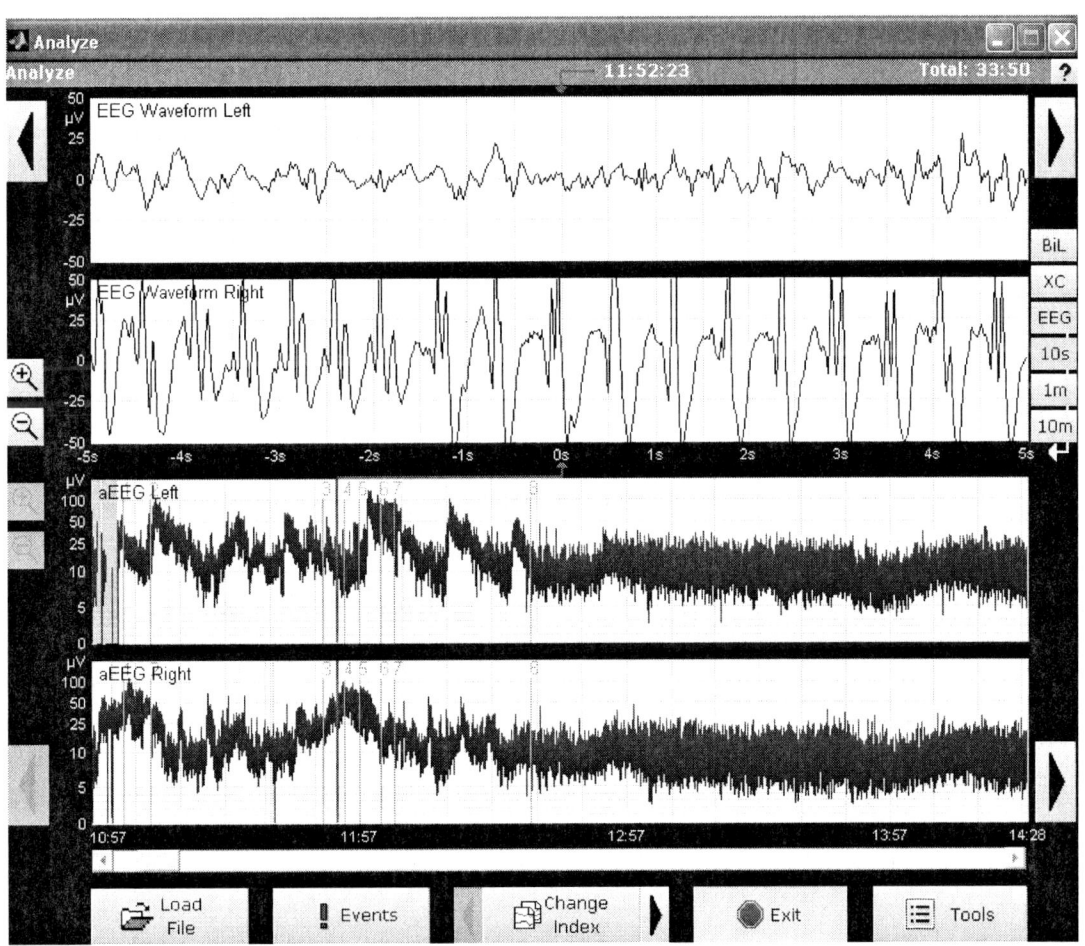

to 20 ng/kg/min (PG 20) and then 50 ng/kg/min (PG 50), following which the baby is artificially ventilated in preparation for a modified Blalock-Taussig shunt.

In the above example the output from a bed-side amplitude-integrated EEG (aEEG) monitor demonstrates the value of both real-time and summary aEEG data in diagnosis and determining the response to a treatment. The user is able to highlight events on the monitor, such as clinical events, handling, and treatments. For this infant, clinical seizures were suspected and are marked as events 1 to 7. A review of the aEEG data demonstrates a raised baseline voltage strongly suggestive of bilateral electrical seizures - indeed, the baseline voltages are high between the time that the EEG is commenced (10:57) and some two hours later. Closer inspection of the raw EEG data between events 3 and 4 shows high-voltage rhythmic electrical discharges over the right cerebral hemisphere, consistent with electrical seizures. No seizures are seen in the 10 second epoch of raw EEG from the left cerebral hemisphere. A loading dose of phenobarbitone is administered (event 8), following which the baseline returns to a normal level around 5 uV. No further electrical seizures are obvious on the aEEG data up until 14:28hr.

As well as data available from cardio respiratory monitoring and EEG systems, trend data can also be viewed and downloaded from ventilators, showing changes in ventilation requirement. For example, our NICU uses Drager Babylog 8000plus ventilators which have a companion computer attached that analyses data collected from the ventilator. Graphical analysis of extracted data using the accompanying software (VentView) allows the clinician to look at a considerable amount of data related to direct patient care, such as the oxygen requirement, tidal volume delivered, and the ventilator pressures required by the baby. Although clinicians may use this information to integrate the support that the baby is receiving with their own clinical analysis of the baby's progress, it is not clear that this amount of information alters clinical outcomes. In a randomized trial of respiratory function monitoring of 35 ventilated newborn infants, where one arm of the study allowed clinicians to view the output of respiratory function monitoring whilst the other arm masked the output, there were no differences in ventilation parameters between the two groups [4]. However, clinicians who were able to see the information provided by the respiratory function monitor did sometimes make clinical decisions around ventilation based on the information that was provided by the monitor, and most clinicians thought that the information was very useful, especially in those infants who were more difficult to ventilate.

There are potentially several major advantages, particularly with regard to safety, associated with the use of the types of informatics tools outlined above. Notably, a web-based data source avoids the need for paper-based copies, which ensures the latest version is the only version available and thus is used at all times. New guidelines and protocols can be updated quickly and efficiently, and multiple copies do not need to be disseminated widely to staff or other stakeholders. However, other systems to inform staff of changes in practice or protocols are useful, such as an email distribution list or a highlighted "update" section on the website. Furthermore, web-based calculators or nomograms assist the clinician in calculations but also may decrease errors and identify areas in which systems and processes may improve efficiency.

Examples of applications that are commonly used in neonatal care include an up-to-date drug formulary and calculators for drugs and clinical guidelines. Although such applications are very useful in saving the clinician time and effort there are important considerations with regard to safety. With the increasing use of computers in medicine, with access to web-based tools or applications based on other platforms, one issue to consider is the use of hand-held devices (for example, personal data assistants, or PDAs) versus networked personal computers. Within our NICU, increasing reliance on web-based applications has seen a marked increase in the availability of personal computers. Therefore, web-based applications have been designed with this platform in mind. Although hypertext pages can be converted to a format for PDAs, the same issues arise around updating webpages and accessing the only version in use within a clinical unit. In addition, some applications that work appropriately on a hypertext markup language web page may not render appropriately in a PDA format, which may lead to problems with the use of the electronic document. Although the role of PDAs in the provision of healthcare is expanding, the use of technology to assist delivery requires caution. One example of poor rendering with conversion of an application from a PC format to a PDA has been reported [5]. In this example, output from a previously performed calculation could not be protected, and a dose of adrenaline seven-times that intended was administered when the previous information was overwritten. It is critical that any information technology system responds safely and reliably in clinical scenarios, and it is the obligation of those developing the software to ensure that the systems are extensively tested by a range of users prior to the widespread adoption of the programs.

It is possible to utilize web-based technology or medical information system to decrease medical errors; a particularly good example of this is the ordering of intravenous nutrition (IVN). Nutritional support is an essential part of neonatal intensive care. Sick or preterm infants often require IVN to meet their metabolic and growth demands. Ordering IVN is a significant task particularly when it needs to be performed on a regular/daily basis. However, it is often left to the most junior member of the team despite the fact that it is a complex activity requiring adjustment of constituents and has potential for errors. A computer system for ordering provides the opportunity to

build in safeguards. This could include limits on individual constituents (such as protein and fat), total osmolality, and ensuring that components are kept below levels that may cause precipitation. Our NICU has adopted this approach, and places some absolute limits on composition (for example, no more than 4 grams/kg of protein per day), but also provides alerts to the person completing the order when intended constituent quantities exceed the usual amounts.

Apart from our anecdotal experience with an IVN calculator, the literature includes examples where a low-cost, pragmatic approach using such technology has been introduced and the effect monitored. Prior to the introduction of such as system an average of 10.8 errors were detected per 100 IVN orders. However after the introduction of an online IVN calculator the rate had fallen to 4.2 per 100 orders. Moreover the system under went a rapid cycle development and after some redesign a further decrease to 1.2 per 100 orders was achieved. Furthermore, the users were positive about use of the system and considered it have merit over the previous paper-based system.

One challenge with the use of extensive information technologies is the integration of data from multiple sources. Whilst a clinical workstation interface, such as that shown above (Figure 1) integrates data from a number of sources, linking multiple data repositories can pose difficulties. Ideally, patients should have a unique identifier and systems should cross-reference this ID so that correct data is pulled across from platform to platform. This allows data be stored in one place (for example, demographic data such as address, contact details, ethnicity, family practitioner) yet used in many documents. Another challenge with such a large amount of data is determining which data is important enough to be included in any documentation or new database. It is all too easy to import data, yet for there to be inadequate interpretation of the meaning of the data. For example, although clinically important data such as the results of a full blood count may give a result such as a hemoglobin of 75 g/L, interpretation of the importance of this result (such as, "The baby is anemic with a hemoglobin of 75g/L. However, she remains asymptomatic and is receiving iron supplementation – we recommend a follow-up full blood count in one week") is often lacking.

CLINICAL NEONATAL DATABASES

Databases have proliferated throughout hospitals over recent years. The best funded, first introduced and best developed ones that tend to be orientated towards hospital finances and management. These are usually followed by systems related to support services such as radiology and laboratories. Databases on clinical units are often developed by the clinicians involved and may or may not integrate with the hospital systems. More recently standardized databases have become available and uptake has been widespread, such as with the Badger system in the UK.

A neonatal database generally includes both demographic and clinical data. Items such as maternal age and ethnicity plus information on pregnancy clinical course and complications would ideally be available from the antenatal record. Postnatal infant data will need to be collected prospectively. Admission data includes gestational age, birth weight, Apgar scores, resuscitation details and initial clinical examination findings and treatment details. Subsequently data can be collected on clinical course, investigations and clinical monitoring such as blood pressure, heart rate, oxygen saturation and blood gas analysis.

Clinical databases are of use in analyzing the workload of a neonatal unit, tracking changes in demographics and clinical presentations, looking at short term outcomes, identifying areas of practice that need reassessing, conducting audits of practice as well as research. Many are well established so giving the potential to review data collected over 20 years previously. They also are used to generate the data to be sent to neonatal

networks. Many databases are fairly limited in their capabilities. For instance many hospital-wide databases will track admissions and discharges and be able to give information on length of stay. However frequently they will not have information on birth weight or gestational age. Such simple information is essential in order to understand workload and interpret length of stay. The lack of basic clinical data limits the usefulness of hospital-wide databases to clinicians.

Neonatal services have tended to develop their own databases using propriety software available on personal computers. The most common system at present is the use of MS Access™, possibly using an SQL server as a data repository. These have advantages of being 'owned' and developed by the clinicians involved. This makes them responsive to clinician needs and they can be adapted quickly as circumstances change. For instance a new field can be added and reports can be generated at short notice. However, the development of the database takes clinician time and effort. Often those involved have limited programming skills. The systems are often not integrated with the hospital systems.

Other clinical databases are set up as web-based databases and are shared by many neonatal units across different hospitals. An example of this is the Pediatrix Medical Group of 220 hospitals in 32 US states and Puerto Rico. Data is entered daily and is used for generating progress notes and billing information. It also provides a valuable repository for generating audit and research[7]. Another example is the database currently being developed for the NICUS Network of all Neonatal Intensive Care Units in New South Wales, Australia. These web-based systems have the advantage of being part of networks, enabling information to be easily exchanged between units and having standardized definitions. They operate in real time with the information from them being available in a timely manner. However, they will often not be linked to hospital systems. Therefore, some data will need to be double-entered, some will be out of date (for instance family doctor addresses or patient demographics). The data will not be available to hospital management or other clinical departments.

Two major issues with all databases are: a) who puts the data in; and b) how easy is it to get data out. The old axiom of 'rubbish in, rubbish out' needs emphasizing. For data input, the choice is generally between clinicians (often residents and nurses, the busiest staff on the Neonatal Unit) or data-entry clerks. Clinicians understand the clinical conditions and the definitions of different diagnoses. However, they often have little motivation or incentive to enter data. To overcome this, it is necessary for them to get some return for entering data. For instance, if the database generates the discharge summary and daily problem list, resident staff will want to enter data in order to avoid prolonged periods in a dictation booth trolling through thick clinical notes to produce the discharge summary. Any database that is being designed for a clinical unit needs to consider who is to input data. If it is to be clinicians, the database must be easy to use, need little training and be considered by them to be useful for them in doing their jobs. Paradoxically, as databases are now so easy to set up many have the fault of collecting too much data. Clinicians in particular tend to ask the developer to add fields that may never be analyzed. It is better to start with the question 'what data and reports do we need to get out' of the database rather than 'what information can we put in'. Even if data is entered by clinicians, there needs to be a system for checking its accuracy and collecting missing data. It is seldom satisfactory to rely sole on multiple clinicians entering data accurately. There is often missing or inaccurate data. Therefore, any setup that is to be used to report important outputs (for instance for hospital planning, reporting to networks or research publications) needs to have regular checking and audit of the data.

Any repository of data requires key identifying features that are unique to the individual, such as a unique hospital identification number, so that data are not erroneously collated for the wrong patient. Allowing for the sensitive nature of clinical data that may be linked to identifying features, security is a critical factor in any system that integrates clinical and demographic data. Notwithstanding these issues for programmers, the portal should ensure availability of clinical data to enable efficiencies in time and integration of health care data. Finally a computerized discharge summary will combine data collection and communication. This allows easy linkage with electronic health records and/or can be distributed by email.

Data Management

Efficient data management is essential in order to provide effective clinical care. Although this is an important aspiration for all fields of clinical care there are some characteristics of neonatology that are particularly relevant to this concept. In common with other intensive care specialties neonatologists often use scoring systems such as CRIB, CRIB II and SNAP scores[8-10] in order to predict outcome or to a lesser extent use in benchmarking exercises. Also like other intensive care specialties neonatology focuses on very unwell individuals and clinical decisions are frequently based on a mixture of clinical and monitoring data. However, in neonatology there is characteristically a more homogeneous population with narrower range of presenting conditions, greater patient numbers and a longer mean stay in the unit[11]. Furthermore, prematurity in general rather than an organ specific clinical condition, such as pulmonary or cardiovascular disease, is the most common indication for neonatal intensive care. Such characteristics increase the need for and utility of a "population" approach to data analysis when compared with adult or pediatric intensive care.

Impact of Data on Clinical Care

Decisions in intensive care are made based on the available clinical information in conjunction with laboratory and imaging data. In addition to the earlier examples reviewing physiological or monitoring data from an individual patient, it may be important to appraise data collected from a larger group or cohort of infants. A classic example of this would be rationalization of antibiotic choice based on microbiological sensitivity data obtained from a single unit or group of units. An example of a very basic data collection system would be a simple spread sheet such as Microsoft Excel with recording of clinical events such as blood-borne infection or pneumothorax in ventilated infants. Simple analysis would include calculating rates for standardized patient groups or identifying trends in organisms and antibiotic sensitivity. Increasing sophistication could be obtained by also collecting data on risk factors and/or associated morbidities and by using either automatic data collection from laboratory systems or the use of computer generated prompts at the point of care. Measures such as these could lead to decreased rates of acquired infection; thus well formatted and accessible data have potential to inform and significantly improve clinical care. A recent example of how surveillance of this sort has contributed to clinical care is the published work on altered rates of early onset sepsis with ampicillin-resistant Escherichia coli associated with the wide spread introduction of antibiotic prophylaxis for newborns at risk of group B streptococcus infection [12,13].

Another way that data can inform and improve clinical care is in the area of medical error. Error is not uncommon in health care [14] and is responsible for a significant amount of morbidity and mortality in hospitalized patients [14]. Newborn infants, especially those in the neonatal intensive care unit are particularly at risk of drug-related adverse events [15]. One major risk factor is the inability to vocalize or comprehend drug orders, a situation in common with the elderly who are another high risk group. Other contributing factors include the fact that drugs may be used for off label indications; drug doses need to be calculated based on weight, with frequent adjustment for weight gain or loss; and the need for pharmacists to make special dilute preparations of drugs, due to small doses [15]. Many adverse events are potentially preventable and better monitoring and education [16] plus more appropriate choice of medication may have a role. However, increasing use of technology in the form of computerized ordering, with appropriate inbuilt checks, is another common prevention strategy suggested [17]. Ideally a system to identify errors and potential errors should be specific to the individual specialty and encourage voluntary reporting of errors by health care professionals. It may also be helpful if the system allowed anonymous reporting as an important method of getting more complete ascertainment. One study examined the feasibility of an Internet-based reporting system for medical errors in neonatal intensive care to identify errors that affect high-risk neonates and their families [18]. A total of 1230 reports were received from 739 health professionals from 54 hospitals in the Vermont Oxford Network. Errors in medication included: wrong dose; schedule; or infusion rate, including nutritional agents and blood products. Other incidents were errors in administration of treatment; patient misidentification; other system failure; error or delay in diagnosis; and error in the performance of an operation, procedure, or test. The contributing factors that were identified were failure to follow policy or protocol (47%), inattention (27%), communications problem (22%), error in charting or documentation (13%), distraction (12%), inexperience (10%), labeling error (10%), and poor teamwork (9%). The study concluded that in addition to identifying a wide range of errors in neonatal intensive care the specialty-based, voluntary, anonymous Internet reporting system promoted multidisciplinary collaborative learning [18].

Role of Data from Neonatal Networks in Quality or Benchmarking Issues

One of the primary reasons to collect and analyze neonatal data is examine variation in both clinical practice and outcomes between centers or services for the purposes of examining quality of the care provided [19]. A common mechanism to do this is subscribing to a neonatal network, which is defined as a collaboration involving more than one clinical site where a common protocol is used for a randomized trial, observational study, or quality improvement project [20]. Data is collected and checked by the individual unit then regularly submitted to the network administration, which collates and processes the data to form a report in a format that allows comparison between the whole network and the individual units. The approach has a proven utility in improving clinical care [21] and has several inherent advantages, particularly, as the quality of data is assured, due to it being checked both at source and by the network. Furthermore, it allows the individual unit to perform comparison over a number of standard outcomes and, using the data from other network centers, can identify any centers that are outliers for each of these outcomes. Finally the combined data from the whole network will have a greater power to examine important questions on the quality of clinical care.

One clinical outcome with important potential adverse long term developmental consequences, which has been examined within a network context, is intraventricular hemorrhage [19, 22, 23]. The incidence of this potentially serious complication of preterm birth may be influenced by both facets of clinical care and case mix; thus adjustment in raw data should be made for this and some disquiet has occurred around creating league tables using data that is not fully adjusted or only recorded over a limited time period [24]. Nevertheless, analysis of network data does suggest that some variation in IVH incidence between units may be dependent on NICU characteristics [22]. Once such

data is available then it can be used to improve outcomes. Although both philosophically and in practice it may be preferable to focus on shifting all centers towards the better centers rather than concentrating on the worst performing hospitals [19]. Examples of further important outcomes that may be studied using large network data sets are chronic lung disease [25], retinopathy of prematurity [26] and death [27].

An example of the benefit of pooled data in a network having an increased power to examine important questions on the quality of clinical care is the topic of sepsis rates, where network data demonstrated the importance of certain intravenous lines as a risk factor [28]. Other important studies based on network outcome data have evaluated the influence of hospital type [29] and time of day when the infant was admitted to neonatal intensive care units at night [30]. Importantly, the first of these studies demonstrated worse outcomes for outborn infants admitted to pediatric hospitals in terms of mortality, nosocomial infection and oxygen dependency at 28 days of age compared to those admitted to perinatal centers. The second study reported a higher neonatal mortality for inborn infants admitted at night. Such information can be used in optimize service provision and clinical outcomes.

One way that services may optimize care is in the appropriate early adaptation of new technologies and proper audit of such developments. Shared network data may be usefully employed to both assess uptake and evaluate the impact on related clinical outcomes from such practices. An example of this is a study of the use of high frequency ventilation in Australia and New Zealand [31]. Data from 3270 infants who received high frequency ventilation between 1996 and 2003 were examined. It revealed that use had doubled over this period but outcome had not improved; in fact there was a higher mortality in the infants receiving this form of ventilation. A further example of new technology assessment is the Vermont Oxford Network of early nasal CPAP (continuous positive airways pressure) [32]. In this study lower rates of adverse outcomes including chronic lung disease and retinopathy of prematurity were associated with CPAP use and associated early respiratory management. The data generated by this type of review of practice are thus useful in informing the collective clinical experience and can generate hypotheses that may be subsequently examined in large randomized multicenter trials.

Provision of Information and Support for Parents

Parents of a sick newborn infant admitted to an intensive care nursery are subjected to a considerable number of potential stresses. Although this fact is well recognized [33,34], the stresses vary between parents, and over time this may make it harder for the health professional to address them fully in one off conversations. Each family will have their own specific fears and worries but there are a number of common and recurring themes. These include uncertain outcome, anxiety about procedures and treatments, financial worries, unfamiliar staff, abnormal appearance of their baby, difficulty understanding complex medical problems, major acute changes in condition and perceived lack of information [33]. Such worries are frequently mixed with feelings of anger and guilt plus concern about the potential adverse impact on the family dynamics. In addition, the situation may be made more difficult if the admission is to a hospital away from the family supports such as transfer to another tertiary neonatal unit due to either bed shortages or the need for specialized services. Finally, the smallest and sickest preterm infants will require prolonged hospital stay often for several months but the mother is often discharged from hospital after a few days resulting in an inevitable separation between the mother and baby that may be quite prolonged. Although visiting is essential for infant attachment or "bonding" and is encouraged by a "family based" approach to neonatal care, it can in itself produce problems for the parents as it is time consuming, tiring, and expensive [33].

Potential ways that informatics may be used to support parents include harnessing web-based technology to "demystify" the NICU environment. This could include the provision of web pages with information on the neonatal unit such as staff names and roles; data on neonatal outcomes, including mortality and morbidity; information on common conditions that may affect their baby, or procedures that may be performed; or may cover more prosaic information such as visiting policies and parking. There could also be the opportunity provide feedback or ask questions of the staff. In addition, particularly where there is geographical separation for any reason, activities that help to form memories such as writing a diary for their baby [35] can be supported by web-based technologies.

In the early days of the NICU admission, despite the efforts of the staff to be supportive and approachable, the parents will be unfamiliar with the potentially complex problems. Thus may find the neonatal unit often "high tech" and intimidating. At this stage the parents are particularly in need of information and a vital aspect of support for the family is orientation to the NICU environment. Although some parents may have had a visit to the neonatal unit as part of routine antenatal education most parents of preterm infants will not have started antenatal classes and so will not have been on a routine visit. In many cases there will have been very little time to prepare the family for a preterm birth. Conversely in some complex pregnancies the mother may be confined to bed rest in hospital for a long period but not be able to visit the NICU. In these situations, one particularly helpful development is the ability to enable a *virtual tour* of the neonatal nursery. In our institution two short video tours are available. One deals with level 3 (intensive care) and the other focuses on level 2 (special care). They are useful to familiarise families, who may potentially use the Newborn Service, and may be viewed by potential parents, on the antenatal or postnatal wards at a mutually convenient time. In many cases a physical tour of NICU is no longer required; although it is not intended that this service replaces fully either medical consultation or orientation to the unit for families who have had a baby admitted to NICU. Once the infant has been admitted for neonatal intensive care they will receive "a package" of measures that may include: respiratory support, such as ventilation; cardiovascular support, including inotropes; antibiotics; intravenous nutrition and in selected cases anticonvulsants or muscle relaxing agents. This type of care is complex and it is not appropriate for written consent to be obtained for each and every therapeutic maneuver or for every medication change to be explained in detail; this would very quickly over burden the families. However, it is very important to include the parents in the care of their baby and the process of consent to neonatal intensive care is based on sharing information. This incorporates explanation of the types of interventions that may be required and the range of outcomes that may be expected. As the family become more familiar with intensive care and understanding increases their need for information may change and they will often require more detailed or complex answers. Thus, providing information that can be accessed by the family in their own time and at their own pace is a vital part of the overall process of consent. In our unit we have a number of resources for families including web-based information sheets covering common conditions, outcome data and procedures performed on the neonatal unit.

Informatics to Support Families

An important principle regarding the provision of information is that it should be available to the intended audience. It is accepted that some information may be needed in printed format such as information sheets and that some items will need to be available in different languages.

Furthermore, it would not be helpful to provide all the information required by families of infants undergoing neonatal care on a website if only a small proportion had regular and easy access to a computer or the internet.

One study from Canada examined access and parent expectations from computer based information and reported that in 100 parents of NICU infants 79% owned a computer, 86% had internet access, and 76% regularly spent more than one to two hours per day on the computer. Of note there were some important socioeconomic factors associated with access. For instance, higher rates of Internet access were associated with higher level of education and fluency in reading English [36]. Similar findings are reported from a US survey of families who have children with congenital heart disease presenting for cardiac surgery [37]. Of 275 families surveyed 160 (58%) had Internet access either from home or work and (93/160) 58% used it to obtain information about their child's cardiac diagnosis. Of the families, who accessed the Internet for material about congenital cardiac disease, 82 % found locating relevant information easy and 95% considered the information to be helpful or very helpful in understanding of their child's condition.

Notwithstanding the fact that most families were able and willing to access the internet, and in one study over 90 % felt the information was helpful [38], many still considered the information as potentially unreliable [36], too distressing or not specific enough [38]. One area of parental information that has been systematically studied is retinopathy of prematurity [39]. Sites were identified using two search engines (MetaCrawler and MSN) and the terms: "retinopathy of prematurity," "premature eye," "premature retina," and "ROP". Each website was classified as academic, organizational, or commercial then graded for readability, general quality of the website and quality of the content specific to ROP. Overall the majority of sites were graded as fair or poor. Several authors [36, 38, 39] have commented that the best way to ensure

that parents have access to good quality and accurate information about their child's condition
or procedure is for the clinician to provide it. It
is important that clinicians should also provide
some time to review and discuss selected material
identified by the family.

The burgeoning use of internet technologies
and increasing acceptability of use in many aspects
of society does not necessarily mean that all families will be confident in the technology or will use
it. Thus, it is important to consider these aspects
with respect particularly to relatively disadvan-
taged families when providing internet based
family supports. Attempts to provide web-based
educational resources for low literacy families in
the NICU include the use of touch-screen platform
with voice-recorded messages to accommodate
varying levels of literacy and computer experience
[40]. Compliance with internet based information
for families is generally good. Current evidence
suggests that if information on a specific webpage,
sometimes called an information prescription,
is provided to a patient or family on how to help
manage a health problem then almost two thirds
of the families will log onto that web site [41]. Also
the probability of logging on is further increased
by 45% if an e-mail reminder is sent [41].

As mentioned above separation is a major
source of stress and web-based technology has
been utilized to attempt to decrease this; using
multimedia communication based on internet
technology to allow parents to view their baby
in neonatal intensive care via the family home
computer is a viable option. Two good examples
of such innovative projects are the *Telebaby* from
University Medical Centre Utrecht and *Baby
CareLink* from Harvard. Experience of using these
systems has been published [42,43]. The *Telebaby*
project used Standard Internet technology and
allowed parents to virtually "visit" their infant.
This system was easily adopted by the parents
and was reported to give parents the feeling of
control. The Baby CareLink system was evaluated in the role of providing *"enhanced medical,
informational, and emotional support to families
of very low birth weight (VLBW) infants during
and after their neonatal intensive care unit (NICU)
stay"*. The system was described as being able to
allow virtual visits and distance learning from
home during the period of hospitalization plus
virtual house calls and remote monitoring after
discharge. It also allowed confidential and efficient
sharing of patient-based data between authorized
hospital and community users. In a randomized
trial conducted in a cohort of VLBW infants,
born between November 1997 and April 1999,
eligible infants were recruited within 10 days of
birth and a computer including internet browser
and videoconferencing equipment was installed in
the family home within three weeks of birth. The
families of intervention group infants were given
access to the *Baby CareLink* telemedicine application and the control group received standard
NICU care. Evaluation was by using a standardized family satisfaction survey and assessment of
the effect on hospital stay, family visitation and
interaction with infant and staff. A total of 30
control and 26 study patients were enrolled from
176 VLBW infants admitted to the unit during
the study period. The two groups were similar
in terms of morbidity and family characteristics.
There were no differences in frequency of family
visits, telephone calls to the NICU, and infant
holding between the groups. However, based on
the survey data the system was considered to
significantly improve family satisfaction including satisfaction with the unit's physical environment and visitation policies. Although the time
to discharge home was similar in the two groups
it was suggested that the system may potentially
lower costs as the infants born weighing <1000
g had a trend toward shorter lengths of stay but
further study would be required to prove this as
there were differences in the process of discharge
between the groups [43].

INFORMATICS TO SUPPORT RESEARCH IN NEONATOLOGY

Informatics may support research and audit in a number of ways. A very simple method is an internet based survey. This could be a satisfaction survey for parents or a simple survey of clinicians on treatments/techniques available in a unit or approaches to medical care [44]. Another example could be analysis of locally held records extracted from a neonatal database specifically set up to prospectively collect data on a given procedure or condition. One centre, from Australia, reporting their experience from 2186 percutaneously inserted silicone central venous catheters over an 18 year period highlighted the value of keeping good prospective records [45]. In reviewing their experience they were able to illustrate the safety of these catheters particularly with reference to catheter tips in the right atrium [45].

However, a real advantage of an internet-based survey over a paper-based survey is that supporting clinical data may be included in an appropriate format. A case in point would be where high quality imaging data is provided. This may then closely mimic the clinical situation and be used to investigate the ability of the subject to interpret the data. There are good examples of this in the neonatal literature. A local study [46] used a series of radiographs demonstrating neonatal long lines and Australian and New Zealand Neonatal Network members and National Women's Hospital NICU staff to identify not just the likely anatomical position but also the desired action. The study provided data on interpretation, including intra and interobserver variation and action taken for a given line tip location. Interobserver and intraobserver reliability using the radiographs was poor and the major determinant of line repositioning was the perceived location. A further example is a web-based assessment of the ability to interpret neonatal cranial ultrasound scans [47]. High resolution scanned images of six important neonatal cranial ultrasound abnormalities were posted as a

questionnaire to the 59 neonatal units. The mean accurate identification of cerebral abnormalities was only 59% (range 45-71%). However, it was noted that there was a difference in experience and training, with only 44% of the neonatal registrars, compared with nearly all the consultant staff, have had any formal training in cranial ultrasonography.

Other potential uses of informatics in neonatal research include the use of web-based technology to record and transmit images for central interpretation. An example of this is a prospective, multicenter, masked, internet-based clinical trial of Retinopathy of Prematurity Study [48]. Pilot data have been collected to evaluate the utility of digital wide-angle photographic fundus screening for retinopathy of prematurity as compared to bedside indirect ophthalmoscopy in premature infants <31 weeks postmenstrual age at birth and <1000 g birth weight. The technology employed in this study is currently available and could be incorporated in to other research studies.

Finally, in common with other fields of medicine, web-based research support is vitally important for conducting large multi-centre randomized trials. The initial screening of patients and ensuring eligible status can easily be supported on a web-based interface. Similarly the randomization process may be performed using this interface and appropriate clinical and demographic data collected without recourse to paper based data entry. This will help to minimize mistakes and also facilitate rapid data analysis. This can also facilitate collaboration between study groups who share similar protocols (such as the BOOST2 group of studies evaluating oxygen saturation in preterm infants), and can allow for a prospective meta-analysis to be performed.

Education

Informatics has considerable potential with regard to education. Electronic textbooks and journals can be made available on a desktop computer.

Other electronic educational resources such as interactive clinical cases using high quality images of x-rays or dermatology slides can be distributed to large groups, viewed on a personal computer and then appropriate interpretation and management discussed, so encouraging interaction. Grand rounds and lectures can be recorded and presented as web casts or Pod casts, so staff unable to attend the original presentation are still able to use the material for learning. Staff training and orientation may include review of material on web pages and training log books may be web-based. However, none of these applications are specific to neonatology so will not be discussed further here.

One area of training and education that is particularly pertinent to neonatology clinical care is the echocardiographic assessment of the newborn infant with congenital cardiac disease [49]. This is a specialized skill usually the domain of highly trained technicians and clinicians and would normally fall to a cardiologist or a neonatologist with specific training in the morphology of congenital heart disease. However, with a widely dispersed population there may be problems in the provision of a nation-wide echocardiographic service. In this case studies may be transmitted by tele-echocardiography and reviewed by a specialist in a referral centre.

Assessment of the Impact of Web-Based Information on Neonatology

There is no doubt that the provision of informatics support is an important development for neonatology. One aspect of this is the ability for a tertiary unit to develop guidelines then share their experience by publishing them on the internet. This activity is likely to improve care not only in the centre developing the clinical guideline but also in the greater neonatal community due to the shared knowledge.

Our neonatal unit has maintained a website, with open access to several sections including clinical guidelines and education pages, since 2002. There has been considerable growth in the amount of activity seen over time such that in one month in 2007 there were 1.3 million total hits with 44,600 hits per day on average. The most common country of origin for the 79,600 visitors per month was USA, followed by UK, Canada, New Zealand and Australia. However, there were up to 800 visits per day from developing countries; this illustrates the important contribution to the wider community.

The most popular pages were educational, particularly those illustrating neonatal dermatological conditions, with 30,000 pages accessed per day. Other popular educational pages deal with neonatal respiratory conditions, including radiographs. There are also frequent requests to use this type of material in other formats such as books or lectures.

FUTURE DIRECTIONS

As described in this chapter, there is already a strong interrelationship between informatics and neonatology. However, it is likely that in the future we will see a further expansion of informatics applications so that these become integral to providing care to newborn infants. There is rich potential to both improve the care delivered and make life for the clinician easier. Key areas for development include the refinement of data analysis to produce appropriate outputs that can be utilized to influence clinical decisions and measures that improve patient safety.

Attempts have already been made to harness informatics systems and data management to provide real time "expert systems" to guide neonatal care. Increased data storage capacity and computer power are likely to be associated with further increases in the data warehousing and mining abilities with which to interrogate data. Important applications of this knowledge would include alteration of respiratory support systems (e.g. ventilator settings) based on physiological monitoring and blood gas parameters. A published example [50] of a rule based expert system, derived from the knowledge of two consultant pediatricians, aimed to provide ventilator settings to maintain the arterial blood gas tensions within an acceptable range. In order to minimize barotrauma the rules were designed to reduce pressures if feasible and increase pressures only as a last resort. Overall, it was able to provide advice on ventilator adjustments that was accepted on 83% of occasions [50]. In another study [51] the artificial ventilation expert system for neonates (AVES-N) made recommendations which were then compared to the decisions made by the expert-physician in 320 newborn infants. Overall, the best agreement (approximately 70 % of the time) was for the parameters: positive end expiratory pressure, inspired oxygen fraction and peak inspiratory pressure. In contrast, there was poor agreement for time related parameters such as frequency (54%), inspiration time (46%) and time of next blood gas analysis (15%). In this study differences were attributed to a) different therapeutic strategies in the two NICU's, b) missing data regarding complications in the database that therefore could not be taken into account by the expert system. Further work is likely required before such systems can be incorporated in to clinical practice and some of this work will need to explore the utility of expert systems with recent developments in respiratory support such as volume guarantee, continuous positive airway pressure and noninvasive ventilation. A third study examined the potential role of expert systems in the stabilization of neonates prior to transport [52]. In this task the computer was considered to be safe, and recommend measures within the guidelines of neonatal clinical practice. Overall, these studies have shown great potential for "expert systems". However, there are still some barriers in practice and further work is required

before an automated analysis is likely to be used as the sole basis for a clinical decision; although currently it may comfortably be used to inform that decision.

There is also enormous potential for the development of algorithms in physiological monitoring systems that can detect subtle changes in physiological measures that may herald a significant alteration in the status of the infant prior to a clinically detectable event. One such important clinical event in the newborn is pneumothorax, which has a significant mortality and morbidity. If an early diagnosis were possible this would likely improve the outcome. In a study of 42 infants with pneumothorax over a 4 year period the mortality before discharge was 45% [53]. Moreover, the median time (range) between onset of pneumothorax and clinical diagnosis was over two hours and in many cases measures such as suctioning the endotracheal tube or reintubation were taken that delayed appropriate action. Computer analysis of data from transcutaneous CO_2 measurements showed good discrimination for a pneumothorax (area under the receiver operating characteristic curve, 89%) and it was concluded that trend monitoring using reference centiles could form the base for automatic decision support. It is likely that in the future we will see more sophisticated forms of monitoring with decision support capability become more frequent in the care of the smallest and sickest infants.

A further area where technology may be utilized to improve infant safety is in identification. Due to their inability to speak, babies are at risk for misidentification errors particularly if there are similarities in standard identifiers such as names or identification/medical record number [54]. There have been frequent calls for increasing the use of information technology to reduce medication errors. It is likely that simple measures such as bar codes for identification and drugs administration purposes will increase. This has already been reported to reduce, and prevent bedside medication errors and to be well accepted by nurses [55]. This type of measure can also potentially be of use in the labeling of expressed breast milk as exposure to the wrong mothers milk can carry risk of disease transmission such as Cytomegalovirus.

There are some general issues including potential barriers that would need to be addressed in order to increase utilization of informatics to the full potential. Some of these issues are similar to other fields of health informatics including alleviation of manual data entry or labor intensive scanning procedures and difficulty with coding of specific clinical conditions. Other general matters are particularly pertinent to neonatology and child birth, where issues around data privacy need to be handled with sensitivity. Apropos the technology, the systems need to be flexible to allow for changes in practice related to new information or local practices. Although there are advantages to proprietary software (in terms of development and support), instituting changes to meet new demands can be challenging. The use of relatively simple software programs (e.g. Microsoft Excel™ or Access™) or programming languages (e.g. JavaScript in web-based applica-

tions) may assist with relatively easy modification and development of IT systems. Frequently, a local "champion" may be required to develop and support local systems. Basic IT skills will be developed over time, but this runs the inherent risk that the support of the system is dependent on the presence, commitment, and activity of a single individual.

Although neonatology is by nature a technology friendly specialty care must be taken to ensure that the first duty of the doctor is care of the baby and their family. If this is not borne in mind, the role of the doctor has the potential to become less humanistic when there is an emphasis on technology! Although heavy dependence on information technology means that medical staff spend less time on the telephone gaining the information they require, it also means that they spend more time in front of a computer screen and less time in direct patient care (Figure4).

At times it is easy to overlook the many developments in informatics that have become part of everyday neonatal care, perhaps because both specialties are relatively young and new develop-

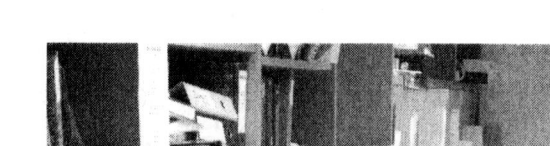

Figure 4. The changing work role of medical staff in a NICU

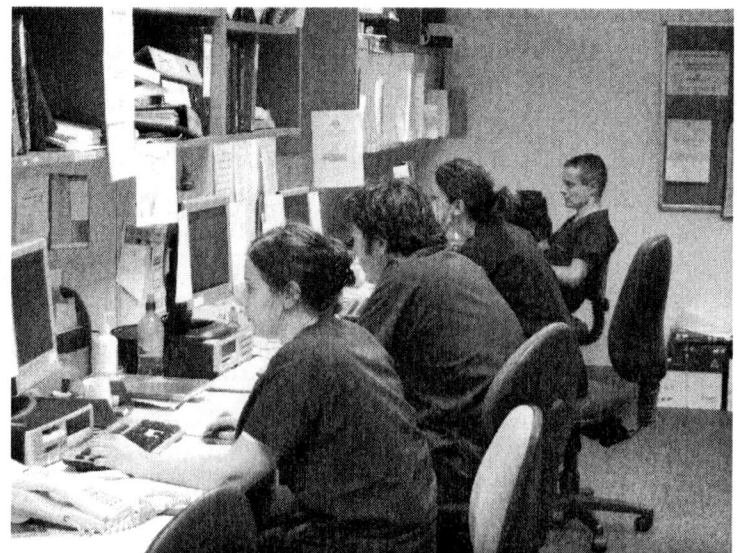

ments are quickly and often seamlessly adopted. However, there remains much that can be learnt not just from other branches of medicine but also other industries, such as aviation which has a strong safety focus. Informatics and neonatology already have a close relationship but in order to see the full benefits of informatics in neonatal care this relationship needs to be nurtured and the role of new applications in clinical care systematically studied.

REFERENCES

1. http://www.merriam-webster.com/dictionary/Neonatology

2. Clinical Guidelines Index. Newborn Services, Auckland City Hospital. http://www.adhb.govt.nz/newborn/Guidelines.htm

3. NICU Tools. A free source of browser-based neonatal and infant calculators. http://www.nicutools.org/

4. Klimek J, Morley CJ, Lau R, Davis PG. Does measuring respiratory function improve neonatal ventilation? J Paediatr Child Health 2006;42:140-2.

5. de Wildt SN, Verzijden R, van den Anker JN, de Hoog M. Information technology cannot guarantee patient safety. BMJ 2007;334;851-852.

6. Lehmann CU, Conner KG, Cox JM. Preventing provider errors: online total parenteral nutrition calculator. Pediatrics. 2004;113(4):748-53.

7. Laughon M, Bose A, Clark R. Treatment strategies to prevent or close a patent ductus arteriosus in preterm infants and outcomes. Journal of Perinatology. 2007;27:164-170.

8. de Courcy-Wheeler RH, Wolfe CD, Fitzgerald A, Spencer M, Goodman JD, Gamsu HR. Use of the CRIB (clinical risk index for babies) score in prediction of neonatal mortality and morbidity. Arch Dis Child Fetal Neonatal Ed. 1995;73(1):F32-6

9. Parry G, Tucker J, Tarnow-Mordi W; UK Neonatal Staffing Study Collaborative Group CRIB II: an update of the clinical risk index for babies score. Lancet. 2003;361(9371):1789-91.

10. Kumar D, Super DM, Fajardo RA, Stork EE, Moore JJ, Saker FA. Predicting outcome in neonatal hypoxic respiratory failure with the score for neonatal acute physiology (SNAP) and highest oxygen index (OI) in the first 24 hours of admission. J Perinatol. 2004;24(6):376-81.

11. Battin M. Health Informatics in Neonatology: What is the Potential to Further Improve Outcomes? http://hcro.enigma.co.nz/website/index.cfm?fuseaction=articledisplay&FeatureID=010707.

12. Stoll BJ, Hansen N, Fanaroff AA, Wright LL, Carlo WA, et al. Changes in pathogens causing early-onset sepsis in very-low-birth-weight infants. N Engl J Med. 2002;347(4):240-7.

13. Jones B, Peake K, Morris AJ, McCowan LM, Battin MR. Escherichia coli: a growing problem in early onset neonatal sepsis. Aust N Z J Obstet Gynaecol. 2004;44(6):558-61

14. To Err Is Human: Building a Safer Health System. Linda T. Kohn, Janet M. Corrigan, and Molla S. Donaldson, Editors; Committee on Quality of Health Care in America, Institute of Medicine 2000.

15. Gray JE, Goldmann DA. Medication errors in the neonatal intensive care unit: special patients, unique issues. Arch Dis Child Fetal Neonatal Ed. 2004;89(6):F472-3.

16. Simpson JH, Lynch R, Grant J, Alroomi L. Reducing medication errors in the neonatal intensive care unit. Arch Dis Child Fetal Neonatal Ed. 2004;89(6):F480-2.

17. Chedoe I, Molendijk HA, Dittrich ST, Jansman FG, Harting JW, Brouwers JR, Taxis K. Incidence and nature of medication errors in neonatal intensive care with strategies to improve safety: a review of the current literature. Drug Saf. 2007;30(6):503-13.

18. Suresh G, Horbar JD, Plsek P, Gray J, Edwards WH, Shiono PH, Ursprung R, Nickerson J, Lucey JF, Goldmann D. Voluntary anonymous reporting of medical errors for neonatal intensive care. Pediatrics. 2004;113(6):1609-18.

19. Simpson JM, Evans N, Gibberd RW, Heuchan AM, Henderson-Smart DJ; Australian and New Zealand Neonatal Network. Analysing differences in clinical outcomes between hospitals. Qual Saf Health Care. 2003;12(4):257-62.

20. Thakkar M, O'Shea M. The role of neonatal networks. Semin Fetal Neonatal Med. 2006;11(2):105-10.

21. Investigators of the Vermont Oxford Network. Horbar JD, Rogowski J, Plsek PE, et al. Collaborative quality improvement for neonatal intensive care. NIC/Q Project. Pediatrics 2001;107(1):14-22.

22. Synnes AR, Macnab YC, Qiu Z, Ohlsson A, Gustafson P, Dean CB, Lee SK; the Canadian Neonatal Network. Neonatal intensive care unit characteristics affect the incidence of severe intraventricular hemorrhage. Med Care. 2006;44(8):754-9.

23. Heuchan AM, Evans N, Henderson Smart DJ, Simpson JM. Perinatal risk factors for major intraventricular haemorrhage in the Australian and New Zealand Neonatal Network, 1995-97. Arch Dis Child Fetal Neonatal Ed. 2002 ;86(2):F86-90.

24. Parry GJ, Gould CR, McCabe CJ, Tarnow-Mordi WO. Annual league tables of mortality in neonatal intensive care units: longitudinal study. International Neonatal Network and the Scottish Neonatal Consultants and Nurses Collaborative Study Group. BMJ. 1998;316(7149):1931-5.

25. Henderson-Smart DJ, Hutchinson JL, Donoghue DA, Evans NJ, Simpson JM, Wright I; Australian and New Zealand Neonatal Network. Prenatal predictors of chronic lung disease in very preterm infants. Arch Dis Child Fetal Neonatal Ed. 2006;91(1): F40-5.

26. Darlow BA, Hutchinson JL, Henderson-Smart DJ, Donoghue DA, Simpson JM, Evans NJ; Australian and New Zealand Neonatal Network. Prenatal risk factors for severe retinopathy of prematurity among very preterm infants of the Australian and New Zealand Neonatal Network. Pediatrics. 2005;115(4):990-6.

27. Evans N, Hutchinson J, Simpson JM, Donoghue D, Darlow B, Henderson-Smart D. Prenatal predictors of mortality in very preterm infants cared for in the Australian and New Zealand Neonatal Network. Arch Dis Child Fetal Neonatal Ed. 2007;92(1): F34-40.

28. Chien LY, Macnab Y, Aziz K, Andrews W, McMillan DD, Lee SK; Canadian Neonatal Network Variations in central venous catheter-related infection risks among Canadian neonatal intensive care units. Pediatr Infect Dis J. 2002 ;21(6):505-11.

29. Shah PS, Shah V, Qiu Z, Ohlsson A, Lee SK; Canadian Neonatal Network. Improved outcomes of outborn preterm infants if admitted to perinatal centers versus free-standing pediatric hospitals. J Pediatr. 2005;146(5):626-31.

30. Lee SK, Lee DS, Andrews WL, Baboolal R, Pendray M, Stewart S; Canadian Neonatal Network. Higher mortality rates among inborn infants admitted to neonatal intensive care units at night. J Pediatr. 2003;143(5):592-7.

31. Tingay DG, Mills JF, Morley CJ, Pellicano A, Dargaville PA; Australian and New Zealand Neonatal Network. Trends in use and outcome of newborn infants treated with high frequency ventilation in Australia and New Zealand, 1996-2003. J Paediatr Child Health. 2007;43(3):160-6.

32. Kirchner L, Weninger M, Unterasinger L, Birnbacher R, Hayde M, Krepler, Pollak A.

Is the use of early nasal CPAP associated with lower rates of chronic lung disease and retinopathy of prematurity? Nine years of experience with the Vermont Oxford Neonatal Network. J Perinat Med. 2005;33(1):60-6.

33. Fowlie PW, McHaffie H. Supporting parents in the neonatal unit. BMJ. 2004;329(7478):1336-8.

34. Singer LT, Salvator A, Guo S, Collin M, Lilien L, Baley J. Maternal psychological distress and parenting stress after the birth of a very low-birth-weight infant. JAMA. 1999;281(9):799-805.

35. Stenson B. Promoting attachment, providing memories. BMJ. 1996;313(7072):1615.

36. Dhillon AS, Albersheim SG, Alsaad S, Pargass NS, Zupancic JA. Internet use and perceptions of information reliability by parents in a neonatal intensive care unit. J Perinatol. 2003;23(5):420-4.

37. Ikemba CM, Kozinetz CA, Feltes TF, Fraser CD Jr, McKenzie ED, Shah N, Mott AR. Internet use in families with children requiring cardiac surgery for congenital heart disease. Pediatrics. 2002;109(3):419-22.

38. Sim NZ, Kitteringham L, Spitz L, Pierro A, Kiely E, Drake D, Curry J. Information on the World Wide Web--how useful is it for parents? J Pediatr Surg. 2007;42(2):305-12

39. Martins EN, Morse LS. Evaluation of internet websites about retinopathy of prematurity patient education. Br J Ophthalmol. 2005;89(5):565-8.

40. Choi J, Starren JB, Bakken S. Web-based educational resources for low literacy families in the NICU. AMIA Annu Symp Proc. 2005;2005:922.

41. Ritterband LM, Borowitz S, Cox DJ, Kovatchev B, Walker LS, Lucas V, Sutphen J. Using the internet to provide information prescriptions. Pediatrics. 2005;116(5):e643-7.

42. Spanjers R, Feuth S. Telebaby videostreaming of newborns over Internet. Stud Health Technol Inform. 2002;90:195-200.

43. Gray JE, Safran C, Davis RB, Pompilio-Weitzner G, Stewart JE, Zaccagnini L, Pursley D. Baby CareLink: using the internet and telemedicine to improve care for high-risk infants. Pediatrics. 2000;106(6):1318-24

44. Taylor RS. Changes in thresholds for prescribing postnatal corticosteroids between 2000 and 2002: are we better educated ? Ped Res 2003;53(4): 103A.

45. Cartwright DW. Central venous lines in neonates: a study of 2186 catheters. Arch Dis Child Fetal Neonatal Ed. 2004;89(6): F504-8.

46. Odd DE, Battin MR, Kuschel CA. Variation in identifying neonatal percutaneous central venous line position. J Paediatr Child Health. 2004;40(9-10):540-3

47. Reynolds PR, Dale RC, Cowan FM. Neonatal cranial ultrasound interpretation: a clinical audit. Arch Dis Child Fetal Neonatal Ed. 2001;84(2):F92-5.

48. Photographic Screening for Retinopathy of Prematurity (Photo-ROP) Cooperative Group, Balasubramanian M, Capone A Jr, Hartnett ME, Pignatto S, Trese MT. The Photographic Screening for Retinopathy of Prematurity Study (Photo-ROP): study design and baseline characteristics of enrolled patients. Retina. 2006;26:S4-10.

49. Groves AM, Kuschel CA, Skinner JR. International Perspectives: The Neonatologist as an Echocardiographer. NeoReviews, Aug 2006; 7: e391 - e399.

50. Snowden S, Brownlee KG, Dear PR. An expert system to assist neonatal intensive care. J Med Eng Technol. 1997;21(2):67–73

51. Michnikowski M, Rudowski R, Siugocki P, Grabowski J, Rondio Z. Evaluation of the expert system for respiratory therapy of newborns on archival data. Int J Artif Organs. 1997;20(12):678–80.

52. Heermann LK, Thompson CB. Prototype expert system to assist with the stabilization of neonates prior to transport. Proc AMIA Annu Fall Symp. 1997;213–7.

53. McIntosh N, Becher JC, Cunningham S, Stenson B, Laing IA, Lyon AJ, Badger P. Clinical diagnosis of pneumothorax is late: use of trend data and decision support might allow preclinical detection. Pediatr Res. 2000;48(3):408-15.

54. Gray JE, Suresh G, Ursprung R, Edwards WH, Nickerson J, Shiono PH, Plsek P, Goldmann DA, Horbar J. Patient misidentification in the neonatal intensive care unit: quantification of risk. Pediatrics. 2006;117(1): e43-7.

55. Anderson S, Wittwer W. Using bar-code point-of-care technology for patient safety. J Healthc Qual. 2004;26(6):5-11.

Chapter X
Computerizing the Cardiotocogram (CTG)

Jenny Westgate
University of Auckland, New Zealand

ABSTRACT

During pregnancy the fetus requires an adequate supply of oxygen and clearance of carbon dioxide which is a waste product of metabolism. In fetal life, the placenta provides this function. After birth the lungs are aerated and perform this. If there is a failure to transport these chemicals across the placenta, the fetus can become hypoxic and acidotic, which can lead to permanent brain damage. In the neonate this can manifest in a number of ways, but most seriously cerebral palsy. Assessment of the fetal heart rate has been shown to identify fetuses where this maybe occurring. However the inter observer variation amongst clinicians assessing the heart rate monitoring is high and interpretation skills are often not good. Computer assessment of the fetal heart rate has been used and developed. Expert system techniques have been used to develop a system. The systems developed have been shown in studies to perform better than humans and to be able to identify subtleties not seen by the human eye. Future research is further assessing the value of these systems.

INTRODUCTION

The cardiotocogram (CTG) is a graphical display of a series of numbers representing fetal heart rate and uterine contraction frequency. The potential to computerize and analyze these signals has been almost irresistible to generations of obstetricians with an interest in mathematics, computers or modelling. Approaches used range from simple archiving of the digital record to highly complex analysis and systems vary from stand alone programs to decision support systems where CTG information is only one of multiple inputs to aid clinical management. This chapter will review the current status of computerization and the CTG.

THE NEED

There is no doubt about the clinical need to standardize and improve clinical use of information contained in the CTG. The aim of recording the fetal heart rate (FHR), however that is done, has always been to detect FHR changes that could indicate that the fetus was at risk of death or damage from oxygen lack so that intervention to rescue the fetus could occur. Continuous recording of the FHR directly from an electrode applied to the fetal scalp or indirectly through the maternal abdomen using the Doppler principle was introduced into clinical practice in the late 1960s and early 1970s. Despite initial optimism that the CTG would prevent intrapartum fetal death and reduce long-term neurological handicap that promise has been difficult to realise. Starting in the late 1970s repeated randomized trials have shown that use of the CTG was associated with an increase in rates of both operative vaginal delivery and caesarean section, especially for deliveries where presumed 'fetal distress' was the indication. The only benefit appears to be a reduction in neonatal seizures (Alfirevic, Devane, & Gyte, 2006). In the early 1980s a number of studies reported large intra- and inter- observer differences in CTG interpretation and by the 1990s there was evidence that interpretation of CTG changes was a major problem in clinical practice. In the United Kingdom the Confidential Enquiry into Stillbirths and Deaths in Infancy reported that nearly 75% of deaths of healthy babies during birth were avoidable and two thirds of intrapartum and early neonatal deaths were attributed to asphyxia (oxygen lack with tissue damage). Most errors were related to interpretation of electronic fetal monitoring traces (*Confidential enquiry into stillbirths and deaths in infancy (CESDI). Fourth Annual Report, 1 January - 31 December 1995.*, 1997). The most frequent criticisms from the Confidential Enquiries have related to delays in recognising or responding to CTG abnormalities (frequently over several hours), failure to appreciate the urgency or severity

of the situation by the obstetric team and lack of senior accountability (CESDI 1997-2000). Other studies have reported similar problems and where examples of abnormal CTGs have been provided it is clear that the abnormalities are severe and the lack of recognition or response is bewildering (J. A. Westgate, Gunn, & Gunn, 1999). It is not surprising that many of these cases become the focus of litigation (Johanson, Newburn, & Macfarlane, 2002) which is immensely stressful for those involved and has significant financial implications for health services.

Closely aligned with these factors is the dramatic rise in caesarean section rates seen worldwide. The reasons for this are not clear but undoubtedly fear of litigation contributes to defensive clinical practice. Mothers themselves are choosing caesarean sections for a number of reasons but fear of labour, loss of confidence in the system of care and fear of bad outcome for mother and baby are all factors which contribute to this growing trend.

It is now recognised that CTG interpretation and management is actually a complex task which requires knowledge of FHR patterns, fetal physiology and labour management applied to the specific clinical aspects of each mother, fetus and labour. Not only is the task difficult, but it is often performed in highly stressful circumstances. High workload, tiredness from long hours or shift work, emotional pressure from dealing with women and families in painful and stressful situations, worries or concerns in their personal lives or the working environment are just some examples of factors which affect the ability of clinicians to function optimally. For example, there is evidence that perinatal mortality or morbidity related to intrapartum asphyxia in low risk pregnancies is more common at night (Heller, Misselwitz, & Schmidt, 2000; Heller, Schnell, Misselwitz, & Schmidt, 2003; Stewart, Andrews, & Cartlidge, 1998; J. Westgate & Gunn, 2001). In one study (Stewart et al., 1998) there was an excess of asphyxial deaths during months when annual leave of labour ward staff was common and less experienced staff were available.

CLINICAL REQUIREMENTS

The fundamental aim of FHR monitoring is to detect a fetus who is suffering oxygen lack and is at risk of death or damage so that intervention to rescue the fetus can occur. Given concerns regarding the rising caesarean section rate, a secondary aim must be to correctly identify the fetus who is not at risk of damage from oxygen lack so as to avoid unnecessary operative intervention. Successful completion of this task has three elements; firstly accurate description of a FHR pattern, secondly correct interpretation of the pattern to assess fetal condition and finally an appropriate course of action within the context of that particular clinical situation and labour ward environment. How can computerising the CTG help clinicians achieve these goals?

Accurate Description of CTG Features

To begin their assessment of a CTG recording, clinicians are taught to first describe five key features of the CTG; baseline heart rate, variability, the presence or absence of accelerations and decelerations and the contraction pattern. In the mid 1990s, standardized definitions of FHR features and FHR patterns were agreed and published (Devoe et al., 2000) and have been adopted into many clinical guidelines for the use of CTG monitoring (Gynaecologists, 2001).

Computerised extraction and presentation of these features is reasonably straightforward where signal quality is adequate. This is a far easier task in the antenatal period as the absence of contractions means less signal artefact related to maternal movement. In addition, there are usually no decelerations of the FHR before labour

allowing easier baseline detection and calculations of variability.

Antenatal

The first commercially available computerised system for CTG feature extraction and display was the Sonicaid System 8000 for antenatal CTGs (Dawes, Moulden, & Redman, 1991). The development and clinical validation of the system and its most recent release as Sonicaid FetalCare has been extensively reported (Pardey, Moulden, & Redman, 2002). The system provides a numerical summary of the five key CTG features and fetal movements as indicated by the mother. It quantifies signal quality as a percentage signal loss and provides feedback to the user if signal loss exceeds 30% in any five minute period. The system also advises the user when the ten specified criteria for a normal recording have been achieved so recording time can be minimised.

A primary function of the Sonicaid FetalCare system is to report gestation specific episodes of low and high fetal heart rate variation exclusive of decelerations (Pardey et al., 2002). The range of FHR excursions around the baseline each minute is reported as the mean minute range and is described as a measure of long term variation (LTV). To calculate a measure of short term variation (STV) each minute of FHR data is divided into sixteen 3.75 second epochs and the difference between the average pulse intervals for each epoch is averaged over each minute and then the 1-minute averages are averaged over the whole recording (See figure 1 below). While it is possible to visually assess variation over each minute of recording, visual assessment of short term variation is impossible, but is highly correlated to the development of fetal academia and intrauterine death (Street, Dawes, Moulden, & Redman, 1991).

Clinical validation of Sonicaid FetalCare and its predecessors has been thorough with a database of over 73,000 recordings collected

Figure 1. Example of CTG Analysis (Sonicaid FetalCare, Huntleigh Healthcare, UK)

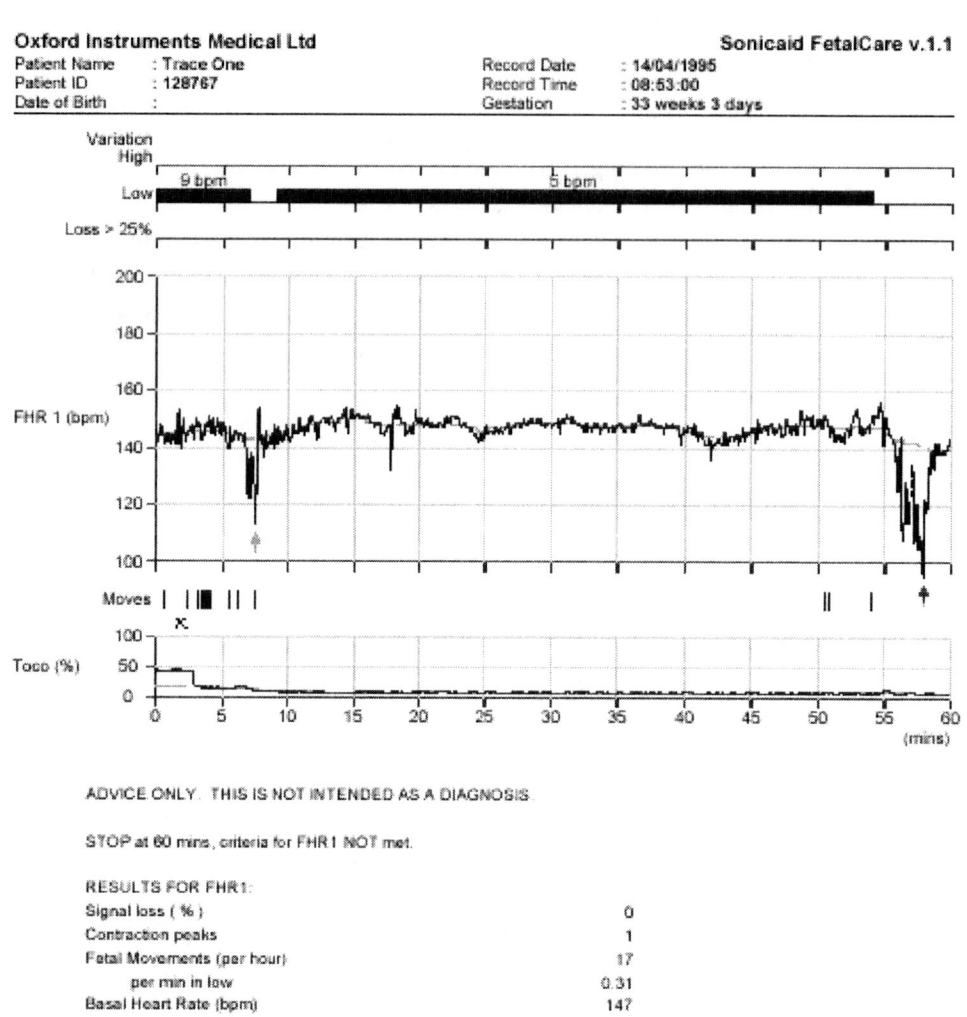

over two decades. Studies have included correlation of LTV and STV immediately prior to (Ribbert, Snijders, Nicolaides, & Visser, 1991) or within 24 hours of (Guzman et al., 1996; Smith et al., 1988; Street et al., 1991) caesarean section delivery with the biochemical status of the fetus at delivery. A randomised trial which compared physician-read antenatal CTGs with the oxford system and compared results with outcome found that women assessed with the system spent less time being monitored and required fewer additional tests (Bracero, Roshanfekr, & Byrne, 2000). Other systems for antenatal CTG analysis have been developed but none can match the extensive clinical database used to develop the Sonicaid system.

There is no doubt that use of computerised antenatal CTGs provides an objective, quantitative and consistent assessment of recordings. It also allows assessment of a measure of short term FHR variation which is impossible to assess visually and has shown to be correlated with outcome as assessed by umbilical cord acid-base status.

Intrapartum

Whilst the Sonicaid systems for antenatal CTGs have been the great success story of computerized CTG applications, it is salutary to realise that the same workers have been singularly unsuccessful in applying the same technology to the intrapartum CTG. Reduced heart rate variation in labour does not carry the same diagnostic significance as it does antenatally (Dawes, Rosevear, Pello, Moulden, & Redman, 1991) and computer derived FHR parameters in the last hour of labour have not been shown to correlate with fetal acid base status at delivery (Agrawal, Doucette, Gratton, Richardson, & Gagnon, 2003; Pello, Rosevear, Dawes, Moulden, & Redman, 1991). The challenges of feature extraction from the intrapartum CTG include signal loss and artefact from maternal and fetal movement. Narcotic drugs administered to the mother and epidural analgesia all affect

FHR parameters (Pello et al., 1991). These factors combined with the presence of decelerations makes reliable identification of the baseline heart rate problematic. There are a number of published methods for baseline detection, each tested with varying degrees of rigor, but no consensus on which methodology is best (Ayres-de-Campos & Bernardes, 2004). Detailed discussion of the advantages and disadvantages of the techniques used is beyond the scope of this publication and probably beyond the interest of most clinicians. What we want to know is do they work? Most publications report off-line validation studies which compare visual assessment and categorisation of CTGs by clinicians with that of a computerised system. Varying levels of agreement are reported. In reality such studies are insufficient to answer the question. What really counts is online testing in real clinical situations in large numbers of women to ensure that the methods used for CTG feature extraction are robust enough to cope with signal noise, artefact and rapid changes in fetal heart rate.

Computerized CTG and Interpretation

The simplest way that computerizing the CTG can facilitate interpretation of FHR patterns is by digitizing and displaying the CTG at a central monitoring station on a labour ward. This allows a number of people, including senior supervising midwifery and medical staff to view the CTG and form their own opinion on its significance. A number of commercial companies offer this technology including the facility for clinicians to dial in from remote sites to view CTGs. There is no evidence as to whether this or similar technology reduces unnecessary intervention or improves outcome. This approach also provides the opportunity to archive digitized CTGs as part of the electronic patient record as discussed elsewhere in this publication.

The next level of sophistication is a CTG feature extraction program with the capacity to set alarms for CTG parameters such as baseline rate or signal quality. Commercial companies such as Hewlett-Packard and Corometrics have had systems with this function since the mid-1980s, but have not been active in marketing them until relatively recently. Even the earliest central monitoring systems had some alarm functions but anecdotal evidence was that midwives found they cried wolf too often and quickly disabled them. The 2000s have seen the release of a number of these commercial systems which digitise the CTG, create an electronic record both for current use and for archiving, allow central and remote monitoring and offer CTG feature extraction and alarm systems. Many offer a further level of CTG analysis by categorising the CTG according to FIGO (http://www.gehealthcare.com/euen/ultrasound/ultrasound-it/viewpoint/trium-ctg.html or NICHHD guidelines (Devoe et al., 2000). There little published data about clinical validation of these programs and none about their clinical efficacy.

The wisdom of using this technology before it has been thoroughly tested in a clinical environment must be questioned.

Computerized CTG and Decision Support

In clinical practice the information about fetal condition gained from the CTG must be added to all the other clinical information about the individual mother, fetus and labour to produce a management or action plan. The same CTG abnormality may precipitate completely different responses depending on clinical factors such as how far on in labour a woman is and whether she has had a successful vaginal delivery before. The ability to integrate all this information and arrive at a correct decision while continuing to support

and care for the woman and her family is the art of intrapartum care.

Computerised decision support systems attempt to assist the clinician in complex decision making. Typically they consist of a medical knowledge base formulated from the knowledge of experts in that field, patient specific data and an inference engine which applies the knowledge to the patient data to generate patient specific advice. The last few decades has seen significant developments in the methods used to represent expert knowledge, the availability of electronic patient records and the ability of different systems to interact with each other (Peleg & Tu, 2006). Whilst it is possible to demonstrate that clinical decision support systems can improve practitioner performance, the effects on patient outcomes remain understudied, and when studied are inconsistent (Garg et al., 2005). For more information on artificial intelligence see chapter fifteen.

The potential for a clinical support decision system to improve clinical outcome was been demonstrated in an off-line study in the early 1990s (Keith et al., 1995). This study demonstrated that a computerised system using CTGs, patient information and fetal blood sampling data was highly consistent and its performance was indistinguishable from 17 clinical 'experts' in the 50 cases studied. A clinical user interface was developed and the system was tested in further on and off-line validation studies. Recordings from over 900 labours were recorded and the performance of the system (although unpublished) was sufficiently promising to obtain funding for a large multicentre randomised trial of an on-line system. Unfortunately, funding was subsequently withdrawn due to inability to obtain insurance to cover clinical risk (Rob Keith, personal communication). The main concern was situations in which there were CTG changes and the system reassured users without recommending action or intervention. A fresh attempt to secure funding for a single centre study with a modified system has been launched.

FUTURE DEVELOPMENTS

Clearly the CTG has the potential to improve perinatal care, but interpretation is key to this. New systems support the decision making process, but in the future there is likely to be further work examining increased technology driven decision support with possible use of alerts or alarms. Clinical trials are needed to assess whether these systems do indeed improve outcome prior to widespread introduction.

SUMMARY

Computerised analysis and clinical decision support of the antenatal CTG has been successfully used for over 20 years. The challenges of CTG feature extraction from intrapartum CTG recordings appear to have been met allowing sophisticated systems to display, record and describe CTG recordings on line in real time. However, there is little, if any, data on the effects of such technology on clinical outcomes. Medicolegal concerns have so far not allowed testing of decision support systems in clinical trials.

REFERENCES

Agrawal, S. K., Doucette, F., Gratton, R., Richardson, B., & Gagnon, R. (2003). Intrapartum computerized fetal heart rate parameters and metabolic acidosis at birth. *Obstet Gynecol, 102*(4), 731-738.

Alfirevic, Z., Devane, D., & Gyte, G. M. (2006). Continuous cardiotocography (CTG) as a form of electronic fetal monitoring (EFM) for fetal assessment during labour. *Cochrane Database Syst Rev, 3*, CD006066.

Ayres-de-Campos, D., & Bernardes, J. (2004). Comparison of fetal heart rate baseline estimation by SisPorto 2.01 and a consensus of clinicians. *Eur J Obstet Gynecol Reprod Biol, 117*(2), 174-178.

Bracero, L. A., Roshanfekr, D., & Byrne, D. W. (2000). Analysis of antepartum fetal heart rate tracing by physician and computer. *J Matern Fetal Med, 9*(3), 181-185.

Confidential enquiry into stillbirths and deaths in infancy (CESDI). Fourth Annual Report, 1 January - 31 December 1995. (1997). London: Maternal and Child Health Research Consortium.

Dawes, G. S., Moulden, M., & Redman, C. W. (1991). System 8000: Computerized antenatal FHR analysis. *J Perinat Med, 19*(1-2), 47-51.

Dawes, G. S., Rosevear, S. K., Pello, L. C., Moulden, M., & Redman, C. W. (1991). Computerized analysis of episodic changes in fetal heart rate variation in early labor. *Am J Obstet Gynecol, 165*(3), 618-624.

Devoe, L., Golde, S., Kilman, Y., Morton, D., Shea, K., & Waller, J. (2000). A comparison of visual analyses of intrapartum fetal heart rate tracings according to the new national institute of child health and human development guidelines with computer analyses by an automated fetal heart rate monitoring system. *Am J Obstet Gynecol, 183*(2), 361-366.

Garg, A. X., Adhikari, N. K., McDonald, H., Rosas-Arellano, M. P., Devereaux, P. J., Beyene, J., et al. (2005). Effects of computerized clinical decision support systems on practitioner performance and patient outcomes: A systematic review. *Jama, 293*(10), 1223-1238.

Guzman, E. R., Vintzileos, A. M., Martins, M., Benito, C., Houlihan, C., & Hanley, M. (1996). The efficacy of individual computer heart rate indices in detecting acidemia at birth in growth-restricted fetuses. *Obstet Gynecol, 87*(6), 969-974.

Gynaecologists, R. C. o. O. a. (2001). *The use of electronic fetal monitoring. The use and interpretation of of cardiotocography in intrapartum fetal surveillance.* London: RCOG Press.

Heller, G., Misselwitz, B., & Schmidt, S. (2000). Early neonatal mortality, asphyxia related deaths, and timing of low risk births in Hesse, Germany, 1990-8: observational study. *Bmj, 321*(7256), 274-275.

Heller, G., Schnell, R., Misselwitz, B., & Schmidt, S. (2003). Why are babies born at night at increased risk of early neonatal mortality?. *Z Geburtshilfe Neonatol, 207*(4), 137-142.

Johanson, R., Newburn, M., & Macfarlane, A. (2002). Has the medicalisation of childbirth gone too far? *Bmj, 324*(7342), 892-895.

Keith, R. D., Beckley, S., Garibaldi, J. M., Westgate, J. A., Ifeachor, E. C., & Greene, K. R. (1995). A multicentre comparative study of 17 experts and an intelligent computer system for managing labour using the cardiotocogram. *Br J Obstet Gynaecol, 102*(9), 688-700.

Pardey, J., Moulden, M., & Redman, C. W. (2002). A computer system for the numerical analysis of nonstress tests. *American Journal of Obstetrics and Gynecology, 186*(5), 1095-1103.

Peleg, M., & Tu, S. (2006). Decision support, knowledge representation and management in medicine. *Methods Inf Med, 45*(Suppl 1), 72-80.

Pello, L. C., Rosevear, S. K., Dawes, G. S., Moulden, M., & Redman, C. W. (1991). Computerized fetal heart rate analysis in labor. *Obstet Gynecol, 78*(4), 602-610.

Ribbert, L. S., Snijders, R. J., Nicolaides, K. H., & Visser, G. H. (1991). Relation of fetal blood gases and data from computer-assisted analysis of fetal heart rate patterns in small for gestation fetuses. *Br J Obstet Gynaecol, 98*(8), 820-823.

Smith, J. H., Anand, K. J., Cotes, P. M., Dawes, G. S., Harkness, R. A., Howlett, T. A., et al. (1988). Antenatal fetal heart rate variation in relation to the respiratory and metabolic status of the compromised human fetus. *Br J Obstet Gynaecol, 95*(10), 980-989.

Stewart, J. H., Andrews, J., & Cartlidge, P. H. (1998). Numbers of deaths related to intrapartum asphyxia and timing of birth in all Wales perinatal survey, 1993-5. *Bmj, 316*(7132), 657-660.

Street, P., Dawes, G. S., Moulden, M., & Redman, C. W. (1991). Short-term variation in abnormal antenatal fetal heart rate records. *Am J Obstet Gynecol, 165*(3), 515-523.

Westgate, J., & Gunn, A. (2001). Early neonatal mortality and timing of low risk births. Data suggest that difficulties in fetal monitoring are magnified at night. *Bmj, 322*(7283), 433-434.

Westgate, J. A., Gunn, A. J., & Gunn, T. R. (1999). Antecedents of neonatal encephalopathy with fetal acidaemia at term. *Br J Obstet Gynaecol, 106*(8), 774-782.

Section IV
Gynecology Applications

Chapter XI
Computer Assisted Cervical Cytology

Liron Pantanowitz
Tufts School of Medicine, Baystate Medical Center, USA

Maryanne Hornish
Tufts School of Medicine, Baystate Medical Center, USA

Robert A. Goulart
Tufts School of Medicine, Baystate Medical Center, USA

ABSTRACT

Automation and emerging information technologies are being adopted by cytology laboratories around the world to augment Pap test screening and improve diagnostic accuracy. Informatics, the application of computers and information systems to information management, is therefore essential for the successful operation of the cytopathology laboratory. This chapter describes how laboratory information management systems can be used to achieve an automated and seamless workflow process. The utilization of software, electronic databases and spreadsheets to perform necessary quality control measures will be discussed. The emerging role of computer assisted screening and application of digital imaging to the field of cervical cytology will be described, including telecytology and virtual microscopy. Finally, this chapter will reflect on the impact of online cytology resources and the emerging role of digital image cytometry.

INTRODUCTION

The Papanicolaou test (Pap test) is a highly successful, widely used, and cost effective method for the early detection of cervical dysplasia and cancer. However, Pap tests are not infallible, and emerging technologies have been developed to help improve diagnostic accuracy. Moreover, the shortage of skilled cytotechnologists to screen and diagnose Pap slides has become a concern, thus driving the goal to develop automated laboratory instruments and screening systems (Kumar and Jain, 2004). There are several steps that occur between obtaining a Pap test from a patient to the issuing of a diagnosis in the form of a useful and timely cytopathology report. These include specimen labeling and tracking, receipt of patient material in the cytology laboratory, accessioning of the specimen along with pertinent patient and clinical information into the laboratory computer system, specimen processing involving instrumentation, the possible performance of special studies, interpretation of prepared material (e.g. slides) by cytotechnologists and cytopathologists, and finally the creation and delivery of an accurate and understandable pathology report.

Laboratory informatics, the application of computers and information systems to information management in the pathology laboratory, is an essential component of this entire process (Pantanowitz, Henricks & Beckwith, 2007). Providing information in a manner that is most effective for patient care is the primary mission of the cytology laboratory. In addition, data from the cytology laboratory is used for documentation of quality control (QC) measures and quality assurance (QA), performance improvement, outcomes studies, and research (Raab et al., 1996; Becich, Gilbertson & Gupta, 2004). Despite the overwhelming interest in the development of several computer based technologies in the last several years, the role of automation in cytology has remained controversial (Masood, Cajulis, Cibas, Wilbur & Bedrossian, 1998). Much of this stems from laboratories not knowing how to incorporate automation in the routine practice of cytology. Around a decade ago, only 12% of cytology laboratories surveyed in the United States were engaged in automated cytology, and they predominantly used it for quality control (QC) measures (Masood et al., 1998). Today, with reduced costs and increased education, there is wider acceptance of these technologies in many different countries, particularly with regard to computer assisted cervical screening (Richards et al., 2007; Palcic, Sun & Wang, 2007).

The aim of this chapter is to demonstrate how cytology laboratories processing, screening, interpreting, and reporting out Pap tests have capitalized on the availability of computers, information systems and digital imaging to ensure quality enhancement, improved productivity, and thereby improved patient care.

LABORATORY INFORMATION SYSTEMS

The laboratory information system (LIS) is the core of many cytology laboratory operations. Its functions include workflow management, specimen tracking, data entry and reporting, assistance with regulatory compliance, code capture, interfacing with other systems, archiving, inventory control, and providing billing information (Pantanowitz et al., 2007; Eleveitch & Spackman, 2001; Cowan, 2005). Components of the LIS include hardware (e.g. servers), peripherals (e.g. instruments, printers), a network, interfaces (hardware and software links) to automated instruments and other information systems (e.g. electronic medical record and financial systems), database(s), and software such as an operating system, database management system, and specific applications required for laboratory operations. The LIS is often leveraged to improve efficiency, enhance productivity, reduce staff needs, facilitate automation (e.g. interface with automatic sample preparation, staining and slide cover slipping machines), and eliminate potential sources of error. The LIS also functions as a database that determines the configuration of system parameters and stores patient-related data (**Figure 1**).

The LIS database provides a flexible and organized way to store, retrieve, and manipulate data to ultimately generate usable information. LIS dictionaries and worksheets define the conventions and logical framework for information

Figure 1. Screen shot of a cytology information system showing its capabilities of connecting a patient's clinical history (fictitious patient), workflow process in the laboratory, diagnostic interpretation (Review tab), billing information, and coding (e.g. SNOMED)

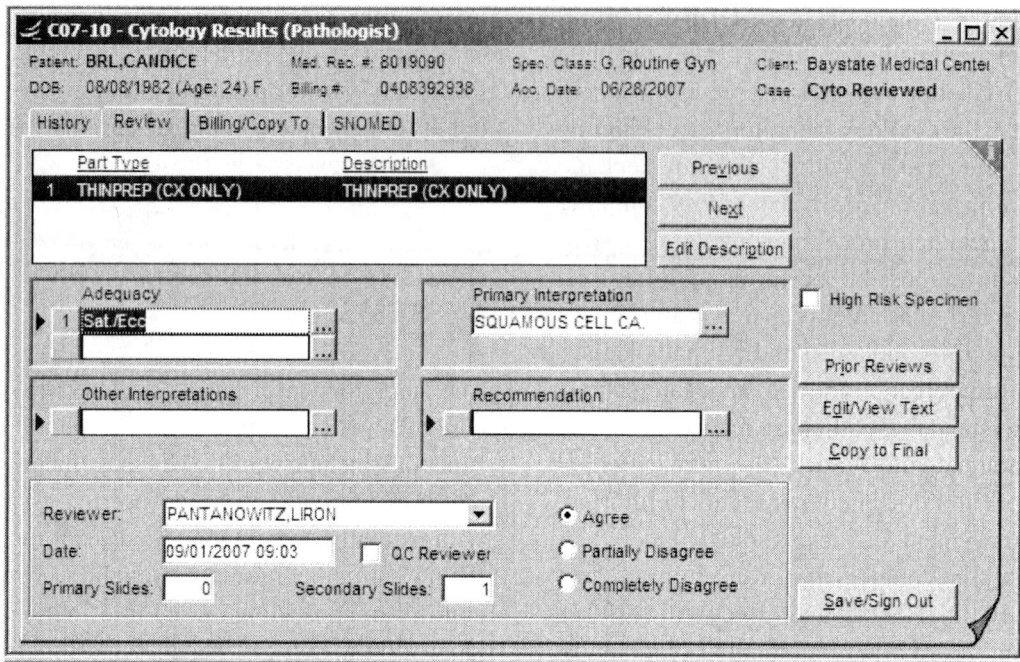

processing and workflow throughout the laboratory. LIS dictionaries (maintenance tables) are database tables or files that store and maintain information used repeatedly during activities such as accessioning of specimens or the ordering of tests. They help standardize and structure protocols, procedures, terminology and codes (e.g. billing codes), control workflow (e.g. logs), provide security features, define rules and limit selections for data fields, improve entry of valid data, define report content/format elements, and automate billing (Pantanowitz et al., 2007). Dictionaries provide choices in look-up windows or drop-down lists. Typically the laboratory defines and maintains the entries within these dictionaries in a manner that meets its specific needs. Dictionaries are typically built in a particular sequence, as some table entries are based on choices from pre-existing tables.

The LIS supports workflow and information flow in all steps (pre-analytic, analytic, and post-analytic) of the laboratory testing process. The pre-analytic phase involves patient registration, test order and selection, specimen collection and labeling, specimen receipt (accession number assignment), and tracking. The analytic phase includes work distribution (worklists) and specimen preparation (e.g. aliquots and bar code labeling), test performance and analysis, test interpretation, possible additional testing (e.g. testing for Human Papilloma Virus DNA or immunocytochemistry), result entry (interfaced, manual, and/or transcription), and verification (manual, automatic release, or via electronic signature). In the post-analytic phase, the LIS allows the generation and delivery of laboratory reports, test results (printing, faxing, electronic transmission), and modification of reports.

QUALITY CONTROL/QUALITY ASSURANCE

Quality control (QC), as applied to the cytology laboratory, is a set of procedures intended to ensure that the preparation, interpretation, and reporting of cytology specimens meets specified quality criteria. It is typically combined with quality procedures focused on the pre-completion tasks (quality assurance, QA), prior to final reporting of the cytologic interpretation or diagnosis.

It is well known that maintenance of quality control (QC) measures help to detect, reduce and correct deficiencies in Pap test analysis (Bonfiglio, 1989; Cibas, 2003; Frable, 2007; Kline, 1997; Marsan, 1995; Rohr, 1990). Although Pap test false negative diagnoses, for example, most often result from the lack of sufficient lesional sampling and cellular representation on the slide, laboratory error does occur, secondary to errors of identification in the screening process, errors of interpretation, or a combination thereof. Therefore, all cytology laboratories should have in place a comprehensive QC/QA program designed to monitor and evaluate the overall quality of the testing process. In the United States, a series of required QC/QA procedures was defined by the federal government in 1988 when Congress passed the Clinical Laboratory Improvement Amendments (CLIA), which established quality standards for all laboratory testing. These standards formed the minimum foundation of modern cytology QC/QA in the US, and with other individualized laboratory measures, are intended to ensure the accuracy, reliability and timeliness of patient test results. This process however cannot be fixed in time and approach, and needs to be ongoing, continually evaluating factors that lead to accurate and reliable test results. With the increasing availability of external QC measures (Cocchi et al., 1996), even cytology laboratories in developing countries can benefit from participating in these procedures (Salvetto & Sandiford, 2004). The opportunity to utilize spreadsheets and databases

to perform such key QC measures is part and parcel of the successful operation of any modern cytology laboratory. Moreover, in order to meet certain regulatory requirements and maintain laboratory accreditation, databases within the LIS are frequently relied upon and manipulated to perform quality measures.

The introduction of electronic record keeping has added a novel dimension to the practice of QA in contemporary cytopathology, and has ushered in a new paradigm of information management. Electronic data extraction and manipulation can be both convenient and complicated, often demanding computer-savvy end users that are willing and able to continually adapt in an environment of rapid change of both software and hardware solutions. Electronic monitoring of quality indicators has provided us with an increased range of opportunities to expose the nuances of the science and art of cytopathology, nuances perhaps most distinctively reflected by the Pap test's unavoidable presence of false negative cases. QA methodologies established and practiced by the laboratory are designed to continually improve diagnostic accuracy of both the cytotechnologist and cytopathologist, with the anticipated reduction, but not elimination of false negative cases.

Electronic Databases

Electronic data has tremendous advantages over paper record keeping, including the ease and efficiency of qualitative and quantitative data analysis, standardizing and structuring the reporting of results, rapid transmission of information, offering efficient integration and consolidation of multiple health records, and timely financial transactions (i.e. billing). Compared to paper record keeping systems, electronic data storage requires far less physical storage space and has the advantage of potentially allowing multiple users remote access to stored information. With regard to disaster recovery of data, electronic backups of data allow for relatively quick re-institution of data. In cases of disaster, the potential for data loss with electronic data is markedly lower than that of paper systems, provided backup of data is performed regularly and securely.

Limitations of electronic data include obsolescence of hardware and software technologies, discontinuation of hardware and software support services, the potential for easy intrusion on patient privacy, lack of end user education on proper use of hardware and software, and the "garbage in, garbage out" (GIGO) principle, because unlike humans, computers will unquestioningly process nonsensical data and accordingly provide a nonsensical output. The above limitations can be mitigated through education and adherence to specific patient privacy and risk management guidelines (e.g. the Health Insurance Portability & Accountability Act of 1996 in the United States).

Storing and retrieving data most commonly involves the utilization of a relational database. Relational databases consist of multiple tables of data each organized into columns (fields) and rows (records). Each table must have a unique indicator or primary key. Primary keys are a column or set of columns that uniquely identify all the rows in a table. Each row has a different primary key value and null values are not allowed. Data is linked through commonly shared fields. The advantage of this relational setup lies in its efficiency. Many tables can refer to one table that contains all the necessary information instead of engaging in the redundant process of having to enter it wherever needed. When considering that in hospital settings the number of tables can be in the hundreds or thousands, use of relational databases results in markedly increased efficiency and reduces the likelihood of data entry errors.

Linking data together is done through queries, which are the software commands that search databases for particular pieces of information. For example, one can search for the result of a patient's Pap test, for all reports associated with a particular patient's medical record number. A valuable application of queries lies in extracting data from across multiple patients' records. An example of this would be to search the past five years for all cases of breast carcinoma. For most laboratory software solutions, if new tables or entries on existing tables are added, future reports will pull data only from the date the change was implemented forward. For this reason, the initial set up of database tables is crucial and time invested in optimizing the database design is time well spent.

Spreadsheet Solutions

Basic spreadsheets are simple to use and allow users great flexibility in terms of data manipulation. Spreadsheets offer a dynamic quality to the data, as data can be charted, sorted, and organized into tables. Most laboratory software solutions accommodate the downloading of data into spreadsheets. Frequently, the cytology laboratory is dependent upon multiple software systems, necessitating the need for interfaces designed specifically to allow for communication and reporting. However, often an inexpensive spreadsheet application (e.g. Microsoft Excel) is all that is required, particularly if data can be downloaded into a common platform, like text (txt) or comma separated value (csv) files. Once downloaded, either macros or if using Excel the VLOOKUP command (a function that searches for value in the left-most column of *table_array* and returns the value in the same row based on the *index_number*) can then be used to match the added fields (columns) into individual patient records (rows) to create a desired data set (**Tables 1-3**). The process of matching data relies on the principles of a relational database, requiring some form of unique indicator for each data set being matched. Once the desired spreadsheet is complete, contingency tables which offer opportunities for further statistical analyses and graphs can be generated.

Tables 1 - 3. Example of a data set generated from disparate computer systems. Table 1 shows

Table 1. Data downloaded from computer system A

Medical Record Number	Cytology #	Patient Last Name	Patient First Name	Patient Date of Birth	Diagnosis
112978	23998	Doe 1	Jane	1/1/65	NEG
499693	3344	Doe 2	Jane	3/15/78	NEG
847347	12576	Doe 3	Jane	12/5/50	ASC
543006	38754	Doe 4	Jane	8/9/77	HSIL
985324	2556	Doe 5	Jane	2/4/49	LSIL

Table 2. Data downloaded from computer system B

Medical Record Number	Patient Last Name	Patient First Name	Patient Date of Birth	HPV Result
112978	Doe 1	Jane	1/1/65	POS
499693	Doe 2	Jane	3/15/78	NEG
847347	Doe 3	Jane	12/5/50	POS
543006	Doe 4	Jane	8/9/77	POS
985324	Doe 5	Jane	2/4/49	NEG

Table 3. Final data set

Cytology #	Patient Last Name	Patient First Name	Patient Date of Birth	Medical Record Number	Diagnosis	HPV Result
23998	Doe 1	Jane	1/1/65	112957	NEG	POS
3344	Doe 2	Jane	3/15/78	499871	NEG	NEG
12576	Doe 3	Jane	12/5/50	847365	ASC	POS
38754	Doe 4	Jane	8/9/77	543687	HSIL	POS
2556	Doe 5	Jane	2/4/49	985467	LSIL	NEG

data downloaded as .txt files from computer system A and Table 2 data downloaded from computer system B. In this example, table 1 and 2 can be matched by the medical record number, a unique identifier shared by both tables. The end result is a complete (combined) data set as shown in Table 3. After adding a column for "HPV Result" to Table 1, data can be matched using Excel's VLOOKUP function by entering the following formula into each row: =VLOOKUP (Table 1, Column 1 (Medical Record Number), Select range of Table 2 (range containing data to be matched, including Medical Record Number), 5 (column # in range that contains HPV results), false.

QC/QA Indicators

Common QC/QA indicators used in the cytology laboratory are often amenable to assessment by electronic methods. Such indicators may include, but are not limited to, test management and reporting systems, electronic data integrity, workflow, cytopreparation, screening and performance, post-analytical monitors (including continuing education and remedial training), and client satisfaction. Electronic tracking of QC/QA indicators can be done either within the LIS, by exporting data from the LIS using common spreadsheet software, or a combination of both.

Test Management and Reporting Systems

This includes several variables that should be electronically monitored as part of a QC/QA program. **Laboratory requisition completeness** can be assessed upon arrival of the specimen in the laboratory and problems documented by the accessioner. Most software solutions have fields where QA comments can be entered. Periodic reports can be run to list occurrences and identify trends with any particular physician office sending Pap tests to the laboratory. If a problem is identified across all offices, this should prompt consideration for clinician education and/or a redesign of the requisition form. **Specimen transportation timeliness** can be assessed by comparing the date of specimen procurement with the date received by the laboratory, both entered electronically into the LIS database. If the delay falls outside a predefined time range (e.g. one business day), documentation and investigation would be indicated.

Specimen rejection incidents should be documented, and quarterly reports run to monitor specimen rejection frequency by clinician office. If patterns that exceed allowable limits are discovered, documented remedial education would be appropriate. Receipt of specimens from clinics and clinician offices with **labeling errors** is unfortunately not uncommon in the cytopathology laboratory. Documentation includes contacting the clinician of note for the corrected information, as well as tracking the transportation of the specimen back to the clinician's office, if required for appropriate identification. This may include a comment within the QA field, which could be included in the final report sent to the clinician. **Lost specimens** must be aggressively investigated. Electronic monitoring for this quality indicator is best accomplished with a simple spreadsheet log, since lost specimens would not be accessioned into the LIS database. Considerations for lost specimen monitors include specimen type, clinician office, courier(s), and specimen sampling dates, amongst others.

Finally, **test reporting** quality indicators may include reporting language accuracy, typographical errors, timely retrieval of reports and slides, and appropriate storage of reports and slides. Electronic monitoring of typographical errors may be achieved, for example, by reviewing amended reports in the LIS due to typographical errors.

Electronic Data Integrity

Electronic data integrity is a quality indicator that includes common network security, and features to ensure that data is entered in a standardized format. Common network security features include password protection and electronic monitoring of access to information, including both data entry and data retrieval. Software solutions typically have the ability to record the who, what, where, and when (i.e. the person logged in, the case they are pulling up, the location of the computer from which they are accessing the network, and the date and time the access is happening) i.e. electronic audit trail. This information can be used as part of a comprehensive QC/QA program that includes monitoring to ensure that users only access information relevant to their job duties, and assigning users different privileges in the LIS (e.g. only a pathologist can sign out abnormal gynecologic diagnoses). Dictionaries can be built to determine which LIS users have privileges to specific fields. Integrity of finalized reports typically entails electronically securing finalized reports so that content cannot be changed except in the form of an addendum to an existing report or an amended report, thereby ensuring preservation of the original report.

When data is entered in a consistent language for each data field (i.e. standardized language), this data can be more efficiently retrieved and easily analyzed. For this reason, the use of standardized language is commonly employed in the cytology laboratory. Standardized data entry for diagnostic interpretations in cytology can be assisted through the use of coded comments, which ensures uniformity of the reporting language. In settings where standardized diagnostic terminology exists and is widely accepted, such as the Bethesda System for the reporting of Pap test results (Solomon et al., 2002; Herbert et al., 2007), coded comments allow for quick data entry and unambiguous results reporting to the clinician. An internationally accepted unified terminology for the reporting of Pap tests is still required (Jones, Valenstein & Steindel, 1999; Collaço, de Noronha, Pinheiro & Bleggi-Torres, 2005). In other settings, such as fine needle aspiration biopsies and non-gynecological specimens, flexibility in the use of language is often necessary, and most software solutions will permit users to manually type in their diagnoses if desired. Reports that queue off of codes provide an efficient means to extract data, enabling swift calculations of abnormal rates and breakdowns by diagnostic categories for comparison against benchmark data. This can be done for the entire laboratory, as well as for individual cytotechnologists and cytopathologists.

Mandatory entries are useful features present in many laboratory software solutions. With regard to Pap test reporting, mandatory entries may include an adequacy statement about the specimen (e.g. if there is sufficient squamous cellularity

and whether cellular evidence of transformation zone sampling is present/absent), primary diagnosis, billing codes, cytotechnologist (primary screener) name and initial diagnosis, and, if the case is sent for pathologist review, their name and final diagnosis. With such a system in place, reports cannot be issued unless all mandatory fields are completed. As mentioned earlier, many software solutions offer the flexibility of entering customized text over mandatory entries. The primary cytology diagnostic code should always remain assigned to the case, regardless of what is typed in lieu of or in addition to the primary coded remark, to ensure that future data analyses based upon retrieval by diagnostic codes are meaningful. Queries based upon the text entered (i.e. natural language search) are possible with many current laboratory information systems. However, something as simple as typographical errors may interfere with searches based on text. This can be avoided by utilizing common built-in software features such as a spell check and automated comments in the LIS.

Workflow Indicators

Timely retrieval of reports and slides in the cytology laboratory can be monitored electronically through a spreadsheet that tracks the length of time it takes to fulfill such requests. Currently, the variable most likely to affect the timely retrieval of slides is its location. When digital imagery become more widely adopted and if whole slide imaging (WSI) replaces glass slides as an archiving medium, the time limitation for retrieving slides would be on par with the retrieval of electronic reports. **Turnaround time** (i.e. the time it takes to provide the patient's caregiver with a cytology report from the time the Pap test specimen was received) provides an possible gauge of workflow management (Jones et al., 1999). As quality in reporting and diagnostic accuracy are often assumed by both clinician and patient, turnaround time unfortunately serves as the major "quality" indicator to both clinical office personnel and the public. As such, the impact of efficiently managing the laboratory to effectively reduce this time cannot be overstated. Reports can be run to calculate turnaround times, identify outliers, investigate the cause of the delay, and implement corrective actions. **Trail sheets** can be used to track locations of specimens should they be sent to different departments or locations outside the laboratory (e.g. to a reference laboratory).

Retrospective reviews may involve randomly selecting a predetermined number of cases from the previous month and checking them for timely retrieval, appropriate storage, and reporting accuracy. Errors should be documented, procedures reevaluated, and if necessary revised. In the United States, CLIA regulations mandate a retrospective review of all negative Pap tests for the last five years for which current cases are diagnosed with a high grade squamous intraepithelial lesion (HSIL) or above (i.e. cancer). Since findings with this review rarely affect current patient care (which would prompt an immediate amended report and verbal discussion with the clinician of note), the value of such a retrospective report is in education (to the cytotechnologist and cytopathologist staff) and in the assessment of past management intervention (e.g. removing telephones from the screening room or adding cytotechnologist cubicles). CLIA also requires the cytology laboratory to provide and document that alerting information (typically in the form of a medical director letter) was sent to providers in regard to all patients with a Pap test diagnosis of HSIL (or carcinoma), in which there is no record of further patient follow-up in the pathology or hospital information system. This ensures that those patients at high risk for cervical cancer get appropriate timely intervention and treatment. In order to meet this requirement, laboratory software can be designed to search for cases of HSIL (or carcinoma) during a specific time period (e.g. prior 3 or 4 months) and then identify any cytology or surgical specimen(s) that have occurred since then. Although a Pap interpretation

of HSIL is the trigger for this federal requirement in the United States, many laboratories include other "lesser" Pap interpretations as triggering events, those which also carry a significant risk of the patient harboring a high-grade precancerous cervical or vaginal lesion, or potentially invasive carcinoma. In this way, the quality monitor can be modified to meet the goals and expectations of one's local medical community (and medico-legal environment). If no such subsequent specimens can be found in the LIS database, letters can be generated that alert the appropriate clinician to this situation, and request follow-up information. These letters can be printed and mailed or electronically distributed to clinician offices.

Cytopreparation Monitors

Exfoliated cells obtained from the uterine cervix by performing a Pap test can either be smeared directly onto a slide (conventional Pap test) or submitted to the cytology laboratory in a vial containing fixative (liquid-based cytology). QC indicators related to the actual preparation of cytologic material in the laboratory may include keeping electronic records of stain quality (monitored daily), changing and filtering of equipment and stains to avoid contamination, logs for the use of automated equipment including preventive maintenance and problem logs, and daily temperature readings of pertinent equipment (e.g. refrigerators and ovens).

Screening and Performance Indicators

Quality indicators related to screening and performance are both subjective and objective in nature. An important component of any accepted QC/QA program in cytology includes provisions for the setting of individual cytotechnologists' maximum workload. This can be determined by evaluating diagnostic accuracy as it compares to productivity, and is typically described in terms of slides per hour. Federal law in the United States requires that cytotechnologists manually document the number of slides screened for each 24 hour period, and the number of hours spent screening each day. Guidelines prohibit screening more than 100 slides (conventional smears) over an eight hour period, and not more than 12.5 slides per hour. Higher per hour and per day slide counts are permissible when screening liquid-based preparations, as they possess a smaller surface area to screen and typically fewer cells than a conventional Pap smear. Slides per hour can be calculated by adding the total number of slides and dividing them by the total hours spent screening, which is determined by subtracting time spent doing non-screening activities from the hours worked. Software solutions can be used to ensure that workload limits are not exceeded. For example, once the daily workload limit has been reached for an individual cytotechnologist, the LIS will not allow them to sign out additional cases.

Common indicators of diagnostic accuracy include rescreening measures. Rescreening is mandated by CLIA in the United States, but has also been implemented as a measure of QC in screening Pap tests in other countries (Collaço, de Noronha, Pinheiro & Bleggi-Torres, 2005). This includes a 10% random rescreen of negative Pap tests and a rescreening of a specified percentage of negative cases defined as "high risk". All rescreening should be performed by a supervisory level cytotechnologist or a pathologist. Several studies have shown that a 100% rapid rescreening method is more efficient at detecting false negative results than 10% random rescreening or rescreening on the basis of clinical criteria, and is recommended as an internal QC method (Amaral et al., 2005; Manrique et al., 2006). However, this may not be practical in a large cytopathology laboratory screening many cases with limited staff. Software can be relied upon to allow the percentage of cases pulled for QC review to be adjusted, and this can be set differently for individual screeners. Situations where this may be useful would include circumstances that mandate closer inspection of

work quality, a tool for remedial training, or for new hirees whose work quality is not yet fully ascertained. QC rescreening is most useful for exposing screening errors, as opposed to diagnostic errors. Accordingly, software often has data entries that allow the degree of error to be defined (e.g. minor disagreement for the missed presence of Candida or major disagreement for a missed squamous intraepithelial lesion or SIL).

A prospective **random 10% rescreen** (re-examination prior to reporting), typically determined by laboratory software, automatically marks for QC 10% of negative cases entered by a primary screening cytotechnologist on a lab-wide basis. If the laboratory has many cytotechnologists signing out cases simultaneously, the 10% should represent a random selection that is unpredictable from the perspective of each cytotechnologist. Once selected for QC, the laboratory software should ensure that the case cannot be modified by the primary screening cytotechnologist. This case must also have a documented review by an appropriate level person defined in the person dictionary (e.g. supervisory cytotechnologist or pathologist). Reports should be generated to verify that each cytotechnologist has indeed met the minimum requirement of 10% QC rescreen of negative Pap test cases.

Cases are designated as **high risk** based upon past and/or current history of abnormal signs, symptoms and/or pathologic findings. The definition of "high risk" varies widely between laboratories, as it is subject to continual adjustment based upon the specific patient population served, evolving scientific data, development of new clinical condition states (e.g. HIV/AIDS), and the judgment of the laboratory medical director. As examples, the "high risk" patient designation is affected by such variables as length of time since past abnormal finding(s), diagnosis associated with past abnormal finding(s), and past or current clinical symptoms and finding(s). Software solutions can automatically designate cases as high risk based on database searches for particular entries within certain fields with consideration for a specific time period (e.g. "History of LSIL" in current field of "clinical history", or a previous specimen coded as abnormal in the primary diagnosis interpretation field within the past three years). Computer-assisted designation of high risk cases greatly increases the likelihood that high risk cases are correctly identified to be part of a secondary review process prior to sign out. Since cases defined as "high risk" are theoretically at higher risk for containing abnormalities, patient care is improved with the (typically small) proportion of negative cases by primary review that are found upon secondary review to contain abnormal findings.

Other indicators that can be easily measured with electronic data include time spent by staff on other activities (e.g. education). These indicators can be monitored to ensure that cytotechnologists are given opportunities to experience a broad range of activities, with the goal of increased job satisfaction and a better-rounded and educated cytology screener and diagnostician. A large part of workload assessment for cytotechnologists involves comparing diagnostic agreement between the cytotechnologist and the reviewing pathologist, for each case forwarded for pathologist review. This is most critical for the negative Pap test by cytotechnologist review. As cytotechnologists function not only as Pap test screeners, but also as Pap test diagnosticians, solely evaluating and reporting the majority of negative Pap tests and thus the overall majority of all patient Pap test results, the evaluation of their ability to accurately determine a Pap slide as negative is crucial. All Pap tests initially deemed negative for intraepithelial lesion or malignancy by cytotechnologist review which then undergo second review due to standard QC practices (10% or high risk rescreen) or pathologist review due to the presence of re-

Table 4. Pivot table comparing the diagnoses of cytotechnologists (cytotech) and pathologists for a series of Pap tests. NEG = negative, ASC = atypical squamous cells of undetermined significance, ASC-H = Atypical squamous cells cannot exclude high grade squamous intraepithelial lesion, LSIL = low grade squamous intraepithelial lesion, LGH = low grade, cannot exclude high grade squamous intraepithelial lesion, HSIL = high grade squamous intraepithelial lesion, CA = carcinoma, UNSAT = unsatisfactory.

Cytotech Diagnoses	Pathologist Diagnoses									Grand Total
	NEG	ASC	ASC-H	AGC	LSIL	LGH	HSIL	CA	UNSAT	
NEG	919	40	1	2	5	0	0	0	6	970
ASC	646	1658	27	0	65	7	1	0	2	2406
ASC-H	6	89	79	1	3	5	8	0	0	191
AGC	50	4	1	26	0	0	0	0	1	82
LSIL	5	181	8	0	698	31	3	0	0	926
LGH	1	22	13	0	65	106	21	0	0	228
HSIL	0	16	41	2	2	45	185	0	0	291
CA	0	0	0	0	0	0	0	6	0	6
UNSAT	44	0	1	0	0	0	0	0	196	241
Grand Total	1671	2110	171	31	838	194	218	6	205	5344

active changes, serve as QA data which must be aggressively analyzed. Pivot tables, created after downloading data into spreadsheets, are useful tools to cross reference diagnoses by cytotechnologists and pathologists and for analyzing diagnostic correlations and discrepancies of Pap tests (**Table 4**), or in addition non-gynecological cases. Areas of cytotechnologist over-interpretation and more importantly under-interpretation (potential false negative cases) can be easily assessed on both an individual cytotechnologist basis, or laboratory-wide. Software systems can also allow for individual cases to be easily retrieved for continuing education purposes.

Additional performance monitors that can be tracked include the rates for frequencies of diagnostic categories (e.g. atypical squamous cells of undetermined significance or ASC-US) and the **ASC-US/SIL rates**, which can be tabulated on a monthly, quarterly, and/or six month basis for each cytotechnologist and compared against the department as a whole, as well as benchmark data where available. Remedial action may be taken if an individual average exceeds a predetermined variance from the norm (e.g. two standard deviations from the laboratory average). If rates fall outside this range, this will prompt a review and appropriate continuing education of individual and/or lab performance by the medical director. With the increasing availability of Human Papilloma Virus (HPV) DNA testing of liquid-based Pap test material, the ASC-US/HPV DNA positivity rate can similarly serve as a useful quality indicator. This rate is particularly informative in regard to pathologist performance as to appropriate utilization of the ASC-US category, providing excellent and timely feedback with well-accepted target performance benchmarks. One can also note the proportion of particular diagnostic categories forwarded for pathologist review by each cytotechnologist, and with discrepancy logs observe the percentage of their negative cases signed out by the pathologist as abnormal (Cibas, Dean, Maffeo & Allred, 2001).

Specimen adequacy analysis can serve as a performance monitor both for individual cytotechnologists (particularly if they are assigned Pap tests pending review on a random basis, without clinic or clinician selection bias) and for the clinicians submitting the Pap test.

For QC purposes, cytology laboratories need to compare Pap test and cervical biopsy reports (if available), and determine the cause of any discrepancies (Joste, Crum, Cibas, 1995; Sodhani, Singh, Das & Bhambhani, 1997).

Such **cytologic-histologic correlation** should be compiled at regular (e.g. six month) intervals. This entails comparing Pap test data to database searches of subsequent surgical specimens (e.g. colposcopic biopsies or excisional cone procedures). The tissue specimen is often regarded as the "gold standard", although colposcopic examination, even with the most experienced colposcopist, has relatively limited sensitivity. Based on the previously described QC procedures focused predominantly on negative Pap test (per cytotechnologist) review, specifically 10% and high risk rescreen and cytotechnologist vs. pathologist diagnosis correlation data, coupled with Pap test vs. subsequent biopsy correlation data, potential false negative and false positive Pap tests can be identified and assessed for both individuals and the laboratory as a whole (**Table 5**). The subgroup of potential false negative cases should be examined to assess for issues of sampling (cells representative of the lesion are absent or in very low number), as well as examination of the potential false positive Pap slides for confirmation of the abnormal finding as originally diagnosed (colposcopic biopsies missed the lesion). In the latter situation, if the abnormal Pap finding is confirmed, it is imperative to reinforce this to the clinician so that further biopsy, LEEP excision, or close Pap follow-up can be scheduled. If Pap case selection by the cytotechnologist is random, as well as an equally distributed or random interaction of the cytotechnologist and pathologist pools, then the rates of false negative Pap interpretation can

Table 5. Table showing potential false negative (yellow) and potential false positive (purple) Pap tests

Pap test diagnosis	Surgical Diagnosis				
	NEG	LSIL	HSIL	CA	Grand Total
NEG	130	3	1	0	134
ASC	191	45	75	2	313
ASCH	17	2	32	1	52
AGC	5	0	2	3	10
LSIL	50	103	51	0	214
LGH	17	14	21	0	52
HSIL	17	6	77	1	101
CA	0	0	1	1	2
Total	427	183	260	8	878

be compared and contrasted between individual cytotechnologists. In large cytology laboratories interpreting thousands, if not hundreds of thousands of Pap tests, this can only be accomplished utilizing the LIS through QC/QA software tools. One common method, amongst others, used to calculate the true false negative rate (FNR) (also known as the false negative fraction or false negative proportion) is to determine the proportion of abnormal Paps that are falsely negative i.e. FNR = false negatives/ (true positives + false negatives) (Cibas, 2003).

3.3.6 Continuing Education/Remedial Training

Monitoring of **continuing education** can involve utilizing laboratory software to facilitate quick retrieval of such items as intradepartmental consultations or interesting cases and their surgical correlations. Documentation of review of cases can consist of logging the list of cases, date reviewed, and persons reviewing the cases into a spreadsheet. Similarly, weekly case review conferences, monthly teleconferences, proficiency test slide review programs, national conferences,

and so on, can all be recorded in spreadsheets for easy manipulation and generation of graphs, charts, and tables.

Remedial action, where necessary, can be assisted with laboratory software and/or spreadsheets which document errors and corrections and serve as a means to track these incidents over time. If a cytotechnologist is removed from non-essential duties in order to focus on remedial education, reviews of tutorial material relevant to the identified deficiency, including name and description of cases studied and the time spent reviewing, can be logged into a spreadsheet application. As described earlier, any workload reduction for any particular cytotechnologist can be ensured by constraining the maximum number of cases allowed to be signed out by the particular cytotechnologist, and the percentage of QC cases can be increased. If there exists a concern that a particular time period was suspected to be prone to potentially misinterpreted cases, laboratory software reports can be run to identify all negative cases signed out during that time period for all cytotechnologists or a particular cytotechnologist.

Client Satisfaction

All clinician, patient, and health service provider quality assessments, complaints and suggestions for improvement should be documented and addressed. To be both effective and efficient, the cytopathology laboratory should work closely with marketing and sales representatives. QA practices pertinent to improving client satisfaction may include assisting clinicians in patient management, such as providing statistical data tailored to suit their particular requests. Examples include percentage of abnormal cytology cases by physician or volume of unsatisfactory specimens over a specified time period. Clinicians may elect to receive monthly lists from the laboratory of all their abnormal Pap tests in order to better safeguard that appropriate follow-up is pursued by their offices.

DIGITAL IMAGING

A digital image is represented in a computer by a two-dimensional array of numbers (bitmap or raster image), each element of which represents a small square area of the picture, called a picture element (pixel). Such images can be transmitted or stored in a compressed form (reduced image size). Compression algorithms may be "lossless" (no loss of data) or "lossy" (some detail is lost). Digital images can be created by a variety of input devices, such as a digital camera. The imaging process involves capture, saving (storage), editing (if necessary), and sharing (viewing, displaying, printing). This process as it relates to applications in pathology has yet to be standardized (Yagi & Gilbertson, 2005). In the field of cytology, digital images are used for telecytology, training and education (e.g. publications, conferences, and web pages), proficiency testing, and automated screening of Pap test slides. In many developed countries, pathologists are increasingly integrating digital images into their practice of medicine (Beals, 2001; Pritt, Gibson & Cooper, 2003).

Image-enhanced reports are also a growing trend among pathology practices (Park, 2007). Therefore, LIS vendors have begun integrating digital image acquisition and storage modules into their products.

Virtual Microscopy

Virtual microscopy (VM) and whole slide imaging (WSI), the use of digital imaging to produce digital slides that simulate light microscopy, are being used for telepathology, consultation, archiving, clinical diagnosis, education, proficiency testing, and examinations (Weinstein, 2005; Steinberg & Ali, 2001). Virtual microscopy provides access to all areas of interest on a slide by using a computer or digital device, without the use of a microscope. In other words, the user can view a scanned image of the entire slide on a computer screen. Current systems are capable of complete, high speed digitization of slides at multiple magnifications (Rojo, Garcia & Mateos, 2006). Selected scanning systems can even digitize multiple focal planes (x, y and z axes), to create a virtual slide with the ability to "focus" at different magnifications. Current automated high-speed WSI systems are sufficient for diagnostic purposes and potentially represent a "disruptive technology" in the traditional practice of pathology. Liquid-based Pap tests have smaller areas to scan, and thus are better suited for virtual microscopy compared to conventional Pap test slides with cells smeared over an entire slide. Shortcomings that still need to be overcome include expensive initial setup, inability to maintain an adequate focus in a thick smear with multiple levels, large storage size of the VM slide, and the relatively long time needed to scan a slide (Steinberg & Ali, 2001).

Telecytology

Telepathology, which includes telecytology, is the practice of pathology at a distance by using telecommunication to transmit images, often when the cytologist and slide (containing the patient's cytologic material) are separated by distance. The emergence of technology that supports digital imaging along with greater image quality, and higher processing capacity of computers, has promoted the use of telepathology (Rojo, Garcia & Mateos, 2006). Telepathology can be used for diagnosis, consultation or education (Allen et al., 2001; Mulford, 2006). Earlier studies found the accuracy of telecytology to be less than that of light microscopy (Raab et al., 2005). However, with technological advances more recent stud-

ies have demonstrated improved accuracy and reproducibility of telepathology (Lee, Kim & Choi, 2003; Alli et al., 2001), even despite image compression (Marcelo, Fontelo, Farolan & Cualing, 2000). There are three types of telecytology systems: static, real-time (dynamic), and virtual (whole) slide imaging systems (**Figure 2**). Static image systems are cheaper, but can only capture a selected subset of microscopic fields. The latter two systems permit evaluation of the entire slide, but are more costly, and may be hampered by high network traffic. With certain real-time telepathology systems, the consultant can actively operate a remote microscope with a robotic stage. Around the world, validation (of both system and user), reimbursement, and medicolegal issues surrounding telepathology still need to be re-

Figure 2. Screen capture image of a telecytology system software interface illustrating the ability to remotely annotate or "dot" a cell on interest on a digitized Pap test slide

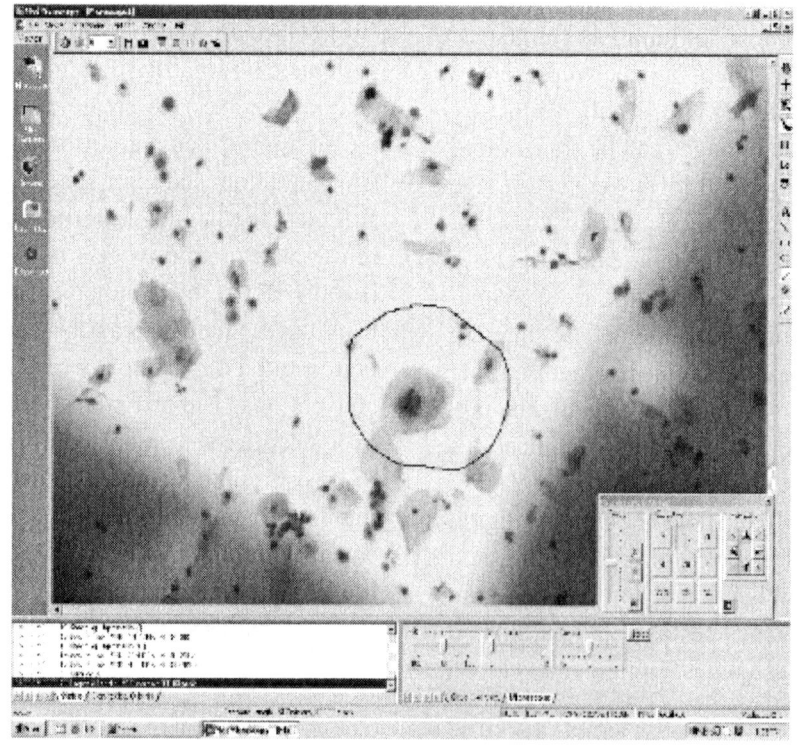

fined (Pantanowitz, Henricks & Beckwith, 2007; O'Brien, Takahashi & Brugal, 1998; Tsuchihashi, Okada & Ogushi, 2000).

Proficiency Testing

Manual screening/review of gynecologic cytology preparations is the current "gold standard" for both training and assessment of proficiency. In certain countries such as the United States of America, the federal government has mandated a national proficiency testing program for gynecologic cytology. This demands that pathologists and cytotechnologists practicing in the USA undertake periodic tests using well-standardized glass slides. To date, the use of virtual microscopy for such proficiency testing has been explored by only a few investigators (Marchevsky et al., 2003; Marchevsky et al., 2006; Gagnon et al., 2004; Stewart et al., 2007). The use of digital images and computer-based methods has been proposed to be more cost effective than glass slides for proficiency testing (Vooijs et al., 1998). This is not surprising, as virtual microscopy allows participants to view digital images representing an entire cytologic glass slide at the same feature resolution currently available with light microscopy. The digital images are able to be stacked along a 3-dimensional z plane, allowing test participants to change focal planes. This is a key feature for the evaluation of cytologic material. However, technical advances are still required, such as improving the time required to examine digitized images. In one study, the individual performance based on glass slides was better than the computer-based test, particularly if individuals did not receive prior training (Gagnon et al., 2004).

Image Cytometry

Cytometry is the measurement of cell properties. As the name implies, image cytometry is an image-based study or measurement of cells.

Such a study usually allows very large populations of cells to be imaged and thereby analyzed. At present, the application of image cytometry to cervical cytology is largely investigational. The most common current applications are for DNA analysis and the evaluation of immunohistochemical staining (Rocher, Gonzalez, Palaoro & Blanco, 2006).

In digital image cytometry, once an image is acquired and objects of interest in the image have been selected (image segmentation), measurements can be made on them. This step, called feature extraction, leads to numerical data that can then be analyzed.

Interpretation of cells in a Pap test based upon defined morphologic criteria is often subjective. Morphological assessment of these cells by digital image analysis is believed to be objective and thus highly reproducible (Watanabe et al., 2004). Static image analysis of the nuclear DNA content (as an indication of aneuploidy) in cytological smears of the uterine cervix has been shown to help distinguish low-grade from high-grade dysplastic lesions (Shirata, Gomes, Garcia & Longatto, 2001; Shirata et al., 2003). In an attempt to improve the positive predictive value for high-risk Human Papilloma Virus (HR-HPV) in primary screening, DNA ploidy was measured by some researchers on the same liquid-based sample by image cytometry in cases showing discrepancies between cytology and HR-HPV testing (Lorenzato et al., 2002).

COMPUTER SCREENING SYSTEMS

As previously noted, the Pap test has been remarkably successful during the past half-century as a cancer screening tool, representing the most cost effective cancer reduction program in history and one of the most significant advances in women's health to date. It is widely accepted and utilized, and is available to hundreds of millions of women worldwide. It is however, as with every other medical technique or device, not perfect. The foundations of its design, a glass slide of smeared and stained cervical-vaginal cellular material to be reviewed by a trained human observer under light microscopy, with strengths in relative simplicity and low technical demands, have also proven to be at the root if its limitations. These limitations were recognized even when initial efforts to automate Pap screening begun shortly after its widespread adoption in the 1950's. However, only as a result of significant technical and computer advances made in the past 10 to 15 years have computer screening systems been routinely utilized.

The task of daily screening cervical cytology (Pap smears/tests) is difficult and repetitive. Screening by a cytotechnologist requires significant training and experience. Moreover, it is labor intensive, requiring up to 5 minutes per slide, with the vast majority of visual fields and cues representing benign or normal findings. Dysplastic squamous and glandular cells are often rare events, admixed with thousands of benign cells. Quite literally, it is the medical counterpart to searching for the needle in the haystack. False negative cases will never reach zero level with unattainable public expectations of perfection, adding to the stress and demands of the profession. It is for these reasons that the field of cytotechnology developed, as an aid and adjunct to the pathologist in the screening and diagnosis of cytologic preparations. However, the growing shortage of skilled cytotechnologists to screen and diagnose Pap slides has become an ever-increasing concern in the field. Automated laboratory instruments and screening systems have developed under two major system designs; (i) those that perform primary screening without cytotechnologist interaction, and (ii) an interactive design that serves as the "cytotechnologist's cytotechnologist", in which both the cytotechnologist and computer depend upon each other for Pap test interpretation.

The Need for a Better "Smear"

In order to have accurate and efficient computer-assisted screening, the cellular material on the slide (the image data) must be prepared in a standardized manner conducive to rapid acquisition and computer processing. The cellular material for Pap smears (or tests) can be obtained from the endocervix, ectocervix and vagina by a number of spatula, brush and broom devices. In the past (and still in many developing countries today), exfoliated cells were physically smeared by the physician or other health care provider onto either one or two glass slides, followed by immediate fixation. Fixation was typically via spray fixative or immersion of the slide directly into liquid fixative. Each of these techniques potentially limits the visual inspection of cells, the goal of the study. Smeared cells were often too thick, with irregular and alternating areas of varied cell dispersion leading to cell clumping. The fixation step, which must be immediate in order to prevent air-drying artifact of the cells, was often only partially successful. By limiting the microscopic evaluation, many Pap smears were unsatisfactory (or non-interpretable). These problems also plagued the development of many early versions of automated screening devices during the 1950 to 1990 period. The solution, and indeed the technique which has at its core allowed the development of computer screening systems, is liquid-based cytology (LBC).

LBC for Pap tests came to fruition in the United States in 1996, when the Food and Drug Administration (FDA) approved the ThinPrep[R](Cytyc Corporation, Boxborough, MA, USA) as an alternative to the conventional Pap smear. This was soon followed by the similar approval of the AutoCyte Prep[R], now BD SurePath[R] (BD Diagnostics - TriPath, Burlington, NC, USA) in 1999, and most recently MonoPrep[R] (MonoGen, Inc., Chicago, Il, USA) in 2006. Although each product is technically different in its approach, the final standardized result for each is a glass Pap slide with its cellular component distributed in a relative monolayer, present over a reduced surface area, largely non-obscured by blood and inflammatory cells. Batch processors with walk-away capability are available for each slide preparation. Although LBC was designed with a major (if not primary) intent of enabling computer screening devices, each preparation has been shown to improve and standardize overall specimen quality, reduce unsatisfactory Pap test rates, and improve the rates of detection of significant and potentially significant cervical-vaginal lesions (Bishop et al., 1998; Hutchinson et al., 1999; Lee et al., 1997; Linder & Zahniser, 1997; Papillo & Zarka, 1998; Wilbur et al., 1994; MonoPrep™, 2007). In addition, the residual liquid vial sample has seemingly endless potential for use in ancillary molecular studies, above and beyond the morphologic Pap test, such as HPV DNA testing (Stevens et al., 2007), with semi-automated computer-assisted HPV testing platforms currently available or in the process of clinical evaluation.

Primary Screening Systems

One of the major screening systems available today is an automated primary slide screener and archiver. The BD FocalPoint[R] Slide Profiler, BD Diagnostics - TriPath (formerly AutoPap[R] System, formerly AutoPap[R] 300 QC System, NeoPath, Redmond, WA) is FDA-approved for both conventional and BD SurePath[R] Pap tests. In the 1990's, the PAPNET[R] system (Neuromedical Systems Inc., Suffern, NY) and the AutoPap 300 QC System were at the forefront of technologic advances in the cervical cytology imaging race, each gaining FDA-approval in the USA for the rescreening of previously manually screened conventional smears. These systems had the potential to greatly improve the yield of detecting false negative cases (Colgan, Patten & Lee, 1995; Mango & Valente, 1998). The AutoPap system subsequently altered its screening algorithm in the mid to late

90's (Patten, Lee & Nelson, 1996; Wilbur, Prey, Miller, Pawlick & Colgan, 1998), gaining FDA-approval as a primary screening device in 1998 (with conventional smears) and in 2001 (with BD SurePath[R] slides), and is currently known as the BD FocalPoint[R] Slide Profiler. PAPNET, a QC system requiring screened glass slides to be sent to central review sites with scanning stations using adaptive computer processing (neural networks), produced images of pertinent cellular fields, which were then transferred to tape cassettes or CD-ROM to be returned to the cytology laboratory for review on high-resolution monitors (Denaro, Herriman Shapira, 1997). It has since ceased to be marketed in the USA, largely due to the associated high costs per additional abnormal case detected and overall logistical issues (Hutchinson, 1996; O'Leary et al., 1998).

Today, the BD FocalPoint[R] Slide Profiler is a self-contained unit, residing entirely on-site within the cytopathology laboratory. Slides are scanned at varying objective levels, including high-resolution field of view (FOV) scans of selected images, with computer processors assigning scores for each FOV based upon single cell, cell group and thick cell group characteristics. These scores are integrated into a final slide score, with the slide ranked (from 0 to 1.0) as to the clinically validated likelihood that it may potentially contain a significant epithelial abnormality (Bibbo, Hawthorne & Zimmerman, 1999), with the slides then sorted into 3 major groups. Up to 25% of successfully processed slides determined to have the lowest probability of containing abnormal cells (below the primary threshold) require no further review and can be directly reported as negative and archived (without human eyes examining the slide). The other 75% of slides designated as requiring human review by the cytotechnologist and/or pathologist, are further ranked in order of potential abnormality. The slide profiler also contains QC measures and checks, meeting CLIA requirements of a 10% random negative case rescreening by selecting 15% of qualified negative cases for an enriched QC population for directed rescreen. It has the ability to automatically generate customizable worklists, slide sorting instructions, result summaries, while alerting one to inadequate Pap test samples.

Interactive Screening Systems

The second major screening design model relies on a close interaction between the computerized primary screener and the cytotechnologist (at a review microscope/station) in the screening interpretation of each Pap test. The major systems (**Figure 3**) today are the ThinPrep Imaging System[R] (Cytyc Corporation), FDA-approved for ThinPrep slides in 2003, and the BD FocalPoint[R] GS (Guided Screening in concert with FocalPoint slide profiler) Imaging System (BD Diagnostics - TriPath). The BD FocalPoint[R] GS Imaging System is currently under FDA review, and not available for sale in the USA. Each incorporates a slide screening system to scan slides, processes the cellular data using a host of predetermined (trained) cues in imaging algorithms, and drives cytotechnologist attention using automated X-Y axis relocation to cellular fields deemed significant with the aid of an automated microscope, or review scope. The scanners and microscopes utilize slide barcodes, with engineered hardware devices incorporated into the microscopes that include: foot switch, mouse, automated stage, and key pad, enabling the cytotechnologist to readily maneuver through the initial review of the fields of interest, with electronic marking capability, and if necessary, the full standard review of the slide.

With such interactive screening systems, the cytotechnologist benefits from improved overall job satisfaction (Miller, Nagel & Kenny-Moynihan, 2007), decreased fatigue, and increased throughput (approximately 70% reduction in cellular dot surface are reviewed per slide). This leads to overall increased laboratory productivity, focused time spent on challenging cases, and focused attention to relevant fields of potential abnormality. The critical importance of human interpretation remains, however, as FOVs directed by the scanner rely on the interpretive skills and diagnostic acumen of the reviewer (cytotechnologist or pathologist) (Schledermann, Hyldebrandt, Ejersbo & Hoelund, 2007). As shown in most studies of these Pap test systems, women's gynecologic health benefits from increased sensitivity, reduction in false negative cases, and/or increased productivity (Miller, Nagel & Kenny-Moynihan, 2007; Lee, Kuan, Oh, Patten & Wilbur, 1998; Biscotti et al., 2005; Dziura, Quinn & Richard, 2006; Chivukula et al., 2007; Lozano, 2007). The increased throughput is of great benefit in

Figure 3. An example of an interactive computer-aided Pap Test screening system: The ThinPrep Imaging System (courtesy of Cytyc Corporation and affiliates).

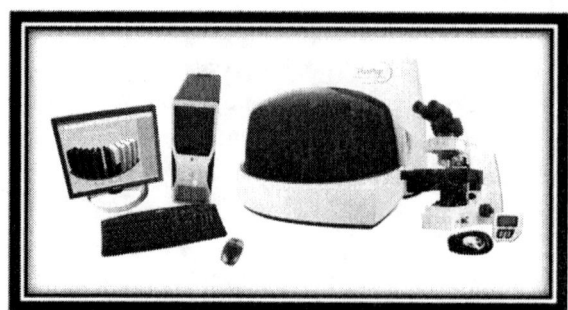

countries where cytotechnologists are not readily available, and cost effectiveness is obtained through a decreased number of inadequate Pap tests and the increase in sensitivity.

ONLINE CYTOLOGY

The Internet is a global network of computer networks that includes international telecommunications infrastructure. Internet functions include e-mail, the World Wide Web (web or www), and file transfer. Information on the web has become increasingly useful to pathologists (DiGiorgio, Richert, Klatt & Becich, 1994; Cowper, 2000; Talmon Abrahams, 2005; Wheeler, 2006), and has provided new opportunity for training and education (Schenck, 2007; Sherman, Dasgupta, Schiffman, Nayar & Solomon, 2007). The Internet is an excellent source of continuing medical education, particularly useful to those individuals that cannot travel. Web-based technology has offered physicians, and even patients, rapid access to laboratory test results. Moreover, the Internet has also provided a mechanism for rural and underserved areas to gain access to healthcare, including cytology. Many cytology society websites are a good resource, as they contain educational content, online publications, newsletters, directories, guidelines, media briefings, facilitate networking with their online community, post job opportunities, certification information, and provide information about meetings and programs. Some society websites are also available as a public (patient) resource. Similarly, vendor supported websites permit laboratories to browse product catalogs, order online, obtain additional information (service, technical, and/or clinical), gain access to question and answer forums, as well as review customer bulletins, press releases, and event information. Most cytology journals now have some online presence, although often full text in HTML or PDF format is restricted to subscribers. BioMed Central, an open access

publisher with around 120 free cyber journals that aims to disseminate new research quickly, does provide free access to the peer reviewed Cytojournal (http://www.cytojournal.com). Several websites are available as resources to aid in the practice of cytology. These include:

- **Medline**, a major medical literature database, searchable via PubMed (http://www.ncbi.nlm.nih.gov/sites/entrez?db=pubmed), which offers access to >15 million citations in several different languages.
- **NCI Bethesda System Atlas** (http://www.cytopathology.org/NIH/), freely available online, consists of around 350 helpful cytology images representing a range of morphologic findings seen on both conventional smears and liquid based preparations.
- **Cytologystuff** (http://cytologystuff.com) is an educational forum that includes several cytology atlases, galleries, and case presentations.
- **Cytopathnet** (http://cytopathnet.org/tiki-read_article.php?articleId=48) is an electronic information center with online forums, news articles, newsletters, and image galleries that provide practical, streamlined access to information on the Internet about the field of cytopathology.

FUTURE TRENDS

Laboratory informatics is critical to meet current and future challenges. These include growing workloads, the shortage of laboratory technologists, patient safety, cost containment, subspecialty centralization, increased demand for molecular testing, and personalized medicine. Many of these challenges can be met by leveraging existing and advancing technologies, such as improving the integration of disparate information systems, specimen tracking, electronic document management systems, telepathology and virtual pathology. Virtual pathology is the practice of diagnostic pathology whereby the technical performance of an analytical technique is performed at one location and the necessary elements are transmitted in electronic form to another site for diagnostic interpretation. The development of better pathology information systems that facilitate data integration and decision support are essential to support laboratories in the future.

The increased use of liquid-based methods for gynecologic cytopathology has provided the platform for several new advances. Laboratory instruments that concentrate liquid-based cells onto slides facilitate automation in the cytology laboratory. These instruments require bidirectional interfaces with laboratory information systems. Screening and digitization is simplified with liquid-based specimens, because the area to work with is considerably smaller than that of a conventional Pap test and the cells are visualized in a largely non-obscured monolayer. There are currently hundreds of computer-assisted Pap screening systems in place in the United States, with the same trend beginning in cytopathology laboratories in Europe and throughout the world. Computer networking will likely develop with the potential of having multiple laboratories, potentially over great distances, interconnected to a remote processing and imaging site. Electronic data could then be downloaded to laboratory-based automated microscopes, for case review and sign-out. As automated interactive computer screening continues to improve Pap test sensitivity, the evolving role of the Pap test warrants re-examination, in particular with further comparison to its potential replacements (e.g. HPV DNA testing) as the primary cervical screening device. In the near future this additional molecular information will need to be generated, integrated, interpreted and coherently reported. Finally, training programs for cytotechnologists and cytopathologists will need to provide formal informatics training and instruction with regard to these new technologies.

REFERENCES

Allen, E., Ollayos, C., Tellado, M., Butler, D., Buckner, S., Williams, B., et al. (2001). Characteristics of a telecytology consultation service. *Hum Pathol, 32*, 1323-1326.

Alli, P., Ollayos, C., Thompson, L., Kapadia, I., Butler, D., Williams, B., et al. (2001). Telecytology: Intraobserver and interobserver reproducibility in the diagnosis of cervical-vaginal smears. *Hum Pathol, 32*, 1318-1322.

Amaral, R., Zeferino, L., Hardy, E., Westin, M., Martinez, E., & Montemor, E. (2005). Quality assurance in cervical smears: 100% rapid rescreening vs 10% random rescreening. *Acta Cytol, 49*, 244-248.

Beals, T. (2001). Digital imaging in Anatomic Pathology. *Lab Med, 32*, 327-330.

Becich, M., Gilbertson, J., Gupta, D., & et al. (2004). Pathology and patient safety: The critical role of pathology informatics in error reduction and quality initiatives. *Clin Lab Med, 24*, 913-943.

Bibbo, M., Hawthorne, C., & Zimmerman, B. (1999). Does use of the AutoPap Assisted Primary Screener improve cytologic diagnosis? *Acta Cytol, 43*, 39622.

Biscotti, C., Dawson, A., Dziura, B., Galup, L., Darragh, T., Rahemtulla, A., et al. (2005). Assisted primary screening using the automated ThinPrep Imaging System. *Am J Clin Pathol, 123*, 281-287.

Bishop, J., Bigner, S., Colgan, T., Husain, M., Howell, L., McIntosh, K., et al. (1998). Multicenter masked evaluation of Autocyte PREP thinlayers with matched conventional smears: including initial biopsy results. *Acta Cytol, 42*, 189-197.

Bonfiglio, T. (1989). Quality assurance in cytopathology. Recommendations and ongoing quality assurance activities of the American Society of Clinical Pathologists. *Acta Cytol, 33*, 431-433.

Chivukula, M., Saad, R., Elishaev, E., White, S., Mauser, N., & Dabbs, D. (2007). Introduction of the ThinPrep Imaging System™ (TIS): Experience in a high volume academic practice. *CytoJournal, 4*, 6.

Cibas, E., Dean, B., Maffeo, N., & Allred, E. (2001). Quality assurance in gynecologic cytology. The value of cytotechnologist-cytopathologist discrepancy logs. *Am J Clin Pathol, 115*, 512-516.

Cocchi, V., Sintoni, C., Carretti, D., Sama, D., Chiari, U., Segala, V., et al. (1996). External quality assurance in cervical/vaginal cytology: Interlaboratory agreement in the Emilia-Romagna region of Italy. *Acta Cytol, 40*, 480-488.

Colgan, T., Patten, S., & Lee, J. (1995). A clinical trial of the AutoPap 300 QC System for quality control of cervicovaginal cytology in the clinical laboratory. *Acta Cytol, 39*, 1191-1198.

Collaço, L., de Noronha, L., Pinheiro, D., & Bleggi-Torres, L. (2005). Quality assurance in cervical screening of a high risk population: A study of 65,753 reviewed cases in Parana Screening Program, Brazil. *Diagn Cytopathol, 33*, 441-448.

Cowper, S. (2000). PathMax: A friendly guide to web pathology (abstract). *Arch Pathol Lab Med, 124*, 822.

Denaro, T., Herriman, J., & Shapira, O. (1997). PAPNET Testing System: Technical update. *Acta Cytol, 41*, 65-73.

DiGiorgio, C., Richert, C., Klatt, E., & Becich, M. (1994). E-mail, the Internet, and information access technology in pathology. *Semin Diagn Pathol, 11*, 294-304.

Dziura, B., Quinn, S., & Richard, K. (2006). Performance of an imaging system vs. manual screening in the detection of squamous intraepithelial lesions of the uterine cervix. *Acta Cytol, 50*, 309-311.

Food and Drug Administration. (2007). *MonoPrepTM. Summary of safety and effectiveness data.* Retrieved Sept 14th, 2007, from http://www.fda.gov/cdrh/pdf4/p040052b.pdf.

Frable, W. (2007). Error reduction and risk management in cytopathology. *Semin Diagn Pathol, 24*, 77-88.

Gagnon, M., Inhorn, S., Hancock, J., Keller, B., Carpenter, D., Merlin, T., et al. (2004). Comparison of cytology proficiency testing: glass slides vs virtual slides. *Acta Cytol, 48*, 788-794.

Herbert, A., Bergeron, C., Wiener, H., Schenck, U., Klinkhamer, P., Bulten, J., et al. (2007). European guidelines for quality assurance in cervical cancer screening: Recommendations for cervical cytology terminology. *Cytopathology, 18*, 213-219.

Hutchinson, M. (1996). Assessing the costs and benefits of alternative rescreening strategies. *Acta Cytol, 40*, 39664.

Hutchinson, M., Zahniser, D., Sherman, M., Herrero, R., Alfaro, M., Bratti, M., et al. (1999). Utility of liquid-based cytology for cervical carcinoma screening. *Cancer, 87*, 48-55.

Jones, B., Valenstein, P., & Steindel, S. (1999). Gynecologic cytology turnaround time. A College of American Pathologists Q-Probes Study of 371 laboratories. *Arch Pathol Lab Med, 123*, 682-686.

Joste, N., Crum, C., & Cibas, E. (1995). Cytologic/histologic correlation for quality control in cervicovaginal cytology. Experience with 1,582 paired cases. *Am J Clin Pathol, 103*, 32-34.

Kline, T. (1997). The challenge of quality improvement with the Papanicolaou smear. *Arch Pathol Lab Med, 121*, 253-255.

Kumar, N., & Jain, S. (2004). Quality control and automation in cervical cytology. *J Indian Med Assoc, 102*, 372, 374.

Lee, E., Kim, I., Choi, J., & et al. (2003). Accuracy and reproducibility of telecytology diagnosis of cervical smears. A tool for quality assurance programs. *Am J Clin Pathol, 119*, 356-360.

Lee, J., Kuan, L., Oh, S., Patten, F., & Wilbur, D. (1998). A feasibility study of the AutoPap System Location-Guided Screening. *Acta Cytol, 421*, 221-226.

Lee, K., Ashfaq, R., Birdsong, G., Corkill, M., McIntosh, K., & Inhorn, S. (1997). Comparison of conventional Papanicolaou smears and a fluid-based, thin-layer system for cervical cancer screening. *Obstet Gynecol, 90*, 278-287.

Linder, J., & Zahniser, D. (1997). The ThinPrep test: A review of clinical studies. *Acta Cytol, 41*, 30-38.

Lorenzato, M., Bory, J., Cucherousset, J., Nou, J., Bouttens, D., Thil, C., et al. (2002). Usefulness of DNA ploidy measurement on liquid-based smears showing conflicting results between cytology and high-risk human papillomavirus typing. *Am J Clin Pathol, 118*, 708-713.

Lozano, R. (2007). Comparison of computer-assisted and manual screening of cervical cytology. *Gynecol Oncol, 104*, 134-138.

Mango, L., & Valente, P. (1998). Neural-network-assisted analysis and microscopic rescreening in presumed negative cervical cytologic smears A comparison. *Acta Cytol, 42*, 227-232.

Manrique, E., Amaral, R., Souza, N., Tavares, S., Albuquerque, Z., & Zeferino, L. (2006). Evaluation of 100% rapid rescreening of negative cervical smears as a quality assurance measure. *Cytopathology, 17*, 116-120.

Marcelo, A., Fontelo, P., Farolan, M., & Cualing, H. (2000). Effect of image compression on telepathology. A randomized clinical trial. *Arch Pathol Lab Med, 124*(11), 1653-1656.

Marchevsky, A., Khurana, R., Thomas, P., Scharre, K., Farias, P., & Bose, S. (2006). The use of virtual microscopy for proficiency testing in gynecologic cytopathology: A feasibility study using ScanScope. *Arch Pathol Lab Med, 130*, 349-355.

Marchevsky, A., Wan, Y., Thomas, P., Krishnan, L., Evans-Simon, H., & Haber, H. (2003). Virtual microscopy as a tool for proficiency testing in cytopathology: A model using multiple digital images of Papanicolaou tests. *Arch Pathol Lab Med, 127*, 1320-1324.

Marsan, C. (1995). Quality control in cytopathology applied to screening for cervical carcinoma. *Pol J Pathol, 46*, 245-248.

Masood, S., Cajulis, R., Cibas, E., Wilbur, D., & Bedrossian, C. (1998). Automation in cytology: a survey conducted by the New Technology Task Force, Papanicolaou Society of Cytopathology. *Diagn Cytopathol, 18*, 47-55.

Miller, F., Nagel, L., & Kenny-Moynihan, M. (2007). Implementation of the ThinPrep imaging system in a high-volume metropolitan laboratory. *Diagn Cytopathol, 35*, 213-217.

Mulford, D. (2006). Telepathology education: reaching out to cytopathology progrmas throughout the country. *ASC Bulletin, 43*, 25-30.

O'Leary, T., Tellado, M., Buckner, S., Ali, I., Stevens, A., & Ollayos, C. (1998). PAPNET-assisted rescreening of cervical smears: cost and accuracy compared with a 100% manual rescreening strategy. *JAMA, 279*, 235-279.

Palcic, B., Sun, X., & Wang, J. (2007). Automated screening for cervical cancer in developing countries (abstract). *Acta Cytologica, 51*(suppl 2), 265.

Pantanowitz, L., Henricks, W., & Beckwith, B. (2007). Medical laboratory informatics. *Clinics in Laboratory Medicine, 27*, 823-843.

Papillo, J., Zarka, M., & St., J., TL. (1998). Evaluation of the ThinPrep Pap test in clinical practice. *Acta Cytol, 42,* 203-208.

Park, R. (2007). Picturing change – enhancing every pathology report with images. *ASC Bulletin, 44,* Sep-22.

Patten Jr., S., Lee, J., & Nelson, A. (1996). NeoPath AutoPap 300 Automatic Screener System. *Acta Cytol, 40,* 45-52.

Pritt, B., Gibson, P., & Cooper, K. (2003). Digital imaging guidelines for pathology: a proposal for general and academic use. *Adv Anat Pathol, 10,* 96-100.

Raab, S., , Z., MS., , T., PA., , N., TH., , I., C., & , J., CS. (1996). Telecytology: diagnostic accuracy in cervical-vaginal smears. *Am J Clin Pathol, 105,* 599-603.

Raab, S., Grzybicki, D., Zarbo, R., Meier, F., Geyer, S., & Jensen, C. (2005). Anatomic pathology databases and patient safety. *Arch Pathol Lab Med, 129,* 1246-1251.

Richards, A., Farnsworth, A., Davey, E., Irwig, L., Macaskill, P., & Chan, S. (2007). The impact of automation on a large Australian cytology laboratory (abstract). *Acta Cytologica, 51*(suppl 2), 264-265.

Rocher, A., Gonzalez, A., Palaoro, L., & Blanco, A. (2006). Usefulness of AgNOR technique and CEA expression in atypical metaplastic cells from cervical smears. *Anal Quant Cytol Histol, 28,* 130-136.

Rohr, L. (1990). Quality assurance in gynecologic cytology What is practical? *Am J Clin Pathol, 94,* 754-758.

Rojo, M., Garcia, G., Mateos, C., & et al. (2006). Critical comparison of 31 commercially available digital slide systems in pathology. *Int J Surg Pathol, 14,* 285-230.

Salvetto, M., & Sandiford, P. (2004). External quality assurance for cervical cytology in developing countries.Experience in Peru and Nicaragua. *Acta Cytol, 48,* 23-31.

Schenck, U. (2007). Web-based training in cytology (abstract). *Acta Cytologica, 51*(suppl 2), 260-261.

Schledermann, D., Hyldebrandt, T., Ejersbo, D., & Hoelund, B. (2007). Automated screening versus manual screening: A comparison of the ThinPrep imaging system and manual screening in a time study. *Diagn Cytopathol, 35,* 348-352.

Sherman, M., Dasgupta, A., Schiffman, M., Nayar, R., & Solomon, D. (2007). The Bethesda Interobserver Reproducibility Study (BIRST): A Web-based assessment of the Bethesda 2001 System for classifying cervical cytology. *Cancer, 111,* 15-25.

Shirata, N., Gomes, N., Garcia, E., & Longatto, F., A. (2001). Nuclear DNA content analysis by static cytometry in cervical intraepithelial lesions using retrospective series of previously stained PAP smears. *Adv Clin Path, 5,* 87-91.

Shirata, N., Longatto, F., A., Roteli-Martins, C., Espoladore, L., Pittoli, J., & Syrjänen, K. (2003). Applicability of liquid-based cytology to the assessment of DNA content in cervical lesions using static cytometry. *Anal Quant Cytol Histol, 25,* 210-214.

Sodhani, P., Singh, V., Das, D., & Bhambhani, S. (1997). Cytohistological correlation as a measure of quality assurance of a cytology laboratory. *Cytopathology, 8,* 103-107.

Solomon, D., Davey, D., Kurman, R., Moriarty, A., O'Connor, D., Prey, M., et al. (2002). The 2001 Bethesda System: Terminology for reporting results of cervical cytology. *JAMA, 287,* 2114-2119.

Steinberg, D., & Ali, S. (2001). Application of virtual microscopy in clinical cytopathology. *Diagn Cytopathol, 25*, 389-396.

Stevens, M., Garland, S., Rudland, E., Tan, J., Quinn, M., & Tabrizi, S. (2007). Comparison of the Digene Hybrid Capture 2 assay and Roche AMPLICOR and LINEAR ARRAY human papillomavirus (HPV) tests in detecting high-risk HPV genotypes in specimens from women with previous abnormal Pap smear results. *J Clin Microbiol, 45*, 2130-2137.

Stewart, J., 3rd., Miyazaki, K., Bevans-Wilkins, K., Ye, C., Kurtycz, D., & Selvaggi, S. (2007). Virtual microscopy for cytology proficiency testing: are we there yet? *Cancer, 111*, 203-209.

Talmon, G., & Abrahams, N. (2005). The Internet for pathologists: A simple schema for evaluating pathology-related Web sites and a catalog of sites useful for practicing pathologists. *Arch Pathol Lab Med, 129*, 742-746.

Tsuchihashi, Y., Okada, Y., Ogushi, Y., & et al. (2000). The current status of medicolegal issues surrounding telepathology and telecytology in Japan. *J Telemed Telecare, 6*(Suppl 1), S143-145.

Watanabe, S., Iwasaka, T., Yokoyama, M., Uchiyama, M., Kaku, T., & Matsuyama, T. (2004). Analysis of nuclear chromatin distribution in cervical glandular abnormalities. *Acta Cytol, 48*, 505-513.

Weinstein, R. (2005). Innovations in medical imaging and virtual microscopy. *Hum Pathol, 36*, 317-319.

Wheeler, D. (2006). Google as a pathology portal. *Adv Anat Pathol, 13*, 275-276.

Wilbur, D., Cibas, E., Merritt, S., James, J., Berger, G., & Bonfiglio, T. (1994). ThinPrep processor clinical trials demonstrate an increased detection rate of abnormal cervical cytology specimens. *Am J Clin Pathol, 101*, 209-214.

Wilbur, D., Prey, M., Miller, W., Pawlick, G., & Colgan, T. (1998). The AutoPap System for primary screening in cervical cytology: comparing the results or a prospective, intended-use study with routine manual practice. *Acta Cytol, 42*, 214-220.

Yagi, Y., & Gilbertson, J. (2005). Digital imaging in pathology: The case for standardization. *J Telemed Telecare, 11*, 109-116.

Chapter XII
Informatics and Ovarian Cancer Care

Laurie Elit
McMaster University, Canada

Susan Bondy
University of Toronto, Canada

Michael Fung-Kee-Fung
University of Ottawa, Canada

Prafull Ghatage
University of Calgary, Canada

Tien Le
University of Ottawa, Canada

Barry Rosen
University of Toronto, Canada

Bohdan Sadovy
Princess Margaret Hospital, Canada

ABSTRACT

Ovarian cancer affects 2,400 women annually in Canada with a case fatality ratio of 0.70. There are several practice guidelines that indicate women with early stage ovarian cancer should be appropriately staged including removal of the gynecologic organs, multiple peritoneal biopsies, and pelvic and para-aortic lymphadenectomy. In advanced disease, removing as much disease as possible and leaving less than a centimeter of residual disease in any one area improves overall duration of survival in cohort studies. Single institution studies and now work using administrative datasets in many high resource countries, show that women are not receiving adequate surgical staging or debulking. Cancer Care Ontario has used the RAND approach for defining quality indicators as a step for evaluating quality of care for several cancers including the management of women with ovarian cancer. The difficulty with current administrative datasets in the province is the lack of specific information such as stage, grade, histology, and size of residual disease. In this chapter, we will elaborate on the research that has brought ovarian cancer care to this juncture. We will highlight the importance of gathering information at the point of procedures and specifically in ovarian cancer at the point of the operation. Problems with the operative note and mechanisms to overcome these using templates, checklists, and synoptic notes will be reviewed. We will provide examples of pilot studies in Canada using synoptic operative notes in Cancer Care Alberta and Princess Margaret Hospital. We will also provide examples of computerized data entry across the spectrum of care from three projects in Ontario, Canada. Issues in building a disease site-specific electronic medical record will be discussed. The problems experienced in attempting to generalize such a system provincially will be addressed. We will elaborate on the potential benefits to the individual patient, the hospital and the province from such information system.

INTRODUCTION

Ovarian cancer (OC) is the fifth leading cause of cancer death in women and the leading cause of gynecologic cancer mortality. In 2007, there were estimated to be 2400 new cases diagnosed in Canada (Marrett, L., Dryer, D., Logan, H. et al., 2007) with a case fatality ratio of 0.70. The most common form of OC arises from the epithelial surface cells of the ovary.

The standard of care for malignant epithelial OC is surgery followed by adjuvant chemotherapy. Surgery plays a key role in the management of OC. Surgery is necessary for diagnosis, which includes determining the origin of the disease (i.e., ovary, colon, pancreas) and defining the histologic type of disease (i.e., epithelial, germ cell, or stromal type tumors) (A-1). This information influences a patient's prognosis and choice of adjuvant therapy. Surgery defines the extent of intra-abdominal disease; this is otherwise known as staging (A-2). The extent of disease spread or stage of disease at diagnosis is a major determinant of prognosis. Chemotherapy is administered after surgery when the disease has spread beyond the ovary. Surgery

is also the means by which tumor is debulked to the smallest size possible. The size of the smallest tumor bulk in any one site in the abdomen at the completion of surgery influences the patient's prognosis. A standard operation to stage and debulk the tumor has been defined (National Institute of Health, 1994-1995; Trimbos, J. B., & Bolis, G., 1994; Allen, D. G., Baak, J., Belpomme, D., et al., 1993; Hoskins, W., Rice, L., & Rubin, S., 1997; Morgan, R. J., Copeland, L., Gershenson, D., et al., 1996; Trimbos, J. B., Schueler, J. A., van Lent, M., Hermans, J., & Fleuren, G. J., 1990).

Unfortunately, there is evidence that women are not being appropriately staged or optimally debulked and this can impact on their survival. Various efforts are a foot to improve the care of women diagnosed with ovarian cancer. In this chapter we will build the case for the use of informatics as a tool to reinforce completion of certain aspect of the operation and by collecting accurate detailed information, improving the data from which decisions are made concerning quality assurance. This will optimize the operative care to women with ovarian cancer by improving the accuracy and completeness of data collection at surgery.

OVARIAN CANCER CARE

Surgery

Guidelines

The Program in Evidence based Care for Cancer Care Ontario has reviewed the existing guidelines for the surgical management of a suspicious ovarian mass ("Gynecologic Disease Site Group Program in Evidence-based Care," 2007).

They document nine guidelines and four reviews, which because of the lack of randomized trials, are recommendations based on lesser quality studies and consensus (Table 1). The most frequent surgical recommendations include peritoneal washings, total hysterectomy (TAH), bilateral salpingo-oophorectomy (BSO), biopsy of suspicious lesions, and omentectomy.

Early Stage Disease

In early stage ovarian cancer, the surgical recommendation include the procedures described above and sampling of the pelvic and para-aortic nodes. Several series have shown that there is a prognostic impact of identifying disease in the pelvic and para-aortic nodes (Hacker, N. F. , 1995; Kikkawa, F., Ishikawa, H., Tamakoshi, K., Suganuma, N., Mizuno, K., Kawai, M. et al., 1995; Petru, E., Lahousen, M., Tamussino, K., Pickel, H., Stranzl, H., Stettner, H. et al., 1994; Chan, J. K., Munro, E. G., Cheung, M. K., Husain, A., Teng, N. N., Berek, J. S., & Osann, K., 2007; Munro, E. G., Cheung, M. K., Husain, A., Teng, N. N., Chan, J. K., Leiserowitz, G. S., & Osann, K., 2007). There is debate concerning the therapeutic benefit of removing these nodes. Kikkawa showed in 150 women from 1989-1991 that those with a lymphadenectomy survive longer than those without a lymphadenectomy. Chan showed in 6686 women with Stage 1 identified using the SEER (Surveillance Epidemiology and End Result) database from 1988-2001 that the lymphadenectomy and extent of lymphadenectomy was an independent prognostic factor in survival of women with non-clear cell ovarian cancer (Petru, E., Lahousen, M., Tamussino, K., Pickel, H., Stranzl, H., Stettner, H. et al., 1994; Chan, J. K., Munro, E. G., Cheung, M. K., Husain, A., Teng, N. N., Berek, J. S., & Osann, K., 2007).

There are 5 retrospective studies, one prospective cross-sectional study and one randomized controlled study, which describe in detail the aspects of the surgery and provide outcome information (Table 2). The studies cannot be pooled as the endpoints vary. However, they all recommend TAH+BSO, biopsies of suspicious lesions and pelvic and para-aortic node sampling. The Adjuvant Chemotherapy in Ovarian Neoplasm Trial (ACTION) (Trimbos, J. B., Vergote, I., Bolis, G., Vermorken, J. B., Mangioni, C., Madronal, C., Franchi, M., Tateo, S., Zanetta, G., Scarfone, G., Giurgea, L., Timmers, P., Coens, C., & Pecorelli, S., 2003). involved randomizing women with stage 1 ovarian cancer to no further treatment after surgery versus chemotherapy. The quality of the surgery was classified into 4 types depending on the extent of surgical staging. Trimbos detected a significant overall and recurrence-free survival advantage for women in the observation group who had undergone complete surgical staging compared to those who did not (p=0.03 and p=0.009). Women who did not receive optimal surgical staging benefited from adjuvant therapy however optimally surgically staged women did not benefit from adjuvant therapy.

The outcomes of surgery as defined in Table 2 are shown in Table 3. Complete surgical staging in early stage ovarian cancer appears to confer a survival benefit. It is likely that complete surgical staging better defines those patients with disease localized to the ovary. Incomplete surgical staging likely misses microscopically more advanced disease and this is the reason for a poorer survival in the incompletely staged group.

Advanced Disease

Optimal debulking implies that removing as much tumor as possible (in other words leaving behind the least amount of disease possible) will result in a survival benefit for the patient. The theoretical arguments for optimal debulking are that cancer has an exponential growth rate. As the tumor enlarges, the tumor's doubling time increases. Removal of large masses means fewer malignant cells require eradication i.e., less risk of drug resistance. Also, the remaining tumor nodules have a high proportion of cells in the active growth phase. Thus, these cells are more sensitive to the benefits of chemotherapy. A second hypothesis is that removal of large tumor masses means a removal of tumor with a poor blood supply that might not receive adequate doses of chemotherapy. A third hypothesis is that patients with ascites and a large tumor burden results in compromised oral intake which is important for immunocompetence.

The European Organization for Research and Treatment of Cancer (EORTC) is currently conducting a trial where women with ovarian cancer are randomized to immediate surgery followed by chemotherapy versus chemotherapy followed by interval surgery. Recruitment is completed. Survival results will be available within the year (Vergote, I., & Stuart, G., n/a).

There are 3 meta-analyses on the survival benefit of debulking surgery using lower quality study designs. Bristow conducted a meta-analysis and showed that for every 10% increase in optimal cytoreduction, survival increased by 5.5% (Bristow, R. E., Tomacruz, R. S., Armstrong, D. K., Trimble, E. L., & Montz, F. J., 2002). Allen used the criteria of no visible disease, <2cm or >2cm disease. In his report women with <2cm residual disease at the end of surgery survived longer with an OR 3.98 (95%CI 3.31-4.79) at 2 years, and 5.51 (95%CI 4.4-6.9) at 5 years (Allen, D. G., Heinta, A. P. M., & Touw, F. W. M. M.,

1995). . Hunter reported on 58 studies and 6962 patients with advanced epithelial ovarian cancer that shows that exposure to platinum chemotherapy was the most important factor linked to survival. However, maximum cytoreduction did have a small contribution to median survival time Hunter, R. W., Alexander, N. D. E., & Soutter, W. P., 1992). Several population-based studies confirm this finding (Eisenkop, S. M., Frieman, R. L., & Wang, H. J., 1998; Aletti, G. D., Dowdy, S. C., Gostout, B. S., Jones, M. B., Stanhope, R. C., Wilson, T. O., Podrzta, K. C., & Cliby, W. A., 2006; & Crawford, S. C., Vasey, P. A., Paul, J., Hay, A., Davis, J. A., Kaye, S. B., 2006).

There are 2 randomized controlled trials, which address the debulking question indirectly (Van Gorp, T., Amant, F., Neven, P., Berteloot, P., Leunen, K., & Vergote, I., 2006). THE EORTC-GCG Trial randomized women to chemotherapy versus an operation after 3 cycles of chemotherapy; this is known as interval debulking surgery (IDS) and the completion of the chemotherapy. The group receiving chemotherapy alone had a median survival of 20 mos; the group receiving chemotherapy and IDS had a median survival of 25 months (p=0.01). In contrast, Gynecologic Oncology Group (GOG52) patients could have an initial operation usually done by gynecologic oncologists and chemotherapy with or without a second operation. In this study there was no survival difference between the two arms. The hypothesis was that in the North American surgical community is more aggressive with initial debulking such that even if more than 2 cm of residual disease is left at the end of the first operation the aggressive initial surgical attempt of removing disease followed by a second operation did not impact the course of the disease.

There are a few case series that describe the feasibility of debulking in a patient deemed inoperable. Piver showed prospectively that in 50 patients with Stage 3 or 4 disease, that debulking to less than 2 cm disease was possible in 77% of the cases referred in as inoperable. When their group saw a new surgical patient with the same stage of disease, they were able to optimally debulk 76% of them (Piver, N., & Baker, T., 1986). Various authors have shown that optimal debulking is not only feasible but can be performed with minimal morbidity or mortality (Hacker, N. F., Berek, J. S., Lagasse, L. D., Nieberg, R. K., & Elashoff, R. M., 1983; & Heintz, A. P., Hacker, N. F., Berek, J. S., Rose, T. P., Munoz, A. K., & Lagsse, L. D., 1986).

For many years an argument has raged concerning whether the issue is optimal debulking or the biology of the disease making optimal debulking feasible. The EORTC trial should clarify the role of optimal debulking where biology of disease is controlled for by randomization.

Systemic Therapy

Guidelines

There are several guidelines outlining the use of adjuvant systemic therapy for both early and advanced stage disease. Based on randomised trials and systematic reviews, survival is improved with the use of an intravenous adjuvant platinum and taxane combination (Elit, L., Chambers, A., Fyles, A., Covens, A., Carey, M., & Fung Yee Fung, M., 2004; Covens, A., Carey, M., Bryson, P., Verma, S., Fung Kee Fung, M., Daya, D., DePetrillo, D., Eisenhauer E., Elit, L., Fyles, Kerr, I., Lukka, H., Malik, S., Rosen, B., Thomas, G., & Yoshida, S.; "Epithelial ovarian cancer" 2003; & National Institute of Health, 2003). More recent work is demonstrating a survival benefit with intraperitoneal disease in Stage 3 small volume or no residual disease patients (Elit, L., Oliver, T. K., Covens, A., Kwon, J., Fung, M. F., Hirte, H. W., & Oza, A. M., 2007).

OPPORTUNITIES TO ASSESS QUALITY OF CARE

Quality Indicators

In an era of limited resources and increasing demands for accountability, performance measures are being used by health care organizations interested in assessing quality of services. Quality of care is defined as the degree to which health services increase the likelihood of desired health outcomes and are consistent with current professional knowledge. Performance data could include an assessment of structures (i.e., hospital factors), processes of care (i.e., how the patient moves from the interaction with the physician for a complaint through diagnostic assessment and treatment) and outcomes (i.e., 5 year survival). This data could be used across institutions to set priorities, assess accountability and inform quality improvement initiatives.

Defining Quality Indicators

Where well-established evidence from controlled clinical trials is lacking, many organizations or research groups are implementing a formal consensus method to develop quality indicators. The Delphi or nominal group technique is a systematic evidence- and consensus-based approach for translating available evidence into objective performance measures. The process begins with a comprehensive literature search to identify all quality indicators. Then members of a multidisciplinary panel independently rate the indicators in terms of how they reflect quality and influence outcomes. This process is iterative. Then the panel comes together to in person to vet the final list of indicators.

Assessing Quality Indicators

In Ontario, a multidisciplinary panel of gynecologic oncologists, medical oncologists, radiation oncologists, nurse, pathologists reviewed 41 articles and 33 possible indicators (Gangliardi, A. R., Fung Kee Fung, M., Langer, B., Stern, H., & Brown, A. D., 2005; & "Care Ontario Web site for Quality Care," 2007). Using a modified Research ANd Development (RAND) methodology, 14 indicators were prioritized by the panel as benchmarks for assessing quality of surgical care. The indicators cover the domains of access to care, outcomes, diagnosis and staging, surgery, pathology, and adjuvant therapy. The indicators represent 3 levels of measurement (provincial/regional, hospital/team, and surgeon/individual provider). The intent is that Cancer Care Ontario will use one or more indicator to assess the quality of ovarian cancer care across the province. This information would be used on a regular basis to evaluate performance in a publicly transparent nature.

Computerized Databases

To facilitate assessment of quality indicators, data must be accurate and easily accessible. There are site-specific databases and provincial or national databases. For ovarian cancer in the province of Ontario Canada, there are examples of both types of database.

Site-Specific Databases

Gynecologic Oncology Surgical Ovarian Cancer System (GOSOCS)

The goal of the GOSOCS project was to develop a multidisciplinary database that is flexible and user friendly to meet the information needs of all health care providers for ovarian cancer patients. To achieve this flexibility, maximum portability of the data gathering mechanism would be required by multiple users imputing data under different clinical environments. We decided to implement a database that was both wirelessly accessible and Internet based to allow for maximal portability and in the process facilitating real time access

for secure data inputs and retrieval. A knowledge management module was also built into the system that would allow for questions and relevant patients' care issues to be sent to the whole group promoting discussion and knowledge transfer among team members. We also built a common reporting template that can quickly examine the database to provide accurate instantaneous statistics on relevant clinical results, accepted quality of care indicators in ovarian cancer as well as frequency of adverse events and treatment outcomes of interest to all care providers. In the design phase of the database, a number of face-to-face meetings were carried out among all health care disciplines including gynecologic oncologists, oncology nurses, pharmacist, psychologist, social workers, and secretarial support staff together with technology information management specialists. Project collaboration with Microsoft, Hewlett Packard, and Hummingbird software companies were sought. The main purpose of these meetings was to identify important relevant variables that should be included in the database to meet the needs of the multidisciplinary group. A relational database was set up based on the information gathered at these meetings. Data were entered in real time after each clinical encounter by all members of the gynecologic oncology team via tablet PC's equipped with wireless cards located at access points strategically placed at common points of clinical patient encounters. Data were securely transmitted to a centrally housed server at the Ottawa Hospital through wireless and wired connections. The front end of the database integrated all relevant clinical data in a single format allowing for easy and accurate recall of pathology, radiology, chemotherapy, and laboratory results (Appendix 3). Prior to implementation, advice was sought from the University of Ottawa research ethics board and the hospital privacy officer to ensure proper level of security and privacy protection of health related information was achieved. Technical supports were also secured from the Ottawa hospital and cancer clinic IT departments.

To build up the database, a medical chart abstractor was hired to retrospectively review all ovarian cancer patients' chart over the past 10 years and relevant clinical information was entered.

Start up funding for the project and ongoing maintenance support was secured from the Ottawa Hospital and Gynecologic Oncology Foundation funds. Hardware costs included tablet PCs', wireless LAN cards, server OS and related licenses together with wireless access points to be installed at locations of clinical encounters. The total software development and enhancements costs include the knowledge management modules. There is an annual maintenance cost for the database.

The GOSOCS system has been in operation since March 2004 after formal training of all team members involved with the care of ovarian cancer patients. Numerous fixes and enhancements were made to achieve maximal user friendliness and to incorporate evolving quality of care indicators. After an initial 6 months of familiarizing and modifications of the database, the data entering and querying process had been streamlined. All team members are currently using the database efficiently to meet their unique needs in clinical care. The apparent benefits after having established the database have been: the ease and accurate retrieval and assimilation of important clinical information in busy clinical settings. Health care providers have found the accurate timeline representation of patients' disease course to be very helpful in patients' counseling. From the secretarial supporting staff points of view, the scheduling of clinics / operating room and clinic preparation has been much more efficient. Furthermore, we can now quickly monitor and report well established ovarian cancer quality indicator variables as defined by Cancer Care Ontario based on the well-established database. At present, the database is being maintained by the Ottawa hospital IT department.

We plan to further expand the functionality of the database by integrating it into the broader Ottawa hospital patients' databases to broaden the scope of GOSOCS. Continued efforts are geared towards revising the system to be cross platform compatible that can be easily modified to individualize results' reporting. New innovative uses of the knowledge management modules of GOSOCS continue to be developed by all team members to further reap its full potential even though this will be a challenge on a busy clinical service. Using the lessons learned and the experience gained, we planned to expand the database to other gynecologic disease sites such as endometrial and cervical cancers. Plans are also being made to expand the database provincially and nationally to facilitate collaborative research and improve on the care of ovarian cancer patients.

The GOSOCS pilot database project has proven effective in providing all heath care providers involved with ovarian cancer patients with an efficient and accurate means of accessing and assimilating clinical data needed to optimize daily patient care. Furthermore, the potentials for the database to facilitate accurate analysis of epidemiology and outcomes data for research purpose can be explored and expanded further. This project will also promote knowledge sharing and the development of community of practice among team members locally and nationally.

Strengths and Limitations of GOSOCS

The strength of the GOSOCS database is that the Ottawa Regional Cancer Centre and affiliated Hospital(s) has information about the quality of ovarian cancer at their hospital site. The limitation of GOSOCS is that similar quality information is lacking for providers at other sites across the province. Unfortunately to obtain GOSOCS a fee is involved at each independent health care facility. Database support is only available through a specific vendor and this makes life complicated if each disease site has a different vendor and database. Data entry into GOSOCS is time over and above the time currently spent caring for the patient. Completeness of the dataset is dependent on vigilance of the staff at each site. Should the same database exist at multiple sites, there will be issues around merging databases due to the provincial privacy act, which protects the confidentiality of patient information.

Administrative Databases

Country or region specific administrative databases have been used to provide quality of care information concerning the management of women with ovarian cancer. These administrative databases were in most cases developed for other purposes. In Ontario, the patient health insurance database was created as a means to reimburse the provider. In Canada, the Canadian Institute for Hospital Information (CIHI) database was created to monitor hospital activity by abstracting admission and discharge information across the nation. Provincial Cancer Registries have been established using hospitalization data and vital statistics records to document incident cases. These databases have variable strengths and weaknesses but, used in combination, can provide important outcome information concerning patients. For example, treatment information can often be associated with survival data and subsequent morbidity data through the use of combinations of Cancer Registry, physician and hospital services, and vital statistics databases. Pulling databases together may require cross provincial and provincial-national collaboration.

Ontario Population Based Project
There are a number of ways to assess the quality of surgical care women with ovarian cancer receive. In 1966, Donabedian (Donabedian, A., 1966). described an approach to measuring the quality of medical care. He used three steps and we will consider these in terms of the delivery

of surgery. First, to determine the benefits that surgery can achieve *outcomes* --such as percent 5-yr survival, progression free interval, and rate of complications -- can be assessed. Second, to determine whether one has applied what is judged to be good medical care, the *process of care delivery* can be evaluated. For example, if guidelines exist for the conduct of ovarian cancer surgery, one can determine how well these are implemented. Finally, to assess the setting in which medical care is provided, *structure* such as facilities and qualifications of the staff can be determined. Volume-outcome studies are an example of assessing structure. Variations in outcomes related to surgical volumes may reflect 1) habitual differences in the way in which medical care is applied and 2) failure to integrate care across boundaries of components of the health care system. If variations are identified, these may point to opportunities where improvements can be brought into the system.

In the Ontario Outcomes for Ovarian Cancer Surgery pilot project (Elit, L., Bondy, S., Paszat, L., Przybysz, R., & Levine, M., 2002). ethics approval was obtained and then we assessed 3815 women with ovarian cancer from 1992 to 1998 just using provincial and national databases. The adjusted relative risk for reoperation within 3 months of the initial surgery showed that patients were less likely to have a repeat operation if the initial operation was done in a high- or intermediate-volume hospital (RR 0.24 95% CI 0.12-0.48, RR 0.29 95% CI 0.20-0.42, respectively), a hospital with a gynecologic oncologist (RR 0.29 95% CI 0.15-0.56), by a gynecologic oncologist (RR 0.04 95% CI 0.01-0.12) or gynecologist (RR 0.37 95% CI 0.21-0.66), or by a high-volume surgeon (RR 0.09 95% CI 0.03-0.23). The adjusted survival was improved if the initial surgery was done by a gynecologic oncologist (HR 0.70 95% CI 0.57-0.85) or gynecologist (HR 0.65 95% CI 0.53-0.79). We concluded that there is a relationship between hospital volume and reoperation rate. Institution type only influenced reoperation rate. Statistically significant associations were found between surgical specialty and all three-outcome variables (operative mortality, reoperation rates, overall survival). The volume of surgery performed by an individual surgeon only influenced reoperation rate. Given the inability to correct for confounders like stage, these results were preliminary and supported the need for further study.

The National Cancer Institute of Canada then funded a population based retrospective cohort study based at the Institute of Clinical Evaluative Sciences (ICES) using the Donabedian model. Included were women with invasive epithelial ovarian cancer who underwent their primary surgery from 1996-1998 in Ontario. After obtaining ethics approval, 1341 women were included in the database. The chart abstraction was completed directly into a computerized database using ACCESS that was password protected and encrypted. As the study was conducted prior to the RAND approach to defining quality indicators, a survey of the Canadian gynaecologic oncology community was used to define the items that would be included in the template (Elit, L., 2005). The template used for this process is included in the Appendix 4. Record linkages were conducted with other Ontario databases such as the hospital discharge data from Canadian Institute for Health Information (CIHI), and the vital statistic data from the Ontario Cancer Registry (OCR) and public health insurance data (RPDP). Analysis was then conducted in SAS and Stata. The analysis showed that re-operation rates were associated with surgeon discipline, younger patient age, well-differentiated tumors and early stage of disease. Survival however, was not associated with surgeon's discipline, but was associated with advancing age, increasing co-morbidities, advancing stage, poorly differentiated tumors, urgent surgery and adjuvant chemotherapy. There was a trend for inadequate surgery being associated with worse survival (Elit, L., Bondy, S., Paszat, L., Chen, Z., Hollowaty, E., Thomas, G., & Levine,

M., 2006; & Elit, L., Bondy, S., Chen, Z., Law, C., & Paszat, L., 2006).

This process allowed us to retrospectively understand the factors influencing surgical staging and debulking and overall survival information for the women in Ontario who had begun their ovarian cancer journey with surgery.

Strengths and Limitations

The strengths of population databases are that they have been established and are supported thru the resources of the provincial and/or national beaurocracies. The providers in the system are obliged to provide the data and there are quality assurance standards and procedures in place. In Ontario access to several administrative datasets is accessible only through the Ministry of Health with special approval or via key research institutes like the Institute for Clinical Evaluative Science. Here there are clear confidentiality agreements, scientific credentialing, with access to the data through experienced and accredited programmers. There are rules that are strictly enforced around data encryption and stripping of personal identifiers for patient and provider information.

One limiting feature of using administrative databases is that, to date, they lack the clinical detail that is needed to adjust for confounders such as stage, grade, and histology. If data are not adjusted for such confounders, this can significantly influence the validity of the final answer. An example of this phenomenon is seen in the two papers by "Elit, et al.", (2002 & 2006). Their initial pilot study using only information from databases suggested an impact of surgical specialty on survival; however, the subsequent work showed that when corrected for confounders through direct chart abstraction showed that the positive association was greatly attenuated and no longer significant. One can argue that a custom-launched prospective cohort study is needed to produce more precise data. However, it is not clear that such an enormous investment in cost and human resources is justifiable.

LITERATURE REVIEW WHERE ADMINISTRATIVE DATABASES ARE USED

Variations in Surgical Care

To show the value of informatics on assessing variations of care in ovarian cancer we will review the work done in several countries around the world. There are many ways to present this information. We have chosen to discuss the issues related to early and late stage ovarian cancer separately. To make clear the impact of structural variables (like, hospital type, hospital volumes of ovarian cancer surgery, surgeon specialty and surgeon volume of ovarian cancer surgery), we will describe the literature in each of these domains as it relates to pertinent outcomes (ie., for early disease the outcomes are lymphadenectomy (or staging surgery) and survival. For advanced disease the outcomes are debulking the tumor to minimal residual disease and survival).

Variations in Care for Early Stage Disease

We have shown that optimal staging is associated with improved survival for patients with early stage disease. The process of achieving optimal staging can be influenced by hospital factors like volume of ovarian cancer cases or type of hospital (i.e., affiliated with a university, affiliated with a cancer center, community hospital) where the surgery takes place and factors related to the surgeon (training ie., gynecologic oncologist, gynecologist, general surgeon; surgical volumes of ovarian cancer cases) who completes the operation.

Lymphadenectomy as a Surrogate Measure for Staging in Early Stage Ovarian Cancer

How Hospital Type impacts Lymphadenectomy rates in early stage disease
Goff reviewed the patterns of surgical care across the USA in 10,432 women with ovarian cancer. She found that node dissection was associated with hospital type (Goff, B., Larson, E., Mathews, B., Andrilla, H., Lishner, D., Baldwin, L., Lackey, M., & Muntz, H., 2006).

How Hospital Volume of Ovarian Cancer Surgery impacts Lymphadenectomy rates in early stage disease
Goff found that node dissection was associated with hospital volume of ovarian cancer surgeries (Goff, B., et al., 2006).

How Surgeon Specialty impacts Lymphadenectomy rates in early stage disease
Using the endpoint of conducting a lymphadenectomy as a component of the surgical staging in early stage ovarian cancer, Giede conducted a meta-analysis that showed that gynecologic oncologists were more likely to stage patients (p=0.001) (Giede, K. C., Kieser, K., Dodge, J., & Rosen, B., 2005). Pul showed in stage 1 patients from Texas and Kentucky that staging was completed by 100% of gynecologic oncologists compared to only 28% of community doctors (Puls, C, R., Morrow, M. S., & Blackhurst, D., 1997). Earle reviewed the medicare claims for women 65 years and older who were diagnosed with Stage 1 and 2 ovarian cancer from 1992-1999. Lymphadenectomies were more likely to be a part of the surgery if it was completed by a gynecologic oncologist (60%), than a gynecologists (36%), or a general surgeon (16%) (Earle, C. C., Schrag, D., Neville, B. A., Yabroff, K. R., Topor, M. Fahey, A. et al., 2006). Engelen et al. (2006) from The Netherlands showed that in Stage 1-2 disease, gynecologic oncologists followed staging procedures in 55% of cases compared to 33% in gynecologists (p=0.01).

How Surgeon's Volume impacts lymphadenectomy rates in early stage disease

Goff's review showed that node dissection was associated with surgeon volumes of ovarian cancer surgeries (Goff, B., et al., 2006).

Survival in Early Stage Ovarian Cancer

How Hospital Type impacts on duration of Survival in early stage disease

Hole showed in 1974 that women with early stage ovarian cancer managed at teaching hospitals survived longer than those managed elsewhere when controlled for age, stage and tumor type (p=0.03) (Hole, D. J., & Gillis, C. R., 1993). Subsequent communication by Gillis suggests this is specifically for women under 65 years of age (Gillis, C. R., Hole, D. J., Still, R. M., & Kaye, S. B., 1991). In contrast, Tingulstad (N/A) completed a historical prospective study matching 2 controls from referral hospitals from 1992-1995 to 1 case referred to the teaching hospital in 1995-1997. Post-operative mortality was no different in the two groups for those with Stage 1-2 ovarian cancer.

How Hospital Volume of Ovarian Cancer Surgery impacts on duration of Survival in early stage disease

No Information

How Surgeon Specialty impacts on duration of Survival in early stage disease

The Giede et al. (2005) meta-analysis concluded that survival was influenced by surgeon's specialty in women with early stage ovarian cancer. The retrospective cohort studies show a lot of variation here. Using the endpoint of survival in early stage ovarian cancer, Mayer and Pul showed that survival was influenced by the specialty of the surgeon (Mayer, A. R., Chambers, S. K., Graves, E., Holm, C., Tseng, P. C., Nelson, B. E. et al., 1992; & Puls, C, R., 1997). In contrast, Junor and Carney showed that surgeon specialty did not influence survival (Junor, E. J., Hole, D. J., McNulty, L., Mason, M., & Young, J., 1999; & Carney, M. E., Lancaster, J. M., Ford, C., Tsodikov, A., & Wiggins, C. L., 2002).

The biologic rationale for this finding likely involves a stage shift for those women with ovarian cancer who are more aggressively staged, thus they truly have early stage disease and do well. Those who are not completely staged may represent a combination of those with truly early stage disease and those with non-identified more advanced disease (false negatives). Thus the overall survival rate is poorer. As well, more aggressively staged women with early disease but poor prognostic factors that are defined by staging could have subsequent treatment decisions such as adjuvant chemotherapy which may improve survival.

How Surgeon's Volume impacts on duration of Survival in early stage disease

Goff showed that comprehensive surgical care was superior if surgeon volumes were medium (2-9 cases/year) to high as compared to low (1 or less cases/year) (Goff, B. A., Matthews, B. J., Larson, E. H., Andrilla, C. H., Wynn, M., Lishner, D. M., & Baldwin, L. M., 2007).

Variations in Care for Advanced Stage Disease

We have shown that optimal debulking is associated with improved survival for patients with advanced stage disease. The process of achieving optimal debulking can be influenced by hospital factors like volume of ovarian cancer cases or type of hospital (ie., affiliated with a university, affiliated with a cancer center, community hospital) where the surgery takes place and factors related to the surgeon (training ie., gynecologic oncologist, gynecologist, general surgeon; surgical volumes of ovarian cancer cases) who completes the operation. We discuss first those studies that show process factors associated with optimal debulking surgery. Then we review those studies that comment on the relationship between process factors and survival.

Debulking to Minimal Residual Disease in Advanced Stage Ovarian Cancer

How Type of Hospital Impacts on Debulking Surgery in Advanced Stage Ovarian Cancer
"Wolfe, C. D., Tilling, K., and Raju, K. S." (1997). prospectively assessed women with ovarian cancer in 7 districts of Southeast Thames, UK. They found that 66% of women at teaching centers, 45% of women at nonteaching centers with oncology support and 28% of women at non-teaching facilities had surgery according to guidelines (p=0.02). There were many centers that averaged fewer than 1 ovarian cancer operation per year.

How Volume of Ovarian Cancer Operations at the Hospital impacts Debulking in Advanced Ovarian Cancer
"Olaitin, A., Weeks, J., Mocroft, A., Smith, J., Howe, K., and Murdoch, J. (2001) showed that if the hospital's annual rate of ovarian cancer surgeries was less than 10 cases, this was associated with a two fold higher likelihood of suboptimal debulking. Goff, B. A., Matthews, B. J., Wynn, M., Muntz, H. G., Lishner, D. M., & Baldwin, L. M. showed that volume of ovarian cancer operations was a factor in non-teaching hospitals but was not important in teaching hospitals. In moderate (10-19 operations/year) to high volume (>20 operations/year) non-teaching settings, more patients received debulking surgeries, lymph node dissections than in low volume settings (1-9 operations/year) (p<0.001).

Type of Surgeon Impacts on Debulking in Advanced Ovarian Cancer
The following studies commented on how the type of surgical training or surgical specialty influences rates of optimal debulking. "Vernooij, F., Peter, A., Heintz, M., Witteveen, E., & van der Graff, Y." (2007) completed a systematic review and showed that gynecologic oncologists perform more debulking operations to less that 2 cm disease (RR 1.4, 95%CI 1.2-1.5), and to no macroscopic

disease (RR 2.3 95% CI 1.5-3.5). There are a number of retrospective cohort studies from various countries in North America and Europe that have confirmed this relationship (Earle, C. C., et al., 2006; Engelen, M. J., 2006; Olaitin, A., 2001; Eisenkop, S. M., Spirtos, N. M., Montag, T. W., Nalick, R. H., & Wang, H. J., 1992; Junor, E. J., Hole, D. J., & Gillis, C. R., 1994.; & Wimberger, P., Lehmann, N., Kimmig, R., Burges, A., Meier, W., & Du Bois, A., 2007).

How Surgeon's Volumes impacts on Debulking in Advanced Ovarian Cancer
No information

Survival in Advanced Ovarian Cancer
How Hospital Type Impacts on Survival in Advanced Ovarian Cancer
Liberati, A., Mangioni, C., Bratina, L., Carinelli, G., Marsoni, S., Parazzini, F. et al." (1885) from Italy reviewed the ovarian cancer cases from 31 centres and showed that there was no difference in the quality of the diagnostic and therapeutic measures between specialized and nonspecialized centers. There was no survival difference. "Hole et al." (1993) from Scotland also showed no impact of type of hospital on women's survival when they presented with advanced disease. In contrast studies from the UK and Finland have shown that when an operation is conducted at a teaching centre, survival for women with advanced disease is extended (Tingulstad, S; & Kumpulainen, S., Grenman, S., Kyyronen, P., Pukkala, E., & Sankila, R., 2002). "Shylasree, T. S., Howells, R. E., Lim, K., Jones, P. W., Flander, A., Adams, M. et al." (2006) showed that prior to guideline introduction in Wales, women managed at a cancer center had improved survival at 1 and 3 years (p=0.022).

How Hospital Volume of Ovarian cancer impacts on Survival in Advanced Ovarian Cancer
Investigators from Japan (Ioka, A., Tsukuma, H., Ajiki, W., & Oshima, A., 2004), USA (Bristow, R.

E., Zahurak, M. L., del Carmen, M. G., Gordon, T. A., Fox, H. F., Trimble, E. L. et al., 2004; Schrag, D., Earle, C., Xu, F., Panageas, K. S., Yabroff, K. R., Bristow, R. E., Trimble, E. L., & Warren, J. L., 2006), and Oberaigner, W., & Stuhlinger, W., 2006) have shown that showed that small departments or low volume centers have a poorer survival compared to patients receiving surgery a high volume centers.

4.01223 How Surgeon Specialty Impacts on Survival in Advanced Ovarian Cancer

Using the endpoint of survival, "Giede, K. C., et al." (2005) meta-analysis showed a 6-9 month median survival advantage for women operated on by a gynecologic oncologist (p=0.009 general surgeon to 0.01 gynecologist). All of the retrospective cohort studies confirmed this finding (Earle, C. C., et al., 2006; Engelen, M. J., 2006; Vernooij, et al., 2007; Eisenkop, S. M. et al., 1992; Wimberger, P., 2007; Nguyen, H. N., Averette, H. E., Hoskins, W., Penalver, M., Sevin, B. U., & Steren, A., 1993;,Kehoe, S., Powell, J., Wilson, S., & Woodman, C., 1994; Woodman, C., Baghdad, A., Collins, S., & Clyma, J-A., 1997; Junor, E. J., Hole, D. J., McNulty, L., Mason, M., & Young, J., 1999; Oksefjell, H., Sandstad, B., & Trope, C., 2006).

The rationale for improved survival when a gynecologic oncologist is involved in care is rooted not only in aggressive cytoreduction to less that 2 cm of disease, but also in more aggressive cytoreduction even if the residual is larger than 2cm and the more frequent use of platinum taxane based chemotherapy (Junor, E. 2000). Higher use of adjuvant chemotherapy by gynecologic oncologists also appears to impact on survival.

How Surgeon's Volumes Impacts on Survival in Advanced Ovarian Cancer

"Woodman et al. (1997)" in Northwestern UK showed that surgeon volume of ovarian cancer surgery did not impact on survival. "Bristow et al. (2004)" showed that high volume surgeons appear to work at high volume centers. Women live longer when surgery was done by high volume surgeons. "Schrag et al. (2006)" showed that surgeon's volume was an important factor in 2-year mortality in the univariate analysis but not in the multivariate analysis (p=0.062). "Goff et al. (2007)" showed that comprehensive surgical care was associated with annual surgeon volumes of than 2-9 cases annually when compared to 1 or less cases per year.

Guideline Adherence

The population-based studies show variations in the uptake of care as defined in guidelines. "Grilli, R., Alexanian, A., Apolone, G., Fossati, R., Marsoni, S., Nicolucci, A. et al. (1990)" showed that the Italian national Research Council education program had a 10 year history of preparing and disseminating ovarian cancer guidelines to community hospitals. However, only 44% of responders were aware of the guidelines. In terms of complying with the surgical recommendations only 45% of physicians document the size of residual disease and only 10% did random biopsies as a component of staging. "Harlan, L. C., Clegg, L.X., and Trimble, E. L. (2003)" in the USA showed that in Stage 1 and 2 patients there was an improvement in guideline adherence in 1996 compared to 1991. Unfortunately, this was not the case in those with stage 3 disease. "Munoz, K. A., Harlan, L. C., and Trimble, E. L. (1997)" showed that using 1991 SEER date, only 10% of stage 1 and 2 patients had lymphadenectomy for early stage disease and only 71% of stage 3 and 53% of stage 4 patients had the recommended staging and chemotherapy. "Sengupta, P. S., Jayson, G. C., Slade, R. J., Eardley, A., and Radford, J. A. (1999)" showed that surgical guidelines for ovarian cancer are widely available. In their retrospective audit of Christie Cancer Centre in Manchester in 1996, less than half the patients had the recommended surgery. Thus population based databases have shown where the uptake of recommended guidelines has improved and where problems still exist.

Variations in Systemic Therapy Care

There are 2 studies that have shown no impact of hospital type or volume, provider specialty or volume on the outcome of women with ovarian cancer. "Elit, L., Cartier, C., Oza, A., Hirte, H., Levine, M., and Paszat, L. (2006)" conducted a retrospective cohort of 2502 women from 1996-2002. They showed that the only factors predictive of improved survival in the multivariate model were younger age, absence of comorbidities and absence of metastasis. "Silber, J. H., Rosenbaum, P. R., Polsky, D., Ross, R. N., Even-Shoshan, O., Schartz, J. S. et al. (2007)" used the SEER data base for women over age 65 years from 1991-2001 showing that in 344 patients with ovarian cancer, prescriber specialty did not affect survival.

OPPORTUNITIES TO IMPROVE OVARIAN CANCER CARE

Operative Reporting

Dictated Operative Notes

All Canadian hospitals mandate a written operative note in the chart and a more detailed dictated operative note. There is no consistent style for this note and often it includes a lot of information about the type of suture used and style of tying a pedicle. The key pieces of information for making adjuvant treatment decisions in ovarian cancer are often missing. "Elit, L. (2006)" showed in Ontario that the size of residual disease at the end of the debulking operation in advanced disease was often missing (50% of cases). "Shaw, M., Wolfe, C., Raju, K. S., and Papadopoulos, A. (2003)" did an audit of gynaecological cancer services from 1999-2000 in South East England. One major problem is that of missing data from the medical record such as stage. They advocated for improved quality of notes.

The deficiencies of the operative note includes failing to document the procedure adequately. Although it is unlikely that the missing details correlate with surgery of less quality, without the details, it is not possible to assess the quality of the surgery. In addition, using the operative note to assess quality of care is a tedious process of data abstraction from the original record, and so it is difficult to feed information back to the surgeon to consider personal results to improve their technique. Listed below are other methods of capturing surgical information.

Checklists

Checklists have the benefit of generating reports that consistently incorporate commonly accepted parameters essential for patient management. Checklists tend to provide more complete data. An example of a checklist for ovarian cancer surgery used by the South and West Regional Cancer Organisation was published by "Olaitin, A. et al. (2006)". Some critics feel that checklists lead to cookbook medicine. Their concern is that checklists stifle a more detailed description and rationale for what took place in the operating room.

Templates

Templates are "canned" descriptions and have been shown to assist residents in organizing, recording and dictating a large volume of information (Leslie, K. O., & Rosai, J., 1994). Templates have been described by the orthopods. DeOrio showed that templates saved the surgeon time dictating, reviewing and correcting and saved transcription time in terms of word processing and corrections. Templates have also been used to facilitate the billing process. Unfortunately, critics feel that this approach stifles creativity and problem solving. Other concerns are that the reporter may not read the detailed lists and so fall into the trap of picking the most convenient response (first or last) as opposed to the most accurate response. This leads to incomplete information. As well, if the template has an incomplete list of options and the reporter does not type the information in the text boxes, this may results in lost information.

Synoptic Operative Reports

Synoptic reports are summary reports that present key information in tabular form rather than sentences/paragraphs. This method has become quite popular with our pathology colleagues. In colorectal surgery, "Edhemovic, I., Temple, W. J., de Gara, C. J., & Stuart, G. C. (2004)" in Calgary showed that this technology is twice as likely to capture the specified data elements of interest as compared to the operative note.

The Cancer Care Alberta Web Surgical Medical Record (webSMR)

In 1999, the Alberta Cancer Board established the Cancer Surgery Working Group (CSWG) to promote the use of computer synoptic reports to eliminate deficiencies in reporting and also improve the quality of surgery. This working group consisted of surgeons, surgical oncologists, gynecologic oncologists, information systems specialists with representatives from Alberta Health and Wellness. The first project was a computerized synoptic operative report template in rectal cancer (Edhemovic, I. et al. 2004) to replace the narrative report. It was clearly demonstrated that the synoptic report captured 99% of the relevant data compared to only 45.9% with the narrative reports. This is the first world Web Surgical Medical Records program (WebSMR) developed by Alberta Cancer Surgeons. Extending the program throughout the province has been possible through additional funding from Canada Health Infoway. This tool enables surgeons to fill a standardized electronic report after surgery, allowing for easy accessibility of reports by the entire cancer care team for better decisions

to improve quality of care and hence short and long term outcomes. The College of Physicians and Surgeons of Alberta and the Calgary Health Region have approved the use of the WebSMR to replace the narrative report.

With the success of the rectal cancer template and the subsequent development of templates for liver and breast cancer, the next agenda was the creation of 3 templates for ovarian cancer – surgical staging for early cancer, cytoreductive surgery and palliative surgery. These templates were created with input from my colleagues (Dr. J. Nation, Dr. P, Chu) Dr. GCE Stuart (Dean of Medicine, UBC) and Dr. W. Temple (Director of Cancer Surgery Alberta). This synoptic report not only addresses the important steps of the surgical procedure, which is a powerful educational tool, but also allows for the collection of relevant preoperative workup and wait-time from referral to surgery. Additionally, symptoms of disease at presentation can be captured. Lists of the variables collected are listed below (Appendix 3). The information with regards to demographics, preoperative assessment and clinical evaluation and investigations are similar for the three procedures and therefore not repeated. Although a lot of information is captured, the OR report is only one to two pages. Entering the data usually takes a maximum of ten minutes. Other advantages of this system include automated import of demographic data, easy changes to the structure of the questionnaire, replacement of OR dictations and consistency in reporting with improvement in the quality of surgery. Most importantly, these templates are not copyrighted and therefore can be used, with modifications, by any institute in the world.

In Alberta, the gynecologic oncologists are based in Edmonton [North] and Calgary [South]. These templates for ovarian cancer are now being used by all the gynecologic oncologists in Calgary since January, 2007. To date, twenty patients have been entered. Modifications to the questionnaires have been easy. Entries can be made from the operating room, office and other designated places in the hospital and cancer centre. In the next three months, we plan to expand this program to the Cross Cancer Institute in Edmonton following which it will be extended to all gynecologists in Alberta.

Aside from seeing whether data entry is complete, we hope to look at the surgical procedures being done as part of quality assurance and compare the ability of the various health regions to adhere to recommended protocols and hence identify areas where resources to meet guidelines may be lacking. This applies particularly to surgical staging. The template for cytoreduction will allow us to collect data on different residual sizes of disease and hence see whether this affects prognosis. The palliative surgery template will collect information as to which surgery is most often carried out. We are intentionally collecting data on the instruments used to see if any particular "brand" is better. Additionally, capturing of information related to symptomatology and investigations may allow for improvement in ovarian cancer screening. Data of wait-time from consultation referral to surgery can only improve patient care.

A recent workshop by the Canadian Cancer Control Guidelines Action Group "Cancer Control Guidelines Action Group (2007)" supports the development of a collaborative plan to promote the use of evidence and practice guidelines in cancer control through synoptic reporting tools.

The replacement of narrative reports with the computerized synoptic reports should improve the quality of reports and surgery which should translate to better short and long term outcomes of patients. We hope in the next year to create templates for the other gynecologic malignancies.

eCANCER^ovarian

Healthcare organizations in North America and around the world have been increasingly deploying Electronic Health Records (EHRs) to improve quality of patient care, enhance clinical efficiency and reduce errors (Poissant, L., Perira, J., Tamblyn, R., & Kawasumi, Y., 2005; & "Determinants of success of inpatient clinical information systems: A literature review, 2003"). However, implementation of EHRs has not resulted in broad acceptance of this technology despite being shown to improve the availability, clarity and accuracy of patient information as well as reduce costs "Determinants of success of inpatient clinical information systems: A literature review, (2003)" This, in part, might be due to the limitations associated with the electronic patient records.

Most of the EHRs deployed in hospitals collect generic patient data that is often not structured, difficult to retrieve and hard to use at the point of care. Clinicians spent most of their time providing care to patients and hope that an electronic patient record used in their institution will help them to increase quality of care and patient interaction time (Poissant, L., 2003). In reality, however, this is difficult to achieve. In many cases, clinical documentation such as visit and procedure notes are dictated, transcribed and uploaded into the EHR in a free text format. It is a challenge for clinicians to retrieve relevant information in a timely manner (both in terms of getting the information into electronic form and gleaning information from prose-form).

As a result, many clinical groups are creating custom disease-specific applications to address their professional and care-specific needs. Gynecologic Oncology Division at Princess Margaret Hospital (PMH) in Toronto, Canada teamed up with Health Research Informatics group to develop a database to allow the collection of disease-specific information on all patients with ovarian cancer receiving care at PMH.

To achieve its goals, the ovarian cancer database had to meet the following criteria: (1) collect discrete clinical data on all clinical visits, OR procedures and chemotherapy treatment, (2) replace dictating reports, (3) integrate the new system with the hospital's existing EHR, (4) ensure the system is usable at the point of care, (5) provide trending of tumor markers such as CA125, and (6) ensure easy extraction of data for research and quality of care analysis.

1. Collect discrete clinical data on all clinical visits, OR procedures and chemotherapy treatment

Traditionally, clinical notes have been dictated, transcribed and then printed. This form of charting patient information has a number of limitations. Dictated reports are often incomplete or delayed, can potentially be inaccurate and provide little value for quality analysis and research as they cannot be queried (Laflamme, M. R., Dexter, P. R., Graham, M. F., Hui, S. L., & McDonald, C. J., 2005). The advent of electronic patient record did not provide a real solution to clinicians with regards to clinical notes. Dictating is still a prevalent practice in many institutions with notes being scanned or sent into an EHR, usually retrospectively. These documents are available electronically, but have no individual data elements that can be processed by the computer (Amatayjakul, M., 2005). This limits health professionals in assessing quality indicators and affects treatment decisions.

Electronic forms that contain discrete fields for each disease point allow clinicians and researchers to query the database and extract information on the population of interest. The challenges of implementing electronic forms lie in populating databases with clinical data and providing clinicians with physical access to electronic data (such as input and access terminals) when and where they need it, and without the hardware having a disrupting influence on patient care or work flow. Healthcare professionals will use any electronic documentation only if it fits their workflow and adds value to their care.

2. Replace dictating reports

A solution that was proposed to Gynecologic Oncology Division included replacing the current practice of dictating clinical notes with electronic note automation (ENA) tool. ENA enhanced ovarian database by creating a prose clinical note while still retaining the integrity of the discrete data fields. Physicians are able to check electronic form boxes on the left side of the screen while seeing the clinical note being generated instantly on the right side of the screen. The text of the note in the ENA is generated from templated sentences stored in the database that incorporate form fields chosen by a physician. Templated sentences where created through review of hundreds of dictated clinical notes, finding commonalities in the structure and style of these notes and creating a standard sentence for each clinical point. Physicians were involved in all the stages of the note design and the letter text went through a number of iterations until it reached satisfaction of all members of the Gyne Oncology group. However, a number of challenges were discovered when the ENA when into "production" and physicians started using it to generate clinical visit and operative reports. Clinicians understood and appreciated the value of a synoptic clinical note such as provision of consistently complete and accurate data, immediate availability of the note and the ease of subsequent retrieval of data (Laflamme, M. R., 2005). However, they were not readily embracing ENA use in clinics or operating rooms for two main reasons. It seemed that an electronic note did not provide enough expressive power to describe relevant information and it potentially required more time to complete the note than current reporting method.

To address the first issue, the note was modified to include optional free text fields. A physician had a choice where the comment would appear in a note to ensure it reads logically and sequentially. This modification was very well received and encouraged the use of an ENA. The problem of adding more time to completion of the note was more difficult to address. Clinicians often consider a system to be efficient if it reduces their documentation time (Poissant, L., 2005) and no matter how useful and advanced the technology may be, it has to be fast.

3.   Integrate the new system with the hospital's existing EHR

One way to improve efficiency of ovarian cancer patient database was to ensure it is integrated with an organization's existing EHR. Stand-alone clinical systems require duplication of information, are prone to errors (with potentially less opportunity for correction than dictation), and are not user friendly at the point of care.

At PMH, the ovarian cancer database called eCANCER[ovarian] is connected to a hospital's electronic patient record system that populates a database with patient demographic information eliminating duplication and manual entry of data. eCANCER[ovarian] interoperability with local EHR allows other information to be exchanged between systems. Electronic clinical note generated in eCANCER[ovarian] is submitted instantly into a patient record system eliminating the need for dictation.

Incorporating a disease-specific application such as ovarian cancer database with a legacy EHR system can be a challenging process as it requires cooperation and resources of organization's IT department. IT groups in hospitals are often understaffed, underfunded and overworked. To gain their buy-in requires proving to them the benefits a new system will provide to the organization. In the case of eCANCER[ovarian], the cost-benefit analysis was used to prove that the organization will gain savings by replacing costly and error-prone dictation system.

4.   Ensure the system is usable at the point of care

Lack of electronic patient record system adoption is also due to the stationary design and use of EHRs. Healthcare professionals usually recall patient information using printed notes (Reuss, E., Menozzi, M., Buchi, M., Koller, J., & Krueger, H., 2004). Visit and OR results are entered retrospectively using office or ward station computers. To overcome this obstacle, Health Informatics Research team designed a tool called DePICT – Disease-specific electronic Patient Illustrated Clinical Timeline that summarizes care patients received in the ovarian clinic. It is well-known that a picture is worth a thousand words and DePICT was built on this premise. It displays icons that illustrate specific treatments such as surgery and chemotherapy as well as tests including laboratory and radiology results.   A glimpse at the clinical timeline allows gynecologic oncologists to quickly recall all aspects of patient care and spend more quality time on patient interaction and decision making. Wireless tablets were introduced to the Ovarian Cancer clinic to allow physicians to use the database application to review patients' past history and complete a note at the point of care.

5.   Provide trending of tumor markers such as CA125

Another important aspect of caring for patients with ovarian cancer is the assessment of their response to treatment such as chemotherapy. CA 125 is a tumor-associated antigen that is used clinically to monitor patients with epithelial ovarian carcinomas. The trending of serum CA 125 level is valuable in the follow-up and restaging of patients. The levels of CA 125 are usually recorded in the lab results of a patient chart and are difficult to trend in the traditional form of presentation. As a result, trending graph of CA 125 levels was developed in eCANCER[ovarian] to allow clinicians efficiently asses patient's response to chemotherapy treatment and assist health providers in clinical decision process. The experience of designing eCANCER[ovarian] and other disease specific applications showed that health professionals appreciate when patient information is summarized and graphically represented.

6. Ensure easy extraction of data for research and quality of care analysis.

Extracting clinical data for research and quality of care analysis remains a challenge. Since most of the EHRs store data as free text, extracting data points for research requires manual review of patient charts. This process is costly, time consuming and occasionally inaccurate. The development of electronic patient documentation must include the ability to extract data for statistical analysis. To achieve this, clinical data points must be collected and stored in a database discretely. The design of ovarian cancer database application has successfully met these requirements allowing clinicians and statisticians to accurately analyze patient data and gain knowledge from obtained results to improve care for women with ovarian cancer.

7. Cross Hospital barriers

The Gynecologic Oncology Group of Ontario is beginning to implement eCANCER^ovarian at other major cancer center affiliated hospitals in the province (Rosen, B., Le, T., Elit, L., Goubanova, E., Fung Kee Fung, M., & Sadovy, B., 2007). The SMART Systems for Health Agency (SSHA) has facilitated this process. SSHA electronically connects all Ontario publicly-funded health care organizations and professionals. This electronic connection allows the exchange of patient information in a secure manner. SSHA is an agency of the Ontario Ministry of Health and Long-Term Care and provides products and services free. The difficulties currently being vetted include marrying eCANCER^ovarian to the myriad of EMR systems among the different hospitals. To bring demographic information into eCANCER^ovarian One needs to download this from various other systems like Meditech, CERNER, or MYSIS. To get the operative note out of eCANCER^ovarian into the hospital specific EMR, there also needs to be a bridge created. At the end of the day, whether the

data from various hospitals can be merged across sites depends on where the master data is housed and whether the intention is research or quality of care. The other main issue is the completeness of the data. If all hospital records require an operative note, and operations for all ovarian masses regardless of the surgeon's specialty are entered into eCANCER^ovarian it is more likely that the data will be inclusive.

The strengths of a database/EHR system include: easy access to ongoing patient care parameters regardless of geography or time of day; more reliable data as it is being captured at the time of activity (ie size of residual disease entered at the time of the operation); it may be a teaching tool to reinforce important aspects of surgery (ie., need for nodal assessment during surgery); data will lead to more relevant quality assessment; and the data may be available to other disciplines (such as tumor bank as is proposed in the National Cancer Institute (NCI) project Cancer Biomedical Informatics GRID (CaBIG)). As healthcare organizations move from paper-based to computerized patient records, the need to address the quality and accessibility of patient information stored electrically will become more evident. Care for complex and life threatening diseases such as ovarian cancer will require decision support systems that help to increase patient-interaction time, provide accurate and structured information at the point of care, and, consequently, improve clinician's quality of care.

Pathology Note

Dictated pathology notes suffer from the same inconsistencies in the kind of information pathologists require for reproducing findings, clinicians require for decision making and administrators require for quality assessments. "Leslie, K. O., and Rosai, J. (2004)" points out that "in making a diagnosis, we imply a predictive value of our assessment." However, the reports "show more idiosyncrasy than consistency in the thoroughness of documentation of findings". To this end the College of American Pathologists (CAP) promoted a synoptic pathology reporting format in 2003. The goal is that information would be captured in a standard way so that there is no pertinent information is missing. This will improve the ability to acquiring staging information for those cancers staged pathologically. It would allow for quick and accurate retrieval by a search query. This facilitates quality assurance and research activities. Although the CAP guidelines are not universally applied across the USA, there is a move to role out this system across Ontario, Canada hospitals. Currently the Cancer Care Ontario Quality Index (http://www.cancercare. on.ca/qualityindex2007/measurement/pathologyReports/index.html accessed 24Jan2008) has used breast, colon, prostate and lung cancer as the test sites. Such standardized reporting in ovarian cancer will only enhance the quality of the available information.

Issues Encountered in Computerizing and Sharing the Electronic Patient Medical Record

Privacy

Patient information is sensitive and needs to be handled in a manner that minimizes the risk of loss of privacy while achieving public good through improving patient care. In all countries there exist restrictions on the collection and sharing of personal information. In Canada, federal and provincial laws now define the characteristics of systems that strike the appropriate balance. In all provinces, the use of health information is now governed by legislation, which can be used to determine policies, procedures and formal approvals. This means that any new sharing of information from within one hospital to outside that facility has to achieve formal approval of the Provincial Ministry of Health as tested against those applicable pieces of legislation. For health

data, the one act that matters most in Ontario is the Personal Health Information Protection Act (PHIPA).

With cancer specific informatics, there is a move toward province-wide application instead of regional or ad hoc systems. It is possible but extremely difficult and slow to establish appropriate privacy-protection agreements and procedures between agencies by ad hoc pairing. Achieving agreement on the content and procedures between all hospitals and a central repository is much more efficient.

Effective protection of privacy also means that the hardware, software and Information Technology staff are in place. Ideally this would be handled by one agency as opposed to several different ones. This central unit would be housed at the ministry or in a centre that specifically has the mandate to take on this role and watch over it. Should eCANCER ovarian become a provincial rather than hospital based resource, housed at say Cancer Care Ontario, then the checks and balances and ownership responsibilities will fall under this provincial resource. Within this context, the evaluation focus becomes quality of care as opposed to research.

Currently, when clinical data are brought into ICES, the following procedures apply. First, confidentiality agreements are in place for all members of the research team (e.g., all abstractors, programmers and investigators). Data collected at remote locations are gathered using secure, password encrypted computers or comparable protocols. Data brought centrally to ICES are stripped of personal identifiers and transferred to a mainframe computer which has no connectivity with other local area networks or the internet, and to which access is strictly limited. All record-linkage and analysis of the data then takes place on the mainframe by qualified personnel. Export of individual level data (even if anonymized) is never permitted without separate and explicit agreements in place involving the originators of the data and the Provincial Ministry of Health.

Data Ownership

There are three possible owners of health data: the patient, the government and the provider (and this can be further subdivided into clinician and institution). The individual patient's ownership rights over health data are defined by the privacy legislation. In Canada, the provincial and federal government can require some movement of data to central repositories for the public good including evaluation and research provided certain principles are followed. These principles are legislated federally by the the Personal Information Protection and Electronic Documents Act (PIPEDA) and provincial by the PHIPA.

The federal and provincial governments can also claim ownership rights in a sense that they have a mandate to offer good value-for-money in health care. The Canadian Health Act ensures universal access to hospital care and there is mandatory data provision to the Canadian Institutes of Health Information (CIHI). The provinces are entitled to get data from care providers under their plans for physician, laboratory and drug benefits. These levels of government have legislative authority to require that providers give comprehensive data, meeting defined standards for timeliness and quality. The Health Ministries can withhold financial transfers in the event of non-compliance.

From time to time, these agencies expand their 'minimum required data'. For example, CIHI has national discussions about expanding their databases, and the provinces may opt in or out of additional CIHI fields. Provinces will periodically revise the mix of billing codes and associated dollars in their fee-for-service schedule in order to provide incentives toward good care and to more accurately track the type of care provided.

A thorny issue is the degree to which health care institutions and individual providers have any rights in terms of ownership over the data. Under the hospitals act, the hospital should use information for quality assurance and can use it for research for approved purposes and under approved procedures. However, the hospital does not have an absolute right to withhold data from the province if those data are required for approved for evaluation, monitory or research. Currently the province is trying to establish mechanisms whereby, in the context of a health crisis, it can get data expeditiously in order to affect care in a timely manner for others.

Benefits of Better Quality Data

Patient Information at the Point Of Care Delivery

Cancer Care Ontario currently hosts a number of datasets such as the Waiting times project which reports quarterly on the time from consult at a cancer centre to the time of treatment (ie., radiation therapy or surgery). Identifying wait times that are beyond benchmarks allow for system adjustments through initiatives or financial incentives. Having a resource like the eCANCER[ovarian] module or webSMR would allow better quality data such as size of residual disease at the end of surgery which could inform immediate issues like treatment decision making.

Using Variations in Care to Optimise Care Delivery

The ultimate goal of improving databases or the EMR is to improve the medical care of women with ovarian cancer. We have tried to outline in this chapter that in many countries, extensive work using databases show that variations in ovarian cancer care exist. Quality indicators have been developed to identify good care. These need to be implemented in a more timely fashion through a process like webSMR or eCANCER[ovarian] where higher quality information is obtainable. However, potential solutions to improving the quality of care must be designed, implemented and evaluated.

Centralization of oncologic surgical procedures has been one approach to improving quality of care. In pancreatic cancer, this approach has been shown to improve 30-day post-operative mortality "ESMO minimum clinical recommendations for diagnosis, treatment and follow-up of ovarian cancer," 2001, Given the imbalance in the number of trained subspecialists and resources in cancer hospitals compared to the volume of ovarian cancer patients a solution of centralizing ovarian cancer operations is not feasible and probably not necessary. Thus a knowledge transfer process needs to be developed. "Kerbrat, P., Lhomme, C., Fervers, B., Guastalla, J. P., Thomas, L., Tournemaine, N., et al. (2001)" has suggested that an ideal organizing framework for a knowledge translation strategy has 5 elements. These are: message, target audience, messenger, method of delivery and evaluation of the process. The message in ovarian cancer is an evidence-defined algorithm of situations and who and where is the best place for delivering operative care. The target audience are the gynecologists and surgeons who see women with pelvic masses and the administrators of hospitals in which operative care is delivered. The messenger is not clear (ie., the provincial cancer care body – Cancer Care Ontario, or a national society like the Society of Obstetrics and Gynecology). No one method of delivering a message has been found to be superior ie., audit and feedback, educational sessions by a respected peer, one on one mentoring to mention a few. Likely a multimethods approach is necessary. Once all of this is defined and implemented, it must then be evaluated to determine if ovarian cancer care has been improved or whether further system adjustments are necessary.

FUTURE

To improve the quality of ovarian cancer care will require on going evaluation of outcomes (ie., survival), structural factors (ie., physician and hospital parameters) and processes of care. Currently in Ontario the quality of care is monitored using the Cancer Care Ontario Quality Index (http://www.cancercare.on.ca/qualityindex2007). Here 6 areas are assessed: prevention, access, outcomes (ie., death after surgery, incidence, survival and death), compliance with evidence guidelines, efficiency and measurement.

Sufficiently detailed information is required so as to control for confounding. Systems like the webSMR or eCANCER[ovarian] have been developed with this in mind. The information must be available in a timely fashion so as to understand the impact of implementing a knowledge transfer strategy. All of this must be accomplished while upholding the tenants of privacy and ownership at the patient, provider, provincial and federal level.

ACRONYMS

- ACTION: Adjuvant chemotherapy in ovarian Neoplasm Trial
- CaBIG: Cancer Biomedical Informatics GRID
- CAP: College of American Pathologists
- CIHI: Canadian Institute for Hospital Information
- DePICT: Disease Specific Electronic Patient Illustrate Clinical Timeline
- EHR: Electronic Health Records
- ENA: Electronic note Automation
- EORTC: European Organization for Research and Treatment of Cancer
- GCG: Gynecologic Cancer Group
- GOG: Gynecologic Oncology Group
- GOSOCS: Gynecologic Oncology Surgical Ovarian Cancer System
- ICES: Institute for Clinical Evaluative Sciences
- IDS: Interval Debulking Surgery
- IT: Information technology

- NCI: National Cancer Institute
- OC: Ovarian Cancer
- PMH: Princess Margaret Hospital
- PFS: Progression Free Survival
- PHIPA: Personal Health Information Protection Act
- PIPEDA: Personal Information Protection and Electronic Documents Act
- RAND: Research ANd Development
- SEER: Surveillance Epidemiology and End Result
- SSHA: SMART System for Health Agency
- TAH+BSO: Total Abdominal Hysterectomy and Bilateral Salpingo-opphorectomy
- webSMR: Web Surgical Medical Record

REFERENCES

(2000). Guidelines for referral to a gynecologic oncologist: Rationale and benefits. The Society of Gynecologic Oncologists. *Gynecologic Oncology, 78*(3 Pt 2), t-13.

(2001). ESMO minimum clinical recommendations for diagnosis, treatment and follow-up of ovarian cancer. *Annals of Oncology, 12,* 1205-7.

(2003, May, June). Determinants of success of inpatient clinical information systems: A literature review. *JAMIA: 10,3,* 235-243.

Aletti, G. D., Dowdy, S. C., Gostout, B. S., Jones, M. B., Stanhope, R. C., Wilson, T. O., Podrzta, K. C., & Cliby, W. A. (2006). Aggressive surgical effort and improved survival in advanced-Stage Ovarian Cancer. *Obstet Gynecol, 107*(1), 1-11.

Allen, D. G., Baak, J., Belpomme, D., et al. (1993). Advanced epithelial ovarian cancer: 1993 consensus statements. *Ann Oncol, 4,* S83-S88.

Allen, D. G., Heinta, A. P. M., & Touw, F. W. M. M. (1995). A meta-analysis of residual disease and survival in stage 3 and 4 carcinoma of the ovary. *Eur J Gyn Oncol* 349-356.

Amatayjakul, M. (2005, November). Are you using an EHR – really? *Healthcare Financial Management, 59*(11), 126 .

Bondy, S., Elit, L., Chen, Z., Law, C., & Paszat, L. (2006). Prognostic factors for women with Stage 1 ovarian cancer with or without adhesions. *Eur Journal Gyn Onc, 27*(6), 585-588.

Bristow, R. E., Tomacruz, R. S., Armstrong, D. K., Trimble, E. L., & Montz, F. J. (2002). Survival effect of maximal cytoreductive surgery for advanced ovarian carcinoma during the platinum era: a meta-analysis. *J Clin Oncol, 20*(5), 1248-1259

Bristow, R. E., Zahurak, M. L., del Carmen, M. G., Gordon, T. A., Fox, H. F., Trimble, E. L. et al. (2004). Ovarian cancer surgery in Maryland: volume-based access to care. *Gynecol Oncol, 93,* 353-360.

Buchsbaum, H. J., Brady, M. F., Delgado, G., Miller, A., Hoskins, W., Manetta, A., et al. (1989). Surgical staging of carcinoma of the ovaries. *Surgery, Gynecology & Obstetrics, 169,* 226-32.

Canadian Partnership Against Cancer, Cancer Control Guidelines Action Group. (2007). *Opportunities for the Inter-Provincial Implementation of Synoptic Reporting Tools to Translate Standards and Guidelines into Practice for Cancer Surgery and Pathology.* Toronto, March 14, 2007.

Cancer Care Ontario Web site for Quality Care

Cancer of the ovary. (1991). ACOG Technical Bulletin Number 141. *Int J Gynecol Obstet, 35,* 359-66.

Carney, M. E., Lancaster, J. M., Ford, C., Tsodikov, A., & Wiggins, C. L. (2002). A Population-based study of patterns of care for ovarian cancer: Who is seen by a gynecologic oncologist and who is not? *Gyn Onc, 84,* 36-42

Chan, J. K., Munro, E. G., Cheung, M. K., Husain, A., Teng, N. N., Berek, J. S., & Osann, K. (2007).

Assocation of lymphadenectomy and survival in stage 1 ovarian cancer patients. *Obstet Gynecol, 109*(1)12-9.

Covens, A., Carey, M., Bryson, P., Verma, S., Fung Kee Fung, M., Daya, D., DePetrillo, D., Eisenhauer E., Elit, L., Fyles, Kerr, I., Lukka, H., Malik, S., Rosen, B., Thomas, G., & Yoshida, S. (N/A). First-line chemotherapy for postoperative patients with Stage II, III, or IV epithelial ovarian cancer. *Cancer Care Ontario Practice Guideline*, 4-1-2.

Crawford, S. C., Vasey, P. A., Paul, J., Hay, A., Davis, J. A., Kaye, S. B. (2006). SCOTROC. Does aggressive surgery only benefit patients with less advanced ovarian cancer? Results from an international comparison within the SCOTROC-1 trial. SGO 2006. *Abstract 5003*, 455s.

DeOrio, J. K. Surgical templates for orthopedics operative reports. *Orthopedics, 25*(6), 639-42.

Earle, C. C., Schrag, D., Neville, B. A., Yabroff, K. R., Topor, M. Fahey. A. et al. (2006, February 1). Effect of surgeon specialty on processes of care and outcomes for ovarian cancer patients. *J Natl Cancer Inst, 98*(3), 172-80.

Edhemovic, I., Temple, W. J., de Gara, C. J., & Stuart, G. C. (2004, October). The computer synoptic operative report--A leap forward in the science of surgery. *Ann Surg Oncol, 11*(10), 941-947.

Eisenkop, S. M., Frieman, R. L., & Wang, H. J. (1998). Complete cytoreductive surgery is feasible and maximizes survival in patients with advanced epithelial ovarian cancer: A prospective study. *Gyn Onc, 69*, 103-108

Eisenkop, S. M., Spirtos, N. M., Montag, T. W., Nalick, R. H., & Wang, H. J. (1992). The impact of subspecialty training on the management of advanced ovarian cancer. *Gynecol Oncol, 47*, 203-209.

Elit, L. (2005). Outcomes for Surgery in Ovarian Cancer. *In Progress in Ovarian Cancer Research*, Bardos, A. P. (Ed.). NY: Nova Science Publishers Inc. ISBN 1-59454-241-4.

Elit, L., Bondy, S., Chen, Z., Law, C., & Paszat, L. (2006, October). The quality of Operative Reports for women with ovarian cancer. JOGC, *28*(10), 892-897.

Elit, L., Bondy, S., Paszat, L., Chen, Z., Hollowaty, E., Thomas, G., & Levine, M. (2006, October). Outcomes in Surgery for Ovarian Cancer. *Submitted to Canadian Journal of Surgery.*

Elit, L., Bondy, S., Paszat, L., Przybysz, R., & Levine, M. (2002). Outcomes in Surgery for ovarian cancer. *Gyn Onc, 87*, 260-267.

Elit, L., Cartier, C., Oza, A., Hirte, H., Levine, M., & Paszat, L. (2006, May). Outcomes for Systemic therapy in ovarian cancer. *Gyn Onc, 103*(2), 554-8.

Elit, L., Chambers, A., Fyles, A., Covens, A., Carey, M., & Fung Yee Fung, M. (2004). Systematic Review of Adjuvant Care for Newly diagnosed Stage 1 Ovarian Cancer. *Cancer, 101*(9), 1926-35

Elit, L., Oliver, T. K., Covens, A., Kwon, J., Fung, M. F., Hirte, H. W., & Oza, A. M. (2007). Intraperitoneal chemotherapy in the first-line treatment of women with stage III epithelial ovarian cancer: A systematic review with meta-analyses. Cancer, *109*(4), 692-702. Review.

Elit, L., Plante, M., Bessette, P., DePetrillo, D., Ehlen, T., Heywood, M., et al. (2000). Surgical management of an adnexal mass suspicious for malignancy. *J Soc Obstet Gynecol Can, 22*, 964-8.

Engelen, M. J., Kos, H. E., Willemse, P. H., Aalders, J. G., de Bires, E. G., Schaapveld, M., Otter, R., & van der Zee, A. G. (2006). Surgery by consultant gynecologic oncologists improves survival in patients with ovarian carcinoma. *Cancer, 106*(3), 589-98.

Gangliardi, A. R., Fung Kee Fung, M., Langer, B., Stern, H., & Brown, A. D. (2005). Development of Ovarian Cancer Surgery Quality Indicators Using a Modified Delphi Approach. *Gyn Onc, 97*(2), 446-456.

Gibbs, D. D., & Gore, M. E. (2001). Pursuit of optimum outcomes in ovarian cancer. *Drugs, 61*, 1103-20.

Giede, K. C., Kieser, K., Dodge, J., & Rosen, B. (2005). Who should operate on patients with ovarian cancer? An evidence-based review. *Gyn Oncol.*

Gillis, C. R., Hole, D. J., Still, R. M., & Kaye, S. B. (1991). Medical audit, cancer registration and survival in ovarian cancer. *Lancet, 337*, 611-612.

Goff, B. A., Matthews, B. J., Larson, E. H., Andrilla, C. H., Wynn, M., Lishner, D. M., & Baldwin, L. M. (2007). Predictors of comprehensive surgical treatment in patients with ovarian cancer. *Cancer, 109(*10), 2031-42.

Goff, B. A., Matthews, B. J., Wynn, M., Muntz, H. G., Lishner, D. M., & Baldwin, L. M. Ovarian cancer: Patterns of surgical care across the United States. *Gyn Oncol, 103*, 383-399.

Goff, B., Larson, E., Mathews, B., Andrilla, H., Lishner, D., Baldwin, L., Lackey, M., & Muntz, H. (2006). What factors predict comprehensive surgical treatment of ovarian cancer patients? *Gyn Onc 101*, (S2), Abstract 1.

Grilli, R., Alexanian, A., Apolone, G., Fossati, R., Marsoni, S., Nicolucci, A. et al. (1990). The impact of cancer treatment guidelines on actual practice in Italian general hospitals: The case of ovarian cancer. *Annals of Oncology, 1*, 112-118.

Gynecologic Disease Site Group Program in Evidence-based Care. *Management of a Suspicious Ovarian Mass. Evidence Summary Report #4-15*, April 29, 2004

Hacker, N. F. (1995). Systematic pelvic and para-aortic lymphadenectomy for advanced ovarian cancer – Therapeutic advance or surgical folly? *Gyn Onc, 56*, 325-327.

Hacker, N. F., Berek, J. S., Lagasse, L. D., Nieberg, R. K., & Elashoff, R. M. (1983). Primary cytoreductive surgery for epithelial ovarian cancer. *Obstet Gynecol, 61*, 413.

Harlan, L. C., Clegg, L. X., & Trimble, E. L. (2003). Trends in surgery and chemotherapy for women diagnosed with ovarian cancer in the United States. *J Clin Oncol 21*(18), 3488-3494.

Heintz, A. P., Hacker, N. F., Berek, J. S., Rose, T. P., Munoz, A. K., & Lagsse, L. D. (1986). Cytoreductive Surgery in Ovarian Carcinoma: Feasibility and morbidity. *Obstet Gynecol, 67*, 783

Hole, D. J., & Gillis, C. R. (1993). Use of cancer registry data to evaluate the treatment of ovarian cancer on a hospital basis. Health Reports, 5(1), 117-119.

Hoskins, W. (1993). Surgical staging and cytoreductive surgery of epithelial ovarian cancer. *Cancer, 71*, 1534-40.

Hoskins, W., Rice, L., & Rubin, S. (1997). Ovarian cancer surgical practice guidelines. *Oncology, 11*, 896-904.

http://www.cancercare.on.ca/pdf/ovarianIndicatorsSummary.pdf (7 July 2007)

Donabedian, A. (1966). Evaluating the quality of medical care. *Milbanks Memorial Fund Quarterly, 44*, 166-206.

Hunter, R. W., Alexander, N. D. E., & Soutter, W. P. (1992). Meta-analysis of surgery in advanced ovarian carcinoma: Is maximum cytoreductive surgery an independent determinant of prognosis? *AJOG, 166*, 504-11.

Ioka, A., Tsukuma, H., Ajiki, W., & Oshima, A. (2004). Influence of hospital procedure volume on ovarian cancer survival in Japan, a country with low incidence of ovarian cancer. *Cancer Sci, 95*(3), 233-237.

Junor, E. (2000). The impact of specialist training for surgery in ovarian cancer. *Int J Gynecol Cancer, 10*(Supp 1), 16-18.

Junor, E. J., Hole, D. J., & Gillis, C. R. (1994). Management of ovarian cancer: Referral to a multidisciplinary team matters. *Br J Cancer, 70*, 363-370.

Junor, E. J., Hole, D. J., McNulty, L., Mason, M., & Young, J. (1999). Specialist gynecologists and survival outcome in ovarian cancer: a Scottish national study of 1866 patients. *Br J Obstet Gynecol, 106*, 1130-1136.

Junor, E. J., Hole, D. J., McNulty, L., Mason, M., & Young, J. (1999). Specialist gynecologists and survival outcome in ovarian cancer: A Scottist national study of 1866 patients. *Br J Obstet Gynecol, 106*(11), 1130-6.

Kehoe, S., Powell, J., Wilson, S., & Woodman, C. (1994). The influence of the operating surgeon's specialization on patient survival in ovarian carcinoma. *Br J Cancer, 70*, 1014-1017.

Kerbrat, P., Lhomme, C., Fervers, B., Guastalla, J. P., Thomas, L., Tournemaine, N., et al. (2001). Ovarian cancer. *British Journal of Cancer, 84*(Suppl2), 18-23.

Kikkawa, F., Ishikawa, H., Tamakoshi, K., Suganuma, N., Mizuno, K., Kawai, M. et al. (1995). Prognostic evaluation of lymphadenectomy for epithelial ovarian cancer. *J Surg Oncol, 60*, 227-231.

Kumpulainen, S., Grenman, S., Kyyronen, P., Pukkala, E., & Sankila, R. (2002). Evidence of benefit from centralized treatment of ovarian cancer: A nationwide population-based survival analysis in Finland. *Int J Cancer, 102*, 541-544.

Laflamme, M. R., Dexter, P. R., Graham, M. F., Hui, S. L., & McDonald, C. J. (2005). Efficiency, comprehensiveness and cost-effectiveness when comparing dictation and electronic templates for operative reports. *AMIA Annu Symp Proc.*, 425-9.

Le, T., Adolph, A., Krepart, G. V., Lotocki, R., Heywood, M. S. (2002). The benefits of comprehensive surgical staging in the management of early-stage epithelial ovarian carcinoma. *Gynecologic Oncology, 85*, 351-5.

Leblanc, E., Querleu, D., Narducci, F., Chauvet, M. P., Chevalier, A., Lesoin, A., et al. (2000). Surgical staging of early invasive epithelial ovarian tumors. *Seminars in Surgical Oncology, 19*, 36-41.

Leslie, K. O., & Rosai, J. (1994, November). Standardization of the Surgical Pathology Report: formats, templates and synoptic reports. *Sem Diag Pathology, 11*(4), 253-257.

Liberati, A., Mangioni, C., Bratina, L., Carinelli, G., Marsoni, S., Parazzini, F. et al. (1885). Process and outcome of care for patients with ovarian cancer. *Br M J 291*, 1007-1012/

Marrett, L., Dryer, D., Logan, H. et al. (2007). *Canadian Cancer Statistics 2007.*

Mayer, A. R., Chambers, S. K., Graves, E., Holm, C., Tseng, P. C., Nelson, B. E. et al. (1992). Ovarian cancer staging: Does it require a gynecologic oncologist? *Gyn Oncol, 47*, 223-227

Morgan, R. J., Copeland, L., Gershenson, D., et al. (1996). NCCN Ovarian Cancer Practice Guidelines. *Oncology, 10*, 293-310.

Munoz, K. A., Harlan, L. C., & Trimble, E. L. (1997). Patterns of care for women with ovarian cancer in the United States. *JCO,15*(11), 3408-3415.

Munro, E. G., Cheung, M. K., Husain, A., Teng, N. N., Chan, J. K., Leiserowitz, G. S., & Osann, K. (2006). The survival benefit of lymph node dissection in stage 1 epithelial ovarian cancer. *Gyn Onc 101*(S27), Abstract 59.

National Institute of Health. (1994). *Ovarian cancer: screening, treatment and follow-up,12,* 1-30.(Abstract).

Nguyen, H. N., Averette, H. E., Hoskins, W., Penalver, M., Sevin, B. U., & Steren, A. (1993). National Survey of ovarian carcinoma Part V. *Cancer, 72,* 3663-70.

NIH Consensus Development Panel on Ovarian Cancer. (1995). Ovarian cancer: screening, treatment, and follow-up. *JAMA, 273,* 491-497.

NIH. (2003). Guidance on the use of paclitaxel in the treatment of ovarian cancer.

Oberaigner, W., & Stuhlinger, W. (2006). Influence of department volume on cancer survival for gynecological cancers-A population-based study in Tyrol, Austria. *103, 527*-534.

Oksefjell, H., Sandstad, B., & Trope, C. (2006). Ovarian cancer stage 3C. Consequences of treatment level on overall and progression-free survival. *Eur J Gynecol Oncol, 27*(3), 209-14.

Olaitin, A., Weeks, J., Mocroft, A., Smith, J., Howe, K., & Murdoch, J. (2001, December 14). The surgical management of women with ovarian cancer in the south west of England. *Br J Cancer, 85*(12), 1824-30.

Ozols, R. F., Morgan, R. J., Copeland, L., & Gershenson, D. (1997). Update of the NCCN Ovarian Cancer Practice Guidelines. *Oncology, 11,* 95-100.

Petignat, P., Vajda, D., Joris, F., & Obrist, R. (2000). Surgical management of epithelial ovarian cancer at community hospitals: A population-based study. *Journal of Surgical Oncology, 75,* 19-23

Petru, E., Lahousen, M., Tamussino, K., Pickel, H., Stranzl, H., Stettner, H. et al. (1994). Lymph-adenectomy in stage 1 ovarian cancer. *AJOG, 170,* 656-62.

Piver, N., & Baker, T. (1986). The potential for optimal (<2cm) cytoreductive surgery in advanced ovarian carcinoma at a tertiary medical center; a prospective study. *Gyn Onc, 24,* 1-8.

Poissant, L., Perira, J., Tamblyn, R., & Kawasumi, Y. (2005). The impact of electronic health record on time efficiency of physicians and nurses: A Systematic Overview. *Journal of the American Medical Informatics Association, 12,* 505-516.

Puls, C, R., Morrow, M. S., & Blackhurst, D. (1997, November). Stage I ovarian carcinoma: Specialty-related differences in survival and management. *South Med J., 90*(11), 1097-100.

Reuss, E., Menozzi, M., Buchi, M., Koller, J., & Krueger, H. (2004). Information access at the point of care: What can we learn for designing a mobile CPR system? *International Journal of Medical Management, 73,* 363-369.

Rosen, B., Le, T., Elit, L., Goubanova, E., Fung Kee Fung, M., & Sadovy, B. (2007, May 23-24). Provincial synoptic Operative reporting. *Celebrating Innovations in Health Care Expo 2007.*

Schrag, D., Earle, C., Xu, F., Panageas, K. S., Yabroff, K. R., Bristow, R. E., Trimble, E. L., & Warren, J. L. (2006). Associations between hospital and surgeon procedure volumes and patient outcomes after ovarian cancer resection. *J Natl Cancer Inst, 98*(3), 163-71.

Scottish Intercollegiate Guidelines Network. (2003). *Epithelial ovarian cancer.*

Sengupta, P. S., Jayson, G. C., Slade, R. J., Eardley, A., & Radford, J. A. (1999). An audit of primary surgical treatment for women with ovarian cancer referred to a cancer center. *Br J Cancer, 80*(3/4), 444-447.

Shaw, M., Wolfe, C., Raju, K. S., & Papadopoulos, A. (2003). National Guidance on gynecological cancer management; an audit of gynecological cancer services and management in the South East of England. *Eur J Gynecol Oncol, 24*(2-4), 246-50.

Shylasree, T. S., Howells, R. E., Lim, K., Jones, P. W., Flander, A., Adams, M. et al. (2006). Survival in ovarian cancer in WalesL Prior to introduction of all Wales guidelines. *Int J Gyn Onc, 16*(5),1770-6.

Silber, J. H., Rosenbaum, P. R., Polsky, D., Ross, R. N., Even-Shoshan, O., Schartz, J. S. et al. (2007, April 1). Does ovarian cancer treatment and survival differ by the specialty providing chemotherapy? *J Clin Oncol., 25*(10),1169-75.

Skirnisdottir, E., & Sorbe, B. (2007). Prognostic factors for surgical outcome and survival in 447 women treated for advanced (FIGO stages 3-4) epithelial ovarian carcinoma. Int J Oncol, (3), 727-34

Tingulstad, S., Skjeldestad, F. E., & Hagen, B. (N/A). The effect of centralization of primary surgery on survival in ovarian cancer patients. *Ob Gyn, 102*, 499-505.

Tingulstad, S., Skjeldestad, F. E., Halvorsen, T. B., & Hagen, B. (2003). Survival and prognostic factors in patients with ovarian cancer. *Obstet Gynecol, 101*(5Pt1), 885-91

Trimbos, J. B., & Bolis, G. (1994). Guidelines for surgical staging of ovarian cancer. *Obstetrical and Gynecological Survey, 49*, 814-816.

Trimbos, J. B., Schueler, J. A., van der Burg, M., Hermans, J., van Lent, M., Heintz, A. P. M., et al. (1991). Watch and wait after careful surgical treatment and staging in well-differentiated early ovarian cancer. *Cancer, 67*, 597-602

Trimbos, J. B., Schueler, J. A., van Lent, M., Hermans, J., & Fleuren, G. J. (1990). Reasons for incomplete surgical staging in early Ovarian Carcinoma. *Gynecol Oncol, 37*, 374-377.

Trimbos, J. B., Schueler, J. A., van Lent, M., Hermans, J., & Fleuren, G. J. (1990). Reasons for incomplete surgical staging in early ovarian carcinoma. *Gynecologic Oncology, 37*, 374-7.

Trimbos, J. B., Vergote, I., Bolis, G., Vermorken, J. B., Mangioni, C., Madronal, C., Franchi, M., Tateo, S., Zanetta, G., Scarfone, G., Giurgea, L., Timmers, P., Coens, C., & Pecorelli, S. (2003). EORTC-ACTION collaborators. European Organisation for Research and Treatment of Cancer-Adjuvant ChemoTherapy in Ovarian Neoplasm. Impact of adjuvant chemotherapy and surgical staging in early-stage ovarian carcinoma: European Organisation for Research and Treatment of Cancer-Adjuvant ChemoTherapy in Ovarian Neoplasm trial. J Natl Cancer Inst., 15, *95*(2), 113-125.

Van Gorp, T., Amant, F., Neven, P., Berteloot, P., Leunen, K., & Vergote, I. (2006). The position of neoadjuvant chemotherapy within the treatment of ovarian cancer. *Minerva Ginecol, 58*(5), 393-403

Vergote, I., & Stuart, G. *Phase 3 study: Upfront debulking surgery versus neo-adjuvant chemotherapy, stage 3c or 4 epithelial ovarian cancer EORTC #55971, NCIC OV13*

Vernooij, F., Peter, A., Heintz, M., Witteveen, E., & van der Graff, Y. (2007, April 11). The outcomes of ovarian cancer treatment are better when provided by gynecologic oncologists and in specialized hospitals: A systematic review. *Gynecol Oncol.*

Williams, S. D., Goulet, R., & Thomas, G. (1996). Early ovarian cancer: A review of its genetic and biologic factors, detection, and treatment. *Curr Probl Cancer, 20*, 83-137.

Wimberger, P., Lehmann, N., Kimmig, R., Burges, A., Meier, W., & Du Bois, A. (2007). For the AGO-OVAR. Prognostic factors for complete debulking in advanced ovarian cancer and its impact on survival. An exploratory analysis of a prospectively randomized phase 3 study of the Arbeitsgemeinschaft Gynaekologische Onkologie Ovarian cancer study group (AGO-OVAR). *Gynecol Oncol, Ma3 28.*

Winter, W. E., Kucera, P. R., Rodgers, W., McBroom, J. W., Olsen, C., & Maxwell, G. L. (2002). Surgical staging in patients with ovarian tumors of low malignant potential. *Obstetrics & Gynecology, 100,* 671-6.

Wolfe, C. D., Tilling, K., & Raju, K. S. (1997). Management and survival of ovarian cancer patients in southeast England. *Eur J Cancer, 33*(11), 1835-40.

Woodman, C., Baghdad, A., Collins, S., & Clyma, J-A. (1997). What changes in the organization of cancer services will improve the outcome for women with ovarian cancer? *Br J Ob Gyn, 104,* 135-139.

Zanetta, G., Chiari, S., Rota, S., Bratina, G., Maneo, A., Torri, V., et al. (2007). Conservative surgery for stage I ovarian carcinoma in women of childbearing age. *British Journal of Obstetrics & Gynaecology, 104,* 1030-5.

APPENDIX 1: HISTOLOGIC TYPES OF OVARIAN CANCER

Epithelial Ovarian Cancer
    Invasive or Borderline or Benign
        Serous
        Mucinous
        Endometrioid
        Clear Cell
        Brenner
        Undifferentiated

Germ Cell Tumors
    Dysgerminoma
    Teratoma
        Immature
        Mature
            Solid
            Cystic
                Dermoid Cyst (mature cystic teratoma)
                Dermoid cyst with malignant transformation
        Monodermal and highly specialized
            Struma ovarii
            Carcinoid
            Struma ovarii and carcinoid
            Others
    Choriocarcinoma
    Endodermal Sinus Tumor
    Embryonal carcinoma
    Polyembryoma
    Mixed forms

Sex cord-Stromal Cell Tumors
    Granulosa-stromal cell
        Granulosa Cell Tumor
        Tumors in the thecoma-fibroma group
            Thecoma
            Fibroma
            Unclassified
    Androblastomas; Sertoli Leydig Cell Tumor
        Well differentiated
            Sertoli cell tumor
            Sertoli-Leydig cell tumor
            Leydig cell tumor; hilus cell tumor
        Moderately differentiated
        Poorly differentiated (sarcomatoid)
        With heterologous elements
    Gynandroblastoma
    Unclassified

APPENDIX 2: FIGO STAGING FOR PRIMARY CARCINOMA OF OVARY

Stage 1   Growth limited to the ovaries

     Stage 1a   Growth limited to one ovary; no ascites containing malignant cells, No tumor on the external surface; capsule intact.

     Stage 1b   Growth limited to both ovaries; no ascites containing malignant cells, No tumor on the external surface; capsule intact.

     Stage 1c   Tumor either Stage 1a or 1b but with tumor on the surface of one or both ovaries; or with capsule ruptured; or with ascites present containing malignant cells or with positive peritoneal washings.

Stage 2   Growth involving one or both ovaries with pelvic extension

     Stage 2a   Extension and/or metastases to the uterus and/or tubes

     Stage 2b   Extension to other pelvic tissues

     Stage 2c   Tumor either Stage 2a or 2b but with tumor on the surface of one or both ovaries; or with capsule(s) ruptured; or with ascites present containing malignant cells or with positive peritoneal washings

Stage 3   Tumor involving one or both with peritoneal implant outside the pelvis and/or positive retroperitoneal or inguinal nodes. Superficial liver metastasis equals Stage 3. Tumor is limited to the true pelvis, but with histologically proven malignant extension to small bowel or omentum.

     Stage 3a   Tumor grossly limited to the true pelvis with negative nodes but with histologically confirmed microscopic seeding of abdominal peritoneal surfaces

     Stage 3b   Tumor of one or both ovaries with histologically confirmed implants of abdominal peritoneal surfaces, none exceeding 2 cm in diameter. Nodes negative

     Stage 3c   Abdominal implants > 2cm in diameter and/or positive retroperitoneal or inguinal nodes

Stage 4   Growth involving one or both ovaries with disease metastasis. If pleural effusion is present, there must be positive cytologic test results to allot a case to Stage 4. Parenchymal liver metastases equals Stage 4.

APPENDIX 3: CALGARY SURGICAL WORKING GROUP: OVARIAN CANCER SURGERY: STAGING

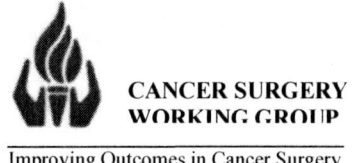

CANCER SURGERY WORKING GROUP

Improving Outcomes in Cancer Surgery

Section 1

DEMOGRAPHIC INFORMATION (AS PER HISCA STANDARDS)

Name:	Date: (yyyy/mm/dd)
DOB: (yyyy/mm/dd)	Date of Surgery:
Hospital number:	Name of Surgeon: CPSA #:
Diagnosis:	Patient's address:

A. PREOPERATIVE ASSESSMENT

Post Menopausal	❑ yes	❑ no	❑ unknown
Weight gain	❑ yes	❑ no	❑ unknown
Weight loss	❑ yes	❑ no	❑ unknown
Ascites present	❑ yes	❑ no	❑ unknown
Abdominal discomfort	❑ yes	❑ no	❑ unknown
Change in bowel habit	❑ yes	❑ no	❑ unknown
Decreased Appetite	❑ yes	❑ no	❑ unknown
Tenesmus	❑ yes	❑ no	❑ unknown
Melena/blood PR	❑ yes	❑ no	❑ unknown
Change in voiding patterns	❑ yes	❑ no	❑ unknown

Patient weight:_____kg
Patient height:_____cm
BMI calculator

FAMILY HISTORY

❑ Significant
❑ Non-significant
❑ Unknown
❑ If significant comment: (text box)

COMORBIDITIES

ASA

- ❑ 1 - healthy patient
- ❑ 11 - mild systemic disease, no functional limitation
- ❑ 111- severe systemic disease, definite functional limitation
- ❑ 1V - severe systemic disease, constant threat to life
- ❑ V - moribund patient, not expected to survive with or without an operation for 24 hours
- ❑ V1 – Clinically dead patients being maintained for harvesting of organs
- ❑ E- an emergency situation (used to modify one of the above classifications)

ECOG Performance Status

- ❑ 0 -Fully active, able to carry on all pre-disease performance without restriction
- ❑ 1 -Restricted in physically strenuous activity but ambulatory and able to carry out work of a light or sedentary nature
- ❑ 2 -Ambulatory and capable of all self care but unable to carry out any work activities. Up and bout > 50% waking hours
- ❑ 3 -Capable of only limited self care, confined to chair or bed >50% waking hours
- ❑ 4 -Completely disabled. Cannot carry on selfcare, totally confined to bed or chair
- ❑ 5 -Dead

B.   CLINICAL EVALUATION AND INVESTIGATIONS

PHYSICAL EXAMINATION

Clinical evidence of disease beyond ovary
- ❑ yes
- ❑ no

If "yes", specify site (branching question) multi select:
- ❑   Pelvis
- ❑   Abdomen
- ❑   Chest

Pleural effusion
- ❑ yes
- ❑ no

If yes,
- ❑   Left
- ❑   Right
- ❑   Bilateral

Preop Tx
- ❑ None
- ❑ Radiotherapy
- ❑ Chemotherapy

Liver disease
- ❑ yes
- ❑ no

If yes, liver disease diagnosis by:
- ❑ CT Scan
- ❑ Ultrasound

Biopsy
- ❑ yes
- ❑ no

INVESTIGATIONS

BLOOD TESTS

	normal	abnormal	not done	absolute level (text box)
CEA	normal	abnormal	not done	absolute level (text box)
AFP	normal	abnormal	not done	absolute level (text box)
HCG	normal	abnormal	not done	absolute level (text box)
LDH	normal	abnormal	not done	absolute level (text box)
Platelets	<150x10(9)L	>150X400(9)L	>400x10(9)L	
Albumin	<30g/L	>30g/L		
Hemoglobin	<100g/L	>100g/L		
SGOT/ AST	normal	abnormal	Not done	Absolute level (text)

Chest XRay
- ❑ yes
- ❑ no

If yes, Thoracentesis:
- ❑ Positive for cells
- ❑ Negative for cells
- ❑ If other specify (text box)

Ultrasound Done
- ❑ yes (branch to disease)
- ❑ no

If yes, disease beyond ovary:
- ❑ None
- ❑ Abdomen
- ❑ Pelvis
- ❑ Retroperitoneal nodes

CT Scan of Abdomen/Pelvis
- ❑ yes (branch to disease):
- ❑ no

If yes, disease beyond ovary:
- ❑ None
- ❑ Abdomen
- ❑ Pelvis
- ❑ Retroperitoneal nodes

MRI Abdomen/Pelvis
- ❑ yes
- ❑ no

If yes, disease beyond ovary
- ❑ None
- ❑ Abdomen
- ❑ Pelvis
- ❑ Retroperitoneal nodes

OTHER TESTS
Specify:_____

Previous Surgery
- ❑ Subtotal Hysterectomy
- ❑ Hysterectomy
- ❑ Left Ovary
- ❑ Right Ovary
- ❑ Appendectomy

End of Generic Section
1. Disease confined to ovary-proceed to (surgical staging)

C. OVARIAN CANCER SURGICAL STAGING

Position
- ❑ supine
- ❑ lithotomy
- ❑ exenteration

If "exenteration", specify (text box)

Anesthetic
- ❑ general
- ❑ regional
- ❑ combined regional and general

Incision
- ❑ midline
- ❑ paramedial
- ❑ transverse
- ❑ endoscopic

If other specify (text box)

Urinary bladder catheter
- ❑ yes
- ❑ no

Specialized instruments
- ❑ CUSA
- ❑ Argon beam laser
- ❑ CO_2 laser
- ❑ Bovie

Ascites present
- ❑ yes
- ❑ no

If yes, specify amount:
- ❑ < 100ml
- ❑ 100-1000ml
- ❑ > 1000ml

Ascites sent for cytology
- ❑ yes
- ❑ no
- ❑ Preoperatively positive

If no Ascites, cytology obtained from washings
- ❑ None
- ❑ Yes – Pelvic area
- ❑ Yes – Left gutter
- ❑ Yes – Right gutter
- ❑ Yes – Left diaphragm
- ❑ Yes – Right diaphragm

Ovarian mass
- ❑ not present
- ❑ left
- ❑ right
- ❑ bilateral

If not present, comment:

Size of mass
- ❑ < 5 cm
- ❑ 5-10 cm
- ❑ 10-15 cm
- ❑ 15-20 cm
- ❑ >20 cm

Clinically significant areas of adhesion
- ❑ yes
- ❑ no

If yes, biopsied
- ❑ yes
- ❑ no

Surface excrescencies
- ❑ yes
- ❑ no

Frozen section in OR
- ❑ yes
- ❑ no

If yes, result:_____

FINDINGS (SITES AND SURFACES) (SHOULD BE MULTI-SELECT)

(L) paracolic gutter
- ❑ examined
- ❑ found to be normal
- ❑ biopsy taken

(R) paracolic gutter
- ❑ examined
- ❑ found to be normal
- ❑ biopsy taken

Anterior abdominal wall
- ❑ examined
- ❑ found to be normal
- ❑ biopsy taken

(L) diaphragm
- ❑ examined
- ❑ found to be normal
- ❑ biopsy taken

(R) diaphragm
- ❑ examined
- ❑ found to be normal
- ❑ biopsy taken

Omentum
- ❑ examined
- ❑ found to be normal
- ❑ biopsy taken
- ❑ removed

If Omentum is removed select: (For Cytoreduction branch to Organs removed)
- ❑ Infracolic with suture/ligature
- ❑ Infracolic with LDS stapling device
- ❑ Supracolic with suture/ligature
- ❑ Supracolic with LDS stapling device

Spleen
- ❑ examined
- ❑ found to be normal
- ❑ biopsy taken

Liver
- ❑ examined
- ❑ found to be normal
- ❑ biopsy taken

Proximal small bowel serosa
- ❑ examined
- ❑ found to be normal
- ❑ biopsy taken

Proximal small bowel mesentery
- ❑ examined
- ❑ found to be normal
- ❑ biopsy taken

Appendix
- ❑ examined
- ❑ found to be normal
- ❑ biopsy taken

Distal small bowel serosa
- ❑ examined
- ❑ found to be normal
- ❑ biopsy taken

Distal small bowel mesentery
- ❑ examined
- ❑ found to be normal
- ❑ biopsy taken

Large bowel serosa
- ❑ examined
- ❑ found to be normal
- ❑ biopsy taken

Large bowel mesentery
- ❑ examined
- ❑ found to be normal
- ❑ biopsy taken

Sigmoid serosa
- ❑ examined
- ❑ found to be normal
- ❑ biopsy taken

Pouch of Douglas
- ❑ examined
- ❑ found to be normal
- ❑ biopsy taken

Bladder peritoneum
- ❑ examined
- ❑ found to be normal
- ❑ biopsy taken

Left Ovary
- ❑ examined
- ❑ found to be normal
- ❑ biopsy taken
- ❑ removed

Right Ovary
- ❑ examined
- ❑ found to be normal
- ❑ biopsy taken
- ❑ removed

Uterus
- ❑ examined
- ❑ found to be normal
- ❑ biopsy taken
- ❑ removed

LYMPH NODES (MUTUALLY EXCLUSIVE CATEGORIES) THIS SELECTION IS FOR STAGING ONLY

Pelvic nodes
- ❑ not assessed
- ❑ assessed by palpation and normal; not biopsied
- ❑ assessed by palpation and normal; biopsied
- ❑ assessed by palpation and abnormal; not biopsied
- ❑ assessed by palpation and abnormal; biopsied

Para-aortic nodes
- ❑ not assessed
- ❑ assessed by palpation and normal; not biopsied
- ❑ assessed by palpation and normal; biopsied
- ❑ assessed by palpation and abnormal; not biopsied
- ❑ assessed by palpation and abnormal; biopsied

Were there clinically significant areas of adhesions?
- ❑ yes
- ❑ no

If yes, were they biopsied?
- ❑ yes
- ❑ no

E.   PROCEDURE PERFORMED

LSO
- ❑ RSO
- ❑ LO
- ❑ RO
- ❑ Subtotal hysterectomy
- ❑ Total hysterectomy
- ❑ If no hysterectomy, endometrial biopsy
  - ❑ yes
  - ❑ no
  - ❑ preoperatively
- ❑ Omentectomy infracolic
- ❑ Omentectomy supracolic
- ❑ Appendectomy
- ❑ Pelvic lymph node dissection
- ❑ Para-aortic lymph node dissection

Catheter for intraperitoneal chemotherapy
- ❑ yes
- ❑ no

If yes, type of catheter:_____

Left ureter
- ❑ identified
- ❑ not identified
- ❑ ureterolysis
- ❑ ureter damaged, please comment

Right ureter
- ❑ identified
- ❑ not identified
- ❑ ureterolysis
- ❑ ureter damaged, please comment

TAH, if this is selected branch to:
retroperitoneal space opened,
- ❑ yes
- ❑ no

Bladder reflected (if this is selected, branch to:)
- ❑ sharp dissection
- ❑ blunt dissection

Uterine vessels skeletonized
- ❑ uterosacral ligaments clamped (if this is selected, branch to:)
- ❑ divided separately,
    - ❑ yes
    - ❑ no

paracervical tissue clamped separately,
- ❑ yes
- ❑ no

vaginal vault
- ❑ open
- ❑ closed

If closed:
- ❑ running whip stitch
- ❑ interrupted sutures

USO (L) If this is selected, (branch to:)
retroperitoneal space opened
- ❑ yes
- ❑ no

USO (R) If this is selected, (branch to:)
retroperitoneal space opened
- ❑ yes
- ❑ no

BSO If this is selected, (branch to:)
retroperitoneal space opened
- ❑ yes
- ❑ no

H.   CLOSURE

Abdominal Irrigation
- ❑ yes (branch)
- ❑ no

If yes, fluid type
- ❑ water
- ❑ saline
- ❑ other specify (text box)

Drains
- ❏ yes
- ❏ no

Drain type
- ❏ Jackson-Pratt
- ❏ Hemovac
- ❏ Blake
- ❏ Sump
- ❏ davol
- ❏ If other specify (text box)

Drain location
- ❏ LLQ
- ❏ RLQ
- ❏ LUQ
- ❏ RUQ
- ❏ subcutaneous

Hemostasis secured
- ❏ yes
- ❏ no
- ❏ oozing

If oozing, hemostatic agent type:_____

Sponge Count completed and correct
- ❏ yes
- ❏ no

Abdominal wall suture technique
- ❏ running
- ❏ interrupted
- ❏ smead jones

Abdominal wall suture type
- ❏ dexon
- ❏ maxon
- ❏ PDS
- ❏ Silk
- ❏ Vicryl

Size
- ❏ 0
- ❏ 1
- ❏ 2

Subcutaneous tissue
- ❑ approximated with suture
- ❑ not sutured

Skin Closure
Staples
- ❑ yes
- ❑ no

Sutures
Suture type
- ❑ absorbable suture
- ❑ non-absorbable suture
- No. of suture (s)
    - ❑ 2-0
    - ❑ 3-0
    - ❑ 4-0
- delayed closure
- ❑ yes
- ❑ no

Estimated Blood Loss (cc) :_____

blood units replaced/number of units?:_____

Operative time (minutes skin-to-skin) (text box)

Status of Patient
- ❑ stable
- ❑ unstable

Unit transferred to:
- ❑ recovery room
- ❑ ICU

H.   OTHER COMMENTS

SECTION II: OVARIAN CANCER SURGERY: CYTOREDUCTION

Known diagnosis of ovarian cancer
- ❑ yes
- ❑ no

Previous laparotomy to confirm diagnosis
- ❑ yes
- ❑ no

Pre-op findings
- ❑ pelvic mass
- ❑ pelvic mass plus ascites

Intent of surgery (mutually exclusive categories)
- ❑ primary cytoreduction
- ❑ interval debulking
- ❑ secondary debulking
- ❑ if secondary, comment:_____

OR positioning
- ❑ supine
- ❑ lithotomy
- ❑ exenteration position
  - If "exenteration position", specify (text box)

Urinary bladder catheter
- ❑ yes
- ❑ no

Anesthesia
- ❑ general
- ❑ regional
- ❑ combined general and regional

Incision (mutually exclusive categories)
- ❑ midline
- ❑ paramedial
- ❑ transverse
- ❑ other
- ❑ if other, specify (text box)

Use of specialized instruments
- ❑ CUSA
- ❑ Argon beam laser
- ❑ CO_2 laser
- ❑ Bovie

Ascites present
- ❑ yes
- ❑ no

If yes, specify amount:
- ❑ < 100ml
- ❑ 100 - 1000ml
- ❑ > 1000ml

Ascites sent for cytology
- ❑ yes
- ❑ no
- ❑ preoperatively positive

If no Ascites, cytology obtained from washings
- ❑ None
- ❑ Yes – Pelvic area
- ❑ Yes – Left gutter
- ❑ Yes – Right gutter
- ❑ Yes – Left diaphragm
- ❑ Yes – Right diaphragm

VISIBLE SITES OF DISEASE UPON OPENING

(L) paracolic gutter
Visible/Palpable Disease:
- ❑ yes
- ❑ no

If yes, specify
- ❑ single
- ❑ multiple

Largest single diameter (cm):
- ❑ < 1cm
- ❑ > 1cm - < 2cm
- ❑ > 2cm - < 5cm
- ❑ > 5cm

Resected:
- ❑ none
- ❑ partial resection
- ❑ complete resection

(R) paracolic gutter
Visible/Palpable Disease:
- ❑ yes
- ❑ no

If yes, specify
- ❑ single
- ❑ multiple

Largest single diameter (cm):
- ❑ < 1cm
- ❑ > 1cm - < 2cm
- ❑ > 2cm - < 5cm
- ❑ > 5cm

Resected:
- ❑ none
- ❑ partial resection
- ❑ complete resection

Anterior abdominal wall
Visible/Palpable Disease:
- ❑ yes
- ❑ no

If yes, specify
- ❑ single
- ❑ multiple

Largest single diameter (cm):
- ❑ < 1cm
- ❑ > 1cm - < 2cm
- ❑ > 2cm - < 5cm
- ❑ > 5cm

Resected:
- ❑ none
- ❑ partial resection
- ❑ complete resection

(L) diaphragm
Visible/Palpable Disease:
- ❑ yes
- ❑ no

If yes, specify
- ❑ single
- ❑ multiple

Largest single diameter (cm):
- ❑ < 1cm
- ❑ > 1cm - < 2cm
- ❑ > 2cm - < 5cm
- ❑ > 5cm

Resected:
- ❑ none
- ❑ partial resection
- ❑ complete resection

(R) diaphragm

Visible/Palpable Disease:
- ❑ yes
- ❑ no

If yes, specify
- ❑ single
- ❑ multiple

Largest single diameter (cm):
- ❑ < 1cm
- ❑ > 1cm - < 2cm
- ❑ > 2cm - < 5cm
- ❑ > 5cm

Resected:
- ❑ none
- ❑ partial resection
- ❑ complete resection

Omentum

Visible/Palpable Disease:
- ❑ yes
- ❑ no

If yes, specify
- ❑ single
- ❑ multiple

Largest single diameter (cm):
- ❑ < 1cm
- ❑ > 1cm - < 2cm
- ❑ > 2cm - < 5cm
- ❑ > 5cm

Resected:
- ❑ none
- ❑ partial resection
- ❑ complete resection

Spleen

Visible/Palpable Disease:
- ❑ yes
- ❑ no

If yes, specify
- ❑ single
- ❑ multiple

Largest single diameter (cm):
- ❑ < 1cm
- ❑ > 1cm - < 2cm
- ❑ > 2cm - < 5cm
- ❑ > 5cm

Resected:
- ❑ none
- ❑ partial resection
- ❑ complete resection

Liver

Visible/Palpable Disease:
- ❑ yes
- ❑ no

If yes, specify
- ❑ single
- ❑ multiple

Largest single diameter (cm):
- ❑ < 1cm
- ❑ > 1cm

Resected:
- ❑ none
- ❑ partial resection
- ❑ complete

Appendix

Visible/Palpable Disease:
- ❑ yes
- ❑ no

If yes, specify
- ❑ single
- ❑ multiple

Largest single diameter (cm):
    ❏   < 1cm
    ❏   > 1cm - < 2cm
    ❏   > 2cm - < 5cm
    ❏   > 5cm

Resected:
    ❏   none
    ❏   partial resection
    ❏   complete

Proximal Small Bowel Serosa

Visible/Palpable Disease:
    ❏   yes
    ❏   no

If yes, specify
    ❏   single
    ❏   multiple

Largest single diameter (cm):
    ❏   < 1cm
    ❏   > 1cm - < 2cm
    ❏   > 2cm - < 5cm
    ❏   > 5cm

Resected:
    ❏   none
    ❏   partial resection
    ❏   complete resection

Proximal Small Bowel Mesentery

Visible/Palpable Disease:
    ❏   yes
    ❏   no

If yes, specify
    ❏   single
    ❏   multiple

Largest single diameter (cm):
    ❏   < 1cm
    ❏   > 1cm - < 2cm
    ❏   > 2cm - < 5cm
    ❏   > 5cm

Resected:
    ❏   none
    ❏   partial resection
    ❏   complete resection

Distal Small Bowel Serosa
Visible/Palpable Disease:
- ❑ yes
- ❑ no
- If yes, specify
  - ❑ single
  - ❑ multiple
  - Largest single diameter (cm):
    - ❑ < 1cm
    - ❑ > 1cm - < 2cm
    - ❑ > 2cm - < 5cm
    - ❑ > 5cm
- Resected:
  - ❑ none
  - ❑ partial resection
  - ❑ complete resection

Distal Small Bowel Mesentery
Visible/Palpable Disease:
- ❑ yes
- ❑ no
- If yes, specify
  - ❑ single
  - ❑ multiple
  - Largest single diameter (cm):
    - ❑ < 1cm
    - ❑ > 1cm
- Resected:
  - ❑ none
  - ❑ partial resection
  - ❑ complete resection

Large Bowel Serosa
Visible/Palpable Disease:
- ❑ yes
- ❑ no
- If yes, specify
  - ❑ single
  - ❑ multiple
Largest single diameter (cm):
    - ❑ < 1cm
    - ❑ > 1cm

Resected:
- ❑ none
- ❑ partial resection
- ❑ complete resection

Large Bowel Mesentary
Visible/Palpable Disease:
- ❑ yes
- ❑ no

If yes, specify
- ❑ single
- ❑ multiple

Largest single diameter (cm):
- ❑ < 1cm
- ❑ > 1cm

Resected:
- ❑ none
- ❑ partial resection
- ❑ complete resection

Sigmoid Serosa
Visible/Palpable Disease:
- ❑ yes
- ❑ no

If yes, specify
- ❑ single
- ❑ multiple

Largest single diameter (cm):
- ❑ < 1cm
- ❑ > 1cm - < 2cm
- ❑ > 2cm - < 5cm
- ❑ > 5cm

Resected:
- ❑ none
- ❑ partial resection
- ❑ complete resection

Pouch of Douglas
Visible/Palpable Disease:
- ❑ yes
- ❑ no

If yes, specify
- ❑ single
- ❑ multiple

Largest single diameter (cm):
- ❑ < 1cm
- ❑ > 1cm - < 2cm
- ❑ > 2cm - < 5cm
- ❑ > 5cm

Resected:
- ❑ none
- ❑ partial resection
- ❑ complete resection

Bladder Peritoneum
Visible/Palpable Disease:
- ❑ yes
- ❑ no

If yes, specify
- ❑ single
- ❑ multiple

Largest single diameter (cm):
- ❑ < 1cm
- ❑ > 1cm - < 2cm
- ❑ > 2cm - < 5cm
- ❑ > 5cm

Resected:
- ❑ none
- ❑ partial resection
- ❑ complete resection

Pelvic Peritoneum
Visible/Palpable Disease:
- ❑ yes
- ❑ no

If yes, specify
- ❑ single
- ❑ multiple

If "pelvic peritoneum", specify
- ❑ bladder
- ❑ pouch of Douglas

Largest single diameter (cm):
- ❑ < 1cm
- ❑ > 1cm - < 2cm
- ❑ > 2cm - < 5cm
- ❑ > 5cm

Resected:
- ❑ none
- ❑ partial resection
- ❑ complete resection

Paraaortic

Visible/Palpable Disease:
- ❑ yes
- ❑ no

If yes, specify
- ❑ single
- ❑ multiple

If "pelvic peritoneum", specify
- ❑ bladder
- ❑ pouch of Douglas

Largest single diameter (cm):
- ❑ < 1cm
- ❑ > 1cm - < 2cm
- ❑ > 2cm - < 5cm
- ❑ > 5cm

Resected:
- ❑ none
- ❑ partial resection
- ❑ complete resection

Ovaries
- ❑ left
- ❑ right
- ❑ other

Uterus
- ❑ no disease on serosa
- ❑ disease on serosa
- ❑ other

Frozen section
- ❑ yes
- ❑ no

If yes,
- ❑ benign
- ❑ malignant

If malignant specify (text box)

Left Ureter
- ❑ identified
- ❑ not identified
- ❑ ureterolysis

If ureter damaged, comment

Right Ureter
- ❑ identified
- ❑ not identified
- ❑ ureterolysis

If ureter damaged, comment

E.   PROCEDURE PERFORMED

LSO
- ❑ RSO
- ❑ LO
- ❑ RO
- ❑ Subtotal hysterectomy
- ❑ Total hysterectomy
- ❑ If no hysterectomy, endometrial biopsy
  - ❑ yes
  - ❑ no
  - ❑ preoperatively
- ❑ Omentectomy infracolic
- ❑ Omentectomy supracolic
- ❑ Pelvic lymph node dissection
- ❑ Para-aortic lymph node dissection

Colon resection
- ❑ None
- ❑ Caecum
- ❑ Ascending colon
- ❑ Hepatic flexure
- ❑ Proximal transverse
- ❑ Mid transverse
- ❑ Distal transverse
- ❑ Splenic flexure
- ❑ Left colon
- ❑ Sigmoid colon
- ❑ Rectosigmoid junction

AP Resection
Stoma
- ❑ loop ileostomy
- ❑ end ileostomy
- ❑ loop colostomy
- ❑ end colostomy
- ❑ other

Stoma site
- ❑ LLQ
- ❑ RLQ
- ❑ RUQ
- ❑ LUQType of suture
- ❑ Dexon
- ❑ Maxon
- ❑ PDS
- ❑ vicryl
- ❑ Silk

Suture Size
- ❑ 4-0
- ❑ 3-0
- ❑ 2-0
- ❑ 0

Anastomosis
- ❑ hand sewn
- ❑ stapled

Staplers
- ❑ linear cutting
- ❑ transverse stapler
- ❑ circular stapler

Enterotomy closed with
- ❑ suture
- ❑ stapler

Comment on complications:_____

Catheter for intraperitoneal chemotherapy
- ❑ yes
- ❑ no

If yes, type of catheter:_____

TAH, if this is selected branch to:
Retroperitoneal space opened,
- ❑ yes
- ❑ no

Bladder reflected (if this is selected, branch to:)
- ❑ sharp dissection
- ❑ blunt dissection

Uterine vessels skeletonized
- ❑ uterosacral ligaments clamped (if this is selected, branch to:)
- ❑ divided separately
  - ❑ yes
  - ❑ no

Paracervical tissue clamped separately,
- ❑ yes
- ❑ no

Vaginal vault
- ❑ open
- ❑ closed

If closed:
- ❑ running whip stitch
- ❑ interrupted sutures
- ❑ other (text box)

Hemostasis secured
- ❑ yes
- ❑ no

USO (L) If this is selected, (branch to:)
Retroperitoneal space opened
- ❑ yes
- ❑ no

USO (R) If this is selected, (branch to:)
Retroperitoneal space opened
- ❑ yes
- ❑ no

BSO If this is selected, (branch to:)
retroperitoneal space opened
- ❑ yes
- ❑ no

G. Residual Disease
- ❑ microscopic
- ❑ macroscopic

SPECIFY SIZE (CM), RESIDUAL DISEASE (MULTI SELECT)

- ❑ (L) paracolic gutter
- ❑ (R) paracolic gutter
    - ❑ anterior abdominal wall
- ❑ (L) diaphragm
- ❑ (R) diaphragm
    - ❑ omentum
- ❑ Liver
- ❑ Appendix
- ❑ proximal small bowel serosa
- ❑ proximal small bowel mesentery
- ❑ distal small bowel serosa
- ❑ distal small bowel mesentery
- ❑ large bowel serosa
- ❑ large bowel mesentery
- ❑ sigmoid serosa
- ❑ Pouch of Douglas
- ❑ bladder peritoneum
- ❑ Pelvic lymph nodes
- ❑ Paraortic lymph nodes
- ❑ Left ovary
- ❑ Right ovary
- ❑ Uterus

H. Closure
Abdominal Irrigation
- ❑ yes (branch)
- ❑ no

If yes, fluid type
- ❑ water
- ❑ saline
- ❑ other specify (text box)

Drains
- ❑ yes
- ❑ no

Drain type
- ❑ Jackson-Pratt
- ❑ Hemovac
- ❑ Blake
- ❑ Sump
- ❑ davol
- ❑ If other specify (text box)

Drain location
- ❑ LLQ
- ❑ RLQ
- ❑ LUQ
- ❑ RUQ
- ❑ subcutaneous

Hemostasis secured
- ❑ yes
- ❑ no
- ❑ oozing

If oozing, hemostatic agent type:_____

Sponge Count completed and correct
- ❑ yes
- ❑ no

Abdominal wall suture technique
- ❑ running
- ❑ interrupted
- ❑ smead-jones

Abdominal wall suture type
- ❑ dexon
- ❑ maxon
- ❑ PDS
- ❑ Silk
- ❑ Vicryl

Size
- ❑ 4-0
- ❑ 3-0
- ❑ 2-0
- ❑ 0

Subcutaneous tissue
- ❑ approximated with suture
- ❑ not sutured

Skin Closure
Staples
- ☐ yes
- ☐ no

Sutures
Suture type
- ☐ absorbable suture
- ☐ non-absorbable suture

No. of suture (s)
- ☐ 2-0
- ☐ 3-0
- ☐ 4-0

Delayed closure
- ☐ yes
- ☐ no

Estimated Blood Loss (cc) :_____

Blood units replaced/number of units?
- ☐ none
- ☐ 1
- ☐ 2
- ☐ 3
- ☐ 4 or greater

Operative time (minutes skin-to-skin) (text box)
Status of Patient
- ☐ stable
- ☐ unstable

Unit transferred to:
- ☐ recovery room

SECTION III: CSWG: OVARIAN CANCER SURGERY: PALLIATIVE

Previous Surgery
- ☐ yes
- ☐ no

Date of diagnosis of cancer
- ❏ month:_____
- ❏ year:_____

FIGO Stage of Cancer
- ❏ I
- ❏ II
- ❏ III
- ❏ IV

Histopathology of Tumour:_____

Previous Chemo
- ❏ yes
- ❏ no

If yes,
- ❏ 1st line only
- ❏ 1,2
- ❏ 1,2,3
- ❏ > 3

Previous radiotherapy
- ❏ yes
- ❏ no

C.   CLINICAL EVALUATION AND INVESTIGATIONS

PHYSICAL EXAMINATION

Clinical evidence of disease beyond ovary
- ❏ yes
- ❏ no

If "yes", specify site (branching question) multi select
- ❏ pelvis
- ❏ abdomen
- ❏ chest

Pleural effusion
- ❏ yes
- ❏ no

If yes,
- ❏ left
- ❏ right
- ❏ bilateral

Liver disease:
- ❑ yes
- ❑ no

If yes, liver disease diagnosis by:
- ❑ CT Scan
- ❑ Ultrasound

Biopsy
- ❑ yes
- ❑ no

INVESTIGATIONS

BLOOD TESTS

	normal	abnormal	not done	absolute level (text box)
CEA	normal	abnormal	not done	absolute level (text box)
AFP	normal	abnormal	not done	absolute level (text box)
HCG	normal	abnormal	not done	absolute level (text box)
LDH	normal	abnormal	not done	absolute level (text box)
Platelets	<150x10(9)L	>150X400(9)L	>400x10(9)L	
Albumin	<30g/L	>30g/L		
Hemoglobin	<100g/L	>100g/L		
SGOT/AST	normal	abnormal	Not done	Absolute level (text)

Chest XRay
- ❑ yes
- ❑ no

If yes, Thoracentesis:
- ❑ positive for cells
- ❑ negative for cells,
- ❑ If other specify (text box)

Ultrasound done
- ❑ yes (branch to disease)
- ❑ no

If yes, disease beyond ovary:
- ❑ yes
- ❑ no

If yes, specify site:
- ❑ abdomen
- ❑ pelvis
- ❑ retroperitoneal nodes

CT Scan of Abdomen/Pelvis
- ❏ yes (branch to disease):
- ❏ no

If yes, disease beyond ovary:
- ❏ yes
- ❏ no

If yes, specify site:
- ❏ abdomen
- ❏ pelvis
- ❏ retroperitoneal nodes

MRI abdomen/pelvis
- ❏ yes
- ❏ no

If yes, disease beyond ovary
- ❏ yes
- ❏ no

If yes, specify site:
- ❏ abdomen
- ❏ pelvis
- ❏ retroperitoneal nodes

GI Studies
- ❏ yes
- ❏ no

If yes, specify
- ❏ Barium enema
- ❏ water soluble enema
- ❏ small bowel follow through
- ❏ Upper endoscopy
- ❏ Lower endoscopy

OPERATIVE DETAILS AND PROCEDURE

Left ureter
- ❏ identified
- ❏ not identified
- ❏ ureterolysis
- ❏ ureter damaged, please comment

Right ureter
- ❑ identified
- ❑ not identified
- ❑ ureterolysis
- ❑ ureter damaged, please comment

Small Bowel Resection
- ❑ yes
- ❑ no

Colon resection
- ❑ None
- ❑ Caecum
- ❑ Ascending colon
- ❑ Hepatic flexure
- ❑ Proximal transverse
- ❑ Mid transverse
- ❑ Distal transverse
- ❑ Splenic flexure
- ❑ Left colon
- ❑ Sigmoid colon
- ❑ rectosigmoid junction

Stoma
- ❑ none
- ❑ loop ileostomy
- ❑ end ileostomy
- ❑ loop colostomy
- ❑ end colostomy
- ❑ other

Stoma site
- ❑ LLQ
- ❑ RLQ
- ❑ RUQ
- ❑ LUQType of suture
- ❑ Dexon
- ❑ Maxon
- ❑ PDS
- ❑ Vicryl
- ❑ Silk

Suture Size
- ❑ 4-0
- ❑ 3-0
- ❑ 2-0
- ❑ 0

Anastomosis
- ❑ hand sewn
- ❑ stapled

Staplers
- ❑ linear cutting
- ❑ transverse stapler
- ❑ circular stapler

Enterotomy closed with
- ❑ suture
- ❑ stapler

Comment on complications:_____

Mucous Fistule
- ❑ yes
- ❑ no

Gastrostomy tube
- ❑ yes
- ❑ no

Bypass for gastrointestinal tract
- ❑ yes
- ❑ no

If yes, comment:_____
  Procedure aborted:
  - ❑ yes
  - ❑ no

  If yes, comment:_____

H. Closure
Abdominal Irrigation
- ❑ yes (branch)
- ❑ no

If yes, fluid type
- ❑ water
- ❑ saline
- ❑ other specify (text box)

Drains
- ❑ yes
- ❑ no

Drain type
- ❑ Jackson-Pratt
- ❑ Hemovac
- ❑ Blake
- ❑ Sump
- ❑ davol
- ❑ If other specify (text box)

Drain location
- ❑ LLQ
- ❑ RLQ
- ❑ LUQ
- ❑ RUQ
- ❑ subcutaneous

Hemostasis secured
- ❑ yes
- ❑ no
- ❑ oozing

If oozing, hemostatic agent type:_____

Sponge Count completed and correct
- ❑ yes
- ❑ no

Abdominal wall suture technique
- ❑ running
- ❑ interrupted
- ❑ smead jones

Abdominal wall suture type
- ❑ dexon
- ❑ maxon
- ❑ PDS
- ❑ Silk
- ❑ Vicryl

Size
- ❑ 0
- ❑ 1
- ❑ 2

Subcutaneous tissue
- ❑ approximated with suture
- ❑ not sutured

Skin Closure
Staples
- ❑ yes
- ❑ no

Sutures
Suture type
- ❑ absorbable suture
- ❑ non-absorbable suture

No. of suture (s)
- ❑ 2-0
- ❑ 3-0
- ❑ 4-0

delayed closure
- ❑ yes
- ❑ no

Estimated Blood Loss (cc) :_____

Blood units replaced/number of units?:_____

Operative time (minutes skin-to-skin) (text box)

Status of Patient
- ❑ stable
- ❑ unstable

Unit transferred to:
- ❑ recovery room
- ❑ ICU

I. OTHER COMMENTS

APPENDIX 4: ONTARIO RETROSPECTIVE POPULATION BASED COHORT (ELIT, L., ET AL. 2006).

1. Screen: Exclusion Criteria

1.1   Health record number

1.2   Patient does not meets inclusion criteria
-no initial surgery
-diagnosis and treatment of ovarian cancer before January 1996
-initial surgery before January 1996
-initial surgery for ovarian cancer after December 1998
-Pathology show low malignant potential epithelial ovarian cancer, germ cell ovarian cancer, stromal ovarian cancer (ie., granulosa cell tumor), or disease metastatic to the ovary

2. Screen: Demographic

2.1   Health Card Number

2.2   Date of Birth

2.3   Postal code

3. Screen: Location and Date of Path Report

3.1   MOH code for institution where pathology performed

3.2   If unknown code, then type name

3.3   Year of initial procedure (should be 1996, 1997, 1998)

3.4   Name of Most responsible surgeon

3.5   Discipline of Most responsible surgeon is a Gynecologist, gynecologic oncologist, general surgeon

3.6   Name of other surgeons attending the OR

3.7   Discipline of other surgeon attending OR ie., gynecologist, gynecologic oncologist, general surgeon, urologist (option to repeat this field twice)

3.8   Date of first Cancer Clinic Appointment

3.9   Date of referral from family doctor

3.10   Date of referral from specialist (gynecologist, general surgeon etc).

4. Screen: Comorbidities

4.1   Charlton Score

4.2   Prior diagnosis of cancer: Yes, no

4.3   What diagnosis: Breast, colon, uterine, cervical

5. Screen: Pre-operative investigations

5.1   Documentation of a pelvic exam (yes, no)

5.2   Pelvic exam shows no mass, mobile mass, fixed hard mass

5.3   Rectal exam (yes, no)

5.4   Abdominal exam (yes, no)

5.5   CXR: (Normal, Small effusion, Large effusion)

5.6   Abdominal and/or Pelvic U/S or CT scan (done or not done)

5.7   CA125 (done or not done and value)

5.8	Date pelvic mass was diagnosed
5.9	Preoperative consult with gynecologic oncology (yes, no)
5.10	Preoperative consult with medical oncology (yes, no)

6. Screen: Clinical Description of the Surgery

6.1	Surgery: emergent, urgent, elective
6.2	Surgery date
6.3	Incision: Vertical, Pfannenstiel, Laparoscopy
6.4	Findings –Assessed yes/no/not assessed in the following areas: Abdominal wall biopsy Ovary: left ovary, right ovary Fallopian Tube: left tube, right tube Intestine: Appendix, Cecum, Colon, Sigmoid colon, small intestine, transverse colon Lymph node: groin, para-aortic, pelvic, external iliac, supraclavicular Omentum Peritoneum: appendix epiploica, bladder peritoneum (urinary bladder serosa), Cul de sac (pouch of Douglas), Hemidiaphragm (right, left), Para-colic gutter (colic gutter –right, left), Pelvic side wall, sigmoid colon (mesentery, epiploica), small bowel mesentery Uterus
6.5	Tumor clinically present: Yes/no/not assessed Abdominal wall biopsy Ovary: left ovary, right ovary Fallopian Tube: left tube, right tube Intestine: Appendix, Cecum, Colon, Sigmoid colon, small intestine, transverse colon Lymph node: groin, para-aortic, pelvic, external iliac, supraclavicular Omentum Peritoneum: appendix epiploica, bladder peritoneum (urinary bladder serosa), Cul de sac (pouch of Douglas), Hemidiaphragm (right, left), Para-colic gutter (colic gutter –right, left), Pelvic side wall, sigmoid colon (mesentery, epiploica), small bowel mesentery Uterus

7 Screen: Intraoperative events

7.1	Date of admission
7.2	Start time for surgery
7.3	End time for surgery
7.4	Estimated blood loss
7.5	Blood transfusion (yes, no, and number of units)
7.6	ASA score
7.7	Date of discharge

8 Screen: Pathology Parameters

8.1   Tissue submitted for histology at initial surgery:

        Binomial response: yes/no/not clear

Ascites or washings
Abdominal wall biopsy
Ovary: left ovary, right ovary
Fallopian Tube: left tube, right tube
Intestine: Appendix, Cecum, Colon, Sigmoid colon, small intestine, transverse colon
Lymph node: groin, para-aortic, pelvic, external iliac, supraclavicular
Omentum
Peritoneum: appendix epiploica, bladder peritoneum (urinary bladder serosa), Cul de sac (pouch of Douglas), Hemidiaphragm (right, left), Para-colic gutter (colic gutter –right, left), Pelvic side wall, sigmoid colon (mesentery, epiploica), small bowel mesentery, Urinary Bladder (Dome of bladder)
Uterus

8.2   Frozen section done at time of OR: yes/no

8.3   Findings in the tissue that was submitted
     Binomial response: was there cancer? yes/no/not clear

9. Screen: Histology

9.1   Epithelial Ovarian Cancer: yes/no/not clear

9.2   Type: Serous carcinoma (Papillary serous), Mucinous cystadenocarcinoma, Endometrioid cystadenocarcinoma, Clear Cell Cystadenocarcinoma, Transitional cell cystadenocarcinoma, Mixed Mesodermal Tumor, Small cell anaplastic, Undifferentiated Unclassified

9.3   Grade: Well differentiated, Moderately differentiated, Poorly differentiated, Undifferentiated, Not stated

10. Screen: Cytology

10.1   Site of cytology: Ascites, Peritoneal fluid, Ovary, Chest (Pleural), Groin Node, Supraclavicular node

10.2   Date of cytology

10.3   Diagnosis: Benign, Suspicious, Malignant

11. Screen: Staging

11.1   Stage 1 – confined to one ovary
        Stage 1A – confined to one ovary
        Stage 1B – involving both ovaries
        Stage 1C – 1A or 1B with tumor on surface of ovary, capsule rupture or malignant ascites
    Stage 2 – confined to pelvis
        Stage 2A – extension or metastases to uterus and or tubes
        Stage 2B – extension to other pelvic tissues
        Stage 2C – 2A or 2B with tumor on surface of ovary, capsule rupture, malignant ascites
    Stage 3 – intra-abdominal spread or involving groin node
        Stage 3A-Tumor limited to pelvis with negative nodes and microscopic seeding of abdominal peritoneal surfaces
        Stage 3B – Tumor of one or both ovaries with histologically confirmed implants on peritoneal surfaces all < 2 cm
        Stage 3C – Abdominal implants greater than 2cm and/or positive retroperitoneal or inguinal nodes
    Stage 4 – into liver. Outside of abdomen

12. Postoperative care

12.1   Lowest serum albumen level while in hospital

12.2   Use of TPN or enteral feeds: yes/no

12.3   Admission to ICU or surgical step down unit: yes or no

13. Second Surgery

13.1 Purpose of second surgery
-prior to chemotherapy for staging/debulking
-prior to chemotherapy due to complication (post operative bleed, bowel obstruction)
-during chemotherapy cycles (interval debulking surgery)
-at the end of chemotherapy

13.2 Date of second surgery

13.3 If second surgery prior to chemotherapy then repeat screen 2 and 3

14. Screen Adjuvant Chemotherapy

14.1 Chemotherapy: yes/no/not clear

14.2 Timing of chemotherapy: Presurgery, Postsurgery, No surgery

14.3 Patient Height (cm)

14.4 Patient Weight (kg)

14.5 Doctor's Discipline: Medical oncology, gynecologic oncology, other

14.6 Name of doctor ordering chemotherapy

14.7 Address of doctor

14.8 Date (for each treatment)

14.9 Agent (first-line chemotherapy): Cisplatin, Carboplatin, Taxol, Adriamycin, VP16 (etoposide), Cyclophosphamide, Topotecan, Caelyx

14.10 Dose for each drug: Repeat Agent, dose and date 8 times

14.11 Derive a total dose for each drug (mg)

14.12 Derive time of treatment (days from first treatment to last)

15. Screen Radiation Therapy

15.1 Radiation therapy given as the initial treatment: Yes/no/not clear

15.2 Site of radiation: pelvic, abdominal, other

15.3 Dose in cGy by the number of treatment days by the number of days from beginning to end of treatment (Start and End date)

16. Outcome Information

16.1 Date of first Recurrence

16.2 Date of Death

Table 1. Guidelines and reviews providing recommendations for the surgical management of a suspicious ovarian mass

Article	TAH + BSO	Laparotomy	Inspection of peritoneal surfaces	Peritoneal washings	Biopsies of suspicious lesions	Pelvic & para-aortic node sampling	Omentectomy	Appendectomy	Debulking
Guidelines									
EORTC, 2003	-	-	✓	✓	✓	✓	✓	-	-
ESMO, 2001	✓	✓	-	✓	✓	✓	✓	-	-
SOR, 2001	✓	-	✓	✓	✓	✓	✓	✓	✓ -- advanced
SGO, 2000*	-	-	-	-	-	-	-	-	-
SOGC, 2000	✓	-	✓	✓	✓	✓	✓	-	✓ -- advanced
NCCN, 1997 & 1996	✓	✓	-	-	-	-	-	-	✓
SSO, 1997	✓	-	-	✓	✓	✓	✓	-	-
NIH, 1994	✓	✓	-	✓	✓	✓	✓	-	✓
ACOG, 1991	✓	-	✓	✓	✓	✓	✓	-	-
Reviews									
Gibbs, 2001**	✓	✓	✓	✓	✓	✓	-	-	-
Leblanc, 2000	✓	-	✓	✓	✓	✓	✓	✓	-
Williams, 1996***	✓	✓	✓	✓	✓	✓	✓	-	-
Hoskins, 1993	✓	-	-	✓	✓	✓	-	-	-

Note: ACOG, American College of Obstetricians and Gynecologists; BSO, bilateral salpingo-oophorectomy; EORTC, European Organisation for Research and Treatment of Cancer; ESMO, European Society for Medical Oncology; NCCN, National Comprehensive Cancer Network; NIH, National Institutes of Health; SGO, Society of Gynecologic Oncologists; SOGC, Society of Obstetricians and Gynaecologists of Canada; SOR, Standards, Options & Recommendations; SSO, Society of Surgical Oncology; TAH, total abdominal hysterectomy

*SGO stressed the importance of surgical staging in their guideline, but did not provide specific recommendations for procedures
**TAH + BSO is optional in early stage patients—dependent upon fertility
***Suspected early stage recommendations
Reprinted with permission from Program in Evidenced Based Medicine – Cancer Care Ontario Guideline Management of Suspicious Ovarian Mass Evidence Summary Report 4-15, Table 6

Table 2. Prospective and retrospective studies' definitions of complete surgical staging

Study	TAH + BSO	Inspection of peritoneal surfaces	Peritoneal washings	Biopsies of suspicious lesions	Pelvic & para-aortic node sampling		Appendec-tomy
Le, 2002	✓	✓	✓	✓	✓	✓	-
Winter, 2002	✓	-	✓	✓	✓	-	-
Petignat, 2000	✓	✓	✓	✓	✓	-	-
Zanetta, 1997	✓	-	-	✓	✓	✓	✓
Trimbos, 1991	✓	✓	✓	✓	✓	✓	-
Buchsbaum, 1989	✓	-	-	✓	✓	-	✓

Reprinted with permission from the Program in Evidence Based Medicine Management of a Suspicious Ovarian Mass. Evidence Summary Report #4-15, April 29, 2004

Table 3. Outcomes from the studies investigating intraoperative management

Study	Type of study	# of patients	Surgical staging	Outcome
Le, 2002	Retrospective	94	Complete	82% disease-free after a median of 58 months
		44	Incomplete	66% disease-free after a median of 58 months
Winter, 2002]	Retrospective	48	Complete	3 (6.3%) patients had recurrences
		45	Incomplete	3 (6.7%) patients had recurrences
Zanetta, 1997	Retrospective	43	Complete	multivariate analysis of disease-free survival p=0.036 (in favour of complete surgery), overall survival p=0.124)
		56	Incomplete	
Trimbos, 1991	Retrospective	24	Complete	100% 5-year disease-free survival
		43	Incomplete	88% 5-year disease-free survival
Trimbos, 1990	Retrospective	46	Complete	15% postoperative complications
		40	Incomplete	30% postoperative complications

Reprinted with permission from the Program in Evidence Based Medicine Management of a Suspicious Ovarian Mass. Evidence Summary Report #4-15, April 29, 2004

Table 4. Factors affecting outcome when assessing debulking surgery

	Era	Type of Study	Number of patients	Definition of groups	Factors that impact on Survival
EORTC		RCT	Pending		Pending
Bristow	1989-1998			For every increase in cytoreduction by 10%	Increases by 5.5%
Hunter		Meta-analysis	6962		Chemotherapy Residual disease
Allen		Meta-analysis		None <2cm >2cm	Residual
Tingulstad	1987-1996 Norway	Retrospective population based	571		Stage Residual Age
Skirnisdottir	Sweden	Retrospective population based	447 stg 3-4		Residual disease
Aletti	1994-1998	Retrospective cohort	194 Stg 3C	<1cm >1cm	Residual disease
Eisenkop	1990-1996	Prospective	263 St 3c-4	<1cm >1cm	Residual Histology Age
Crawford	Scotland		1077		PFS-residual disease

Table 5. Outline for this section

Stage	Structural Variable	Outcome
Early Stage Disease (Stage 1-2)	Type of Hospital	Lymphadenectomy
	Hospital Volume of Cancer Surgery	
	Surgeon Specialty	
	Surgeon's Volume	
	Type of Hospital	Survival
	Hospital Volume of Cancer Surgery	
	Surgeon Specialty	
	Surgeon's Volume	

Table 6. The impact of various structural variables on outcomes in population based studies of early stage ovarian cancer

	Population	Variables found to impact Lymphadenectomy	Variables found to impact Survival
Giede 2005	18 studies	Surgeon specialty	Surgeon specialty
Hole 1974	59 Stage 1-2 Scotland		Hospital Type
Mayer 1992			Surgeon specialty
Pul 1997	54 Stage 1 Texas, Kentucky	Surgeon type	Surgeon Type
Junor 1999	1866 total 1987, 1992-1994		*Not Surgeon specialty*
Carney 2002	848 total 1992-1998 Utah		*Not surgeon specialty*
Engelen 2006	680 (total or stage 1-2) Stage 1-2 1994-1997 Netherlands	Surgeon type	
Earle 2006	1992-1999 women >65yr	Surgeon type	
Goff 2006	10432 women 1999-2002	Hosp type Hosp volume Surgeon volume	

Table 7. The impact of various structural variable on outcomes in population based studies of advanced stage ovarian cancer

Author	Number[a]	Study type	Optimal debulking [b]	Survival [c]
Vernooj 2007		Systematic Review	Surgeon Specialty	
Giede 2005		Systematic Review		Surgeon Specialty
Liberati 1985	1978-1979	Retrospective cohort		*No impact of Hospital type*
Hole 1993	200 total 1974 Scotland	Retrospective cohort		*No impact of Hospital type*
Junor 1987	533 total 1987 Scotland	Retrospective cohort		Surgeon Specialty Residual Disease Platinum Chemotherapy MTD

continued on following page

Table 7. continued

Eisenkop 1992	263 Stage 3C-4A USA	Retrospective cohort	Size of largest metastases Surgeon Specialty	Surgeon Specialty Residual Disease Grade Frozen tumor
Nguyen 1993	12,316 total 1983-1988			Surgeon specialty
Kehoe 1994	1184 total 1985-1987 UK	Retrospective cohort		Surgeon Specialty Stage Age Residual disease
Woodman 1997	UK			Surgeon specialty Referal to oncologist *No impact from surgeon volume*
Wolfe 1997	118 total UK	Prospective Audit	Hospital type	
Junor 1999	Stage 3 1987, 1992-4 Scotland	Retrospective cohort		Surgeon Specialty
Olaitin 2001	682 1997-1998 England		Surgeon type	
Elit 2002	3815 1992-1998 Canada	Retrospective cohort		Surgeon type *Not Hosp Vol* *Not Surg Vol*
Carney 2002	848 Total Stage 3-4 Utah, USA	Retrospective cohort		Surgeon specialty
Kumpulainen 2002	3851 total 1983-1994 Finland	Retrospective cohort		Hospital type
Tingulstad 2003	1992-1997 Norway	Historical prospective cohort		Adjuvant chemotherapy Residual Disease Hospital type
Bristow 2004	2417 total 1990-2000 Maryland	Retrospective cohort		Surgeon Volume
Ioka 2004	2450 total 1975-1995 Osaka	Retrospective cohort		Hospital Volumes
Earle 2006	Stage 3-4 1992-1999 USA	Retrospective cohort	Surgeon Specialty	Surgeon Specialty
Engelen 2006	680 total 1994-1997 Netherlands	Retrospective cohort	Surgeon Specialty	Surgeon Specialty
Oberaigner 2006	Austria	Retrospective cohorts		Hospital volumes

continued on following page

Schrag 2006	2952 1992-1999 USA	Retrospective cohort		Hospital volumes Not surgeon volume
Shylasree 2006	287 total Wales	Retrospective cohort		Hospital Type
Oksefjell 2006	776 Stage 3 1985-2000 Norway	Retrospective cohort		Surgical Specialty Residual Disease
Wimberger 2007		Retrospective cohort	Surgeon Specialty	Surgeon Specialty
Elit 2007	1341 total All stages 1996-1998 Canada	Retrospective cohort		Age Comorbidity Advanced Stage Higher Grade Emergent surgery Adjuvant chemotherapy
Goff 2007		Retropesctive review	Hospital Volume in non-teaching hospitals	

a – Number – where numbers for Stage 3-4 cases were available these were included. When a population study was completed and only conclusions on the whole population were available, given that stage 3 and 4 accounts for 75% of all cases, that study was included in this table of advanced disease.

b - factors that are statistically significantly associated with optimal debulking

c - factors that are statistically significantly associated with survival

MTD – multidisciplinary team

Section V
Knowledge and Information Management and Use

Chapter XIII
Women's Health and Health Informatics:
Perinatal Care Health Education

Jamila Abuidhail
Faculty of Nursing, The Hashemite University, Jordan

ABSTRACT

Information and communication technologies include computers, telecommunication, digital networks, and television. Using informatics in healthcare systems can improve the quality of healthcare through the effective use of information systems. Nursing Informatics (NI) is a component of health informatics, and it has become a widely used tool in the nursing profession. Information technology has begun to be employed in the field of women's health. The perinatal period is one of the topics related to women's health, as well as to that of their newborn infants. Information technology in patients' health education process empowered patients, and enhanced their self-management skills. However, applications of health informatics in perinatal care for women and their newborn infants have not been reported widely in research studies and projects. Thus, there is a gap of knowledge related to this topic on the Internet.

INTRODUCTION

Everywhere in the world the Internet has entered homes, schools, universities, work places, and hospitals, becoming as wide spread as television. Furthermore, the World Wide Web is visited by millions of people daily for various purposes.

Many people use the Internet to search for health information or to provide health education from the health care professionals and organizations.

Using informatics in the health care systems can improve the quality of health care through the effective use of information systems; the facilitation of knowledge and information management by on-line and on-site databases and electronic medical records (EMR); the enhancement of decision making by using computerized decision support systems; and improvements to the communication between patients and providers by sharing access to electronic medical records and using e-mails to further exchange information.

In this chapter, an overview of health informatics and nursing informatics will be presented. Major main concepts of health informatics will be discussed. Then women's health and perinatal care through health informatics will be focused on. After that the relationship between health education and health informatics will be discussed. Finally the major barriers against using health informatics applications in perinatal care area will be highlighted.

HEALTH INFORMATICS/ NURSING INFORMATICS: GENERAL VIEW

Information and communication technologies-computers, telecommunication, digital networks, and television etc.- enhanced the dissemination of information and knowledge through multiple disciplines, such as education, medicine, business, research, and entertainment in many countries of the world (Arunachalam, 2002). E-Health technology is a term used to describe different activities that include any electronic exchange of health- related data, voice, or video. It is defined as an emerging field in the intersection of medical informatics, public health and business. It refers to health services and information delivered or enhanced through the Internet and related technologies (Cashen et al, 2004). However, health informatics (health information system) is defined as the systematic application of information management and technology (IM &T) to the planning and delivery of high- quality and cost- effective health care (Norris, 2002). It is also the application of information processing involving both hardware and software that deals

with the storage, retrieval, sharing, and use of health care information, data, and knowledge for communication and decision- making (Jenkins et al, 2006). The application of computer information systems in the health sector means: a goal system of data gathering, the development of professional terminology, prompter documentation, a way of measuring the work done, support for statistical and analytical work, a facility for financial evaluation, support evidence based studies research, support of the education process in the overall healthcare of patients (Habjanic et al, 1999).

Nurses are the members of the health care team who are most responsible for the education of patients, a role they fulfil in addition to their task of direct patient care in order to improve the quality of patient care.

An informatics nurse can play a key role in the area of patient education and consultation (Meadows, 2002).

Nursing Informatics (NI) is a component of health informatics, and it has become a part of the nursing professional activities. Nursing Informatics has been defined as a combination between three different sciences: computer science, information science and nursing science to manage and communicate data, information and knowledge in nursing practice (American Nurses Association (ANA), 2001; cited in Meadows, 2002). The integration between the three sciences produced a new specialty in nursing that was recognized in 1992 by the American Nurses' Association (ANA) (Meadows 2002). Using computer science to manage the information and knowledge in nursing means that nurses are involved in the application of computer information systems. Therefore nurses are required to use computers daily in the health care environment to access the health information and to utilize it appropriately and efficiently to deliver the health care services. By using clinical information systems, the nurses understand the informational and cognitive foundations of their profession. Additionally, the nurses will have the ability to synthesise nursing knowledge and develop nursing wisdom that affects patient care (Meadows, 2002). Furthermore, Smedley (2005) emphasized that the use of computers and intranet/Internet; familiarity with and understanding of computerized equipment in the clinical environment; and the ability to employ skills appropriate to the nurse's role are essential for competent care delivery and must be promoted throughout nursing workplaces. In a computerized clinical environment nurses are using computers not just for dealing with information management, word processing, electronic mails, but they use computers to review and enter physicians' orders, and to review laboratory and radiology results. Moreover, there is electronic medical equipment that depends on computerization (Hobbs, 2002).

Using informatics can improve the quality of nursing care; it enhances error reduction through an effective use of information systems, facilitation of knowledge and information management by on-line and on-site databases and electronic medical records (Barton, 2005).

HEALTH/ NURSING INFORMATICS CONCEPTS

Basic concepts of health informatics can be applied to nursing informatics. Identifying and understanding these concepts is essential to present examples of health informatics applications later in this chapter. The following concepts are the ones related to the discussion of the chapter, but there are other concepts that may be presented in other chapters

ELECTRONIC MEDICAL RECORDS (EMR)

EMR is a computer based clinical data system designed to replace patients' records (Wyatt & Liu, 2002) that is now the core element of health informatics in health care. These records include the medical history of the patient as well as non-medical information. Health care providers can provide a high quality of care through analysing of electronic medical record data and documenting patient care (Doyle, 2006). Many benefits can be gained by using EMR, for example, a patient's status can be tracked easily; a patient's data can be accessed, tracked easily by multiple end users with proper security clearance and safeguards to prevent medical errors. EMR systems can also be unified with other hospital departments where the patient's data are used, and EMR enables data to be recovered quickly (Doyle, 2006). Furthermore, EMR can enhance patient safety as a framework for processing clinical information and linking various technology applications (McCartney, 2006). However, the electronic patients' data may be at risk for misuse or security breaches. This misuse can be due to the growth of these data and the practice of sharing health data with third parties for clinical, administrative, statistical, and research purposes. Therefore, many regulations, laws and legal actions have been developed to protect the privacy of patients' data in the countries that are implementing the EMR through their health care systems. More discussion about confidentiality issues will be presented in this chapter.

STANDARDISED LANGUAGE

To exchange the paper medical record systems with the electronic medical records (EMR) system, a standardised language needs to be designed. Health care systems demand a large amount of detailed information. Accordingly, a restricted set of phrases (controlled vocabulary) have been enumerated in a list and arranged into a hierarchy to serve as a form of standardised language. Although the lists seem to be simple and attractive, various problems have been associated with these lists. A huge number of phrases would be needed to represent all possible information and data. However, the constraints imposed by the development and by the consultations at the user interface mean that the number of phrases in the controlled vocabulary must be limited (Hardiker et al, 2000). Throughout the field of nursing there are some examples of this language, which are not comprehensive for all types of information such as: North American Nursing Diagnosis Association (NANDA), Nursing Interventions Classification (NIC), and Nursing Outcomes Classification (NOC).

CONSUMER HEALTH INFORMATICS

Consumer health informatics is the use of medical informatics methods to facilitate the study and development of paper or electronic systems that support public access to and the use of health and lifestyle information (Wyatt & Liu, 2002). In addition, it focuses on how consumers access and use health information for decision making (VanBiervliet & Edwards-Schafer, 2004). It helps consumers by putting their health information such as diagnoses, lab results, and prescribed drugs into their hands. Furthermore, it empowers patients and their families by supporting a better understanding of their medical conditions and communication with health professional through direct or indirect ways so they can take a more active role in their treatment (Mullner & Chung, 2006). One example of using internet based health records that are accessible to patients is a system in the USA called SeniorMed that gives elderly patients access to their medication lists through internet (Eysenbach, 2000). Consumer health informatics appeared during 1990s, a period that was characterised by huge growth of the internet. Since then many internet health sites have been developed to provide information about different

kind of diseases, treatments and health promotion (Mullner & Chung, 2006).

Telehealth/Telenursing

Telemedicine is the use of any electronic medium to mediate or augment clinical consultations. It can be simultaneous by telephone, videoconference or store and forward as e-mails and attached images. Telecare is a kind of telemedicine used with patients located in community (Wyatt & Liu, 2002). While telehealth is a broader concept than telemedicine, it refers to the use of telecommunication technologies and computers to exchange health care information and to provide services to clients to another location. Telehealth services are provided by licensed health professionals: physicians, nurses, social workers, psychologists, and nutritionist in various care setting (Park, 2006). Telenursing is the use of telemedicine technology to provide nursing care and conduct nursing practice (Peck, 2005). Telenursing enables the nurse to monitor, educate, and follow up remote data collection, remote interventions, pain management, and family support (Peck, 2005). One of the characteristics of telehealth is the change from provider – centred to patient centred care and from hospital – based care to community – based care, so the patient care services will move to the patients' homes, and this is the current change in the health care system (Park, 2006). Cost saving is an advantage of using telehealth, as it decreases the health care utilization of chronic patients as well as hospital stays. Consequently this advantage plays a role in solving nursing shortage problems by returning experienced and dedicated nurses to the work. More advantages for telehealth include improved access to care, the facilitation of patient-provider communications, and the removal of barriers such as time and distance.

After discussing the main concepts of health informatics used in this chapter, an overview of women's health and its relation to reproductive health will be presented in the following section.

REPRODUCTIVE HEALTH AND WOMEN'S HEALTH

Reproductive health is an essential component of health for individuals, couples and families. Furthermore, it is important for the development of communities and nations worldwide (WHO, 2004). Reproductive health extends before and beyond the years of reproduction and it is associated with socio cultural factors, gender roles, and the protection of human rights in relation to sexuality and personal relationships. It deals with different aspects of health care: improving antenatal, perinatal, postpartum and newborn care; providing high quality services for family planning including infertility; eliminating unsafe abortion; combating sexually transmitted infections including HIV and reproductive track infections; dealing with gender issues, sexual health and reproductive rights; and promoting the sexual and reproductive heath of adolescents (WHO, 2006). Women's health and reproductive health complement each other and deal with similar topics regarding women. However, reproductive health is wider and can be directed to both genders.

Information technology has begun to take its place in the field of women's health (Crandall et al, 2001). Women –as a health informatics consumers- are more frequently visiting the Internet for health information. A study done by the Pew Internet and American Life Project found that women more frequently searched for information about illnesses or symptoms than men. Furthermore, they were more likely to do online health searches after visiting a doctor and to seek health information on behalf of their children (NWHRC, 2001).

Health informatics is a vehicle to produce the technology applications that target the most

vulnerable consumers and promote their health. It is potentially a powerful and dynamic method for providing health education. Information technology can provide education, access to services, promotion of research development, and continuously updated material. Many people are turning to the internet for health education and support. Fox (2005) revealed that more than two thirds of Internet users report that they have searched for information about a specific disease or medical problem. Furthermore, Internet information influences the choice of treatments although the quality of information is variable (Pérez-López, 2004).

Women's health issues are an important online topic for health promotion and education for women. For example, breast cancer and breast self examination are very important areas of women's health issues on the Web. The literature findings indicate that breast cancer patients are among the populations of patients that refer to the Internet for help in coping with health issues (Shaw et al, 2006). Many educational materials for women about early detection of breast cancer by breast self examination have been designed online. Furthermore, breast cancer on- line groups are of particular interest due to their usage. Public Bulletin Boards (BBs) that are characterized by having 100s of members with the same medical condition who are self- directed and peer-led. These boards are available 24 hours a day with no coast to the users (Lieberman and Goldstein, 2005); they allow the user to communicate and seek support from other individuals.

Lieberman and Goldstein (2005) conducted a study to find out whether such self- directed Internet groups are effective in providing help to the participants of BBs and improve their quality of life. The researchers considered decreasing the level of depression, increasing psychological well-being and personal growth as indicators for the effectiveness of the on-line support groups (BBs) of breast cancer women. The tool of the study were three reliable psychological questionnaires used to evaluate the outcome in cancer intervention studies. The sample of the participants in the BBs included 114 women. This study found that the participants improved in all of the three measures of quality of life in a follow up conducted after six month. These results support that participation in a self- directed BB improves the psychosocial quality of life for women with breast cancer. The main limitation to this study is the lack of randomisation that might prevent the generalization of the study results but would not affect the efficacy of the boards. However, the study has been one of the first studies that validate on- line BBs empirically as a form of help for breast cancer women.

Public access computing through computer kiosks placed in a community setting is another way to use technology in patient education. Kiosks are portable, freestanding units containing computer programs that provide information or services to the users through a simplified user interface like a touch screen or keypad (Kreuter et al, 2006). The use of kiosks to provide health information is well known for many diseases as asthma, diabetes, and headache management, and for education about Alzheimer's disease, skin cancer and food safety. Despite the fact that kiosks are familiar tool in health education, studies about its usage have been rare. Women's health kiosks are also used to educate women about their health issues in the form projects. Kreuter et al (2006) conducted one of these projects that examine more complex user profiles and describe kiosk use in a minority population with limited access to technology. It focuses particularly on the use of the *Reflections of You* breast cancer educational kiosk, which is an evidence- based tailored health communication program designed specifically for African American women. This project compares kiosk use, user demographics, users' breast cancer knowledge and screening history among kiosk users at five different community settings: beauty salons, churches, neighbourhood health centres, Laundromats, and social service agencies. The

project's findings revealed that more than 4,500 users interacted with the program in five different community settings over a period of less than 18 month. Furthermore, the findings showed that the kiosk's users would seem to have a need for the information provided by the kiosk.

Another application of health informatics in the area of women's health is the Comprehensive Health Enhancement Support System (CHESS) Living With Breast Cancer Program. It is a computer- based system that provides patients and their families with a wide range of services, information, social support, decision support, and skills training. This program was developed at the University of Wisconsin- Madison's Centre for Health Systems Research and Analysis in the year 1991 to increase health awareness about breast cancer for underserved parts of the population. One of the purposes of CHESS is to help cancer patients to focus on trusted information and resources to alleviate the potential for being overwhelmed by the huge volume of health information available on the Internet, because the uncontrolled nature of the Internet as a source of health information can have detrimental effects on users if used in an unguided manner (Shaw et al, 2006).

The same purpose of evaluating the quality of health information on the Internet or on the Web was the aim of Pérez-López's (2004) study. This study evaluated 100 websites of another issue of women's health- the menopausal stage- where patient self- management is an important component of menopause management. Pérez-López (2004) found in this evaluation that the scientific content and quality of the Web information about menopause is heterogeneous. Further, Pérez-López (2004) highlighted that there are few websites have evaluated topics with well-balanced information. In addition, the study found that the majority of sites have commercial content with very poor, useless or unrelated information to promote sales, although some of these websites are in the top 10 sites and consumers who carry out a general search visit them. Thus, the popularity of the websites is not parallel to the medical quality content and the accuracy of information.

The previous examples show some of the health informatics applications to a number of women's health issues. However, perinatal care is a topic that does not deal with women's health only but extends further to infants' health issues in the critical period of life.

PERINATAL CARE AND HEALTH INFORMATICS

The perinatal period is defined by WHO as a 22 completed weeks (154 days) of gestation (the time when the birth weight is normally 500 g) and ends seven completed days after birth (Zeitlin et al, 2003). However, Burgio et al (2006) specified that the p*erinatal* period was the phase that coincides, at its onset (22nd-23rd week of gestation, according to common acknowledgment), with the possible beginning of an extrauterine life susceptible of protraction. The 1st, or in some definitions the 4th, week of neonatal life marks the conclusion of the *perinatal* phase. Thus, perinatal care is related to women's and their infants' health. According to the above description of the perinatal period, it interacts with both antenatal and postnatal periods, and it is not isolated phase. During this period many serious events can occur either for the woman or her newborn infant. For example 45% of maternal deaths occur within the first 24 hours after birth (AED et al, 2005) and over 60% of maternal deaths occur during the first six weeks after birth (Bhutta et al, 2003). Regarding newborns, 50% to 70% of life threatening illnesses in newborns occur in the first week after birth (AED et al, 2005). Moreover, three million deaths out of 10.8 million cases of child mortality (under five years) occur during the first seven days of the neonatal period (WHO, 2004).

Although most maternal deaths and disabilities occur during postpartum period, the neonatal mortality rate remains high (WHO, 1998). The focus of the strategies to reduce maternal and perinatal morbidity and mortality are on the first and second phase of the reproductive cycle (pregnancy and birth) by providing comprehensive antenatal care and skilled attendance at birth (Ministry of Health, University of Nairobi and Population Council, 2005). This is supported by a WHO (2006) report that presents an overview of reproductive health research work over 2004-2005. In the section of improving maternal health of previous report recommended that the best possible care during pregnancy and childbirth is necessary to reduce the maternal and neonatal mortality rates. However, the providing health care during last phase (postpartum) is ignored, in spite of the common occurrence of fatal events in this phase. Therefore maintaining safety for the women and infants through perinatal period (mainly postpartum phase) is essential to decrease the maternal and neonatal morbidity and mortality in this period.

One of the uses of health informatics is to promote and improve patient safety. However published research between technology and safety is limited. Furthermore, few publications explore the experiences made with information technology in perinatal care (McCartney, 2006). Such IT application are electronic health records (EHR); decision support systems (DSS); medication safety devices as automated drug- dispensing units (ADU), bar code medication administration (BCMA); computerised medication order entry (either for physician or provider); and smart pumps. Although these IT applications enhance patient safety generally and in perinatal care particularly, unintended consequences and errors are still produced by such applications (McCartney, 2006).

The Regional Perinatal Data System is another example of an application of health informatics in the clinical setting. It combines electronic birth certificate information with special quality improvement questions that are asked to all women giving birth to a live infant in one of the 14- county in New York State birthing hospitals.

In addition to the contents of the electronic birth certificate, the data within the system includes selected quality improvement information such as breastfeeding intentions, exercise during pregnancy, and genetic testing offered. Furthermore, the system includes the consent of the women to share the information from the Regional Perinatal Data System electronically with every woman's obstetric provider, her infant's paediatricians, and the Central New York Immunisation Registry (Dye et al, 2002).

All of the previous IT applications in the perinatal care are used in clinical areas. However, there are no IT applications for health education and promotion or any guidance for the consumers to help self treatment and management. It can be rationalized that the health care providers use these applications in health care settings more than the patients. However, Wootton (1999) gives many trusted World Wide Web resources for perinatal care that are suitable both for health care providers (physicians, nurses, and midwives) and for consumers as a method of health promotion and education. For example, electronic publications, online specialist journals, and online journals relevant to perinatal nursing are provided for the professionals. The electronic resources for the consumers are: the website of the Atlanta Reproductive Health Centre, the Maternity Centre Association, and the National Women's Health Information Centre.

The use of the Internet and the World Wide Web in health education has been widely reported (Ginman, 2000). However, applications of health informatics in perinatal care for consumers who are mainly women and their newborn infants have not been reported widely through the research studies and projects. Similarly, general health education using health informatics applications are not widely presented in the literature. However, health informatics has been used for other topics of health education and they have been effective for the consumers. To understand how health informatics can be used for the benefits of the clients, consumes and patients, the next section will discuss some issues of health informatics in health education.

HEALTH EDUCATION AND HEALTH INFORMATICS

Today, people are living longer in most of countries, but they may be living with and adapting to chronic health problems that require their participation in the daily care regimen. For example, hypertension, diabetes mellitus, joints problems or heart diseases are diseases that accompany the patient for a long time. Furthermore, health questions and enquiries are more frequent and wide-spread among people than ever before because health risks and problems are growing too. Ginman (2000) revealed that more than 40 percent of illness and bad health are the direct results of factors that are under the individual's control. It is believed that a patient who is educated about his/ her health related conditions would better comply with treatment plans and has improved health outcomes (Pérez-López 2004). It has been realized that health education does not affect people automatically, although they are loaded with information. On the other hand, health-promoting knowledge is created within a learning process taking place in the interaction between the offered information and the cognitive ability of the receiver. Thus, the quality of knowledge that has been developed depends on the quality of information (offered and received) and on the quality of the learning process (Ginman, 2000).

Information technology in patients' health education process empowers patients and enhances their self-management skills (Cashen et al, 2004). For example, by using the Internet and e-mail, patients can find information on GP services, renew prescriptions, and communicate with their GPs. They can also access the Internet for information about their medical conditions, prognosis and their choices of treatment. Moreover, there are sites with advice, referral sites and activist sites for particular causes. Furthermore, the Internet may offer support for patients by allowing them to meet with others who complain of the same medical problems. Information technology can enable remote treatment or monitoring of patients in their place through telecare or telehealth (Wootton, 1999; Norris, 2002).

However, the huge amounts of existing information are often ineffective. Consumers often find it difficult to differentiate between true and incorrect information when it comes to reviewing health care information. Thus it is necessary to direct the consumers of health informatics to high quality information and to teach them how to assess this quality of information (Eysenbach, 2000; VanBiervliet & Edwards-Schafer, 2004).

Maintaining quality control of electronic health information depends on educating the consumers about ways to determine the quality of information, encouraging the self-regulation of health information providers, having third parties to evaluate the information, and enforcing sanctions in cases of fraudulent or harmful information (Eysenbach, 2000). The ability to distribute information rapidly, cheaply, and anonymously through the Internet has resulted in serious health care fraud online. The concern about the quality of medical advice provided on Web sites led to the development of evaluation guidelines aimed at raising the quality of health information available over the Internet by using self-regulatory and voluntary means (VanBiervliet & Edwards-Schafer, 2004). One example of the evaluation of web information is the web site evaluation guide called: *Guide for Older Adults and Caregivers* that was published by the Spry Foundation. This guide helps consumers to use widely accepted procedures for evaluating the accuracy, completeness, clarity, and usefulness of a health information websites. This guide also provides a simple checklist and tips on finding reliable health Web sites (VanBiervliet & Edwards-Schafer, 2004).

Another example that was designed to combat health fraud on the Internet is the program called *Operation Cure.All*. This program was an enforcement and consumer education program. Many prosecutions have occurred and over 100 web sites have been closed or removed their health bogus since Operation Cure.All was launched in USA in 1999. Furthermore, consumers have been encouraged to report suspicious health claims to either the Federal Trade Commission (FTC) or to the Food and Drug Administration (FDA) who are the designers of this program (VanBiervliet & Edwards-Schafer, 2004).

The World Wide Web can be used as an effective tool for patient health education and promotion, but the quality of the health information on the web should be evaluated regularly to protect the consumers from abuse and health problems.

CHALLENGES FOR HEALTH INFORMATICS APPLICATION IN THE PERINATAL CARE

Although the Internet has become an integral part of life in most societies, and reliance on information technologies has increased, there are changes that may limit applying information technology in the consumers' health education generally and in the perinatal area particularly. Such challenges include the computer literacy of the consumers, funds, security issues, and population distribution (rural and urban), all of which have great influence on the application of IT in perinatal care patient's education.

Computer and Health Literacy

Technologies are effective only if there are skilled and knowledgeable users, communities practicing appropriate health- promoting health seeking behaviours and functioning health care systems (Tsu, 2005).

To take use of the information technologies, the consumers should have the basic computer and Internet skills, and they should -at least- have basic health information that may be used to take decisions (VanBiervliet & Edwards-Schafer, 2004).

Health literacy refers to the degree to which individuals have the capacity to obtain, process, and understand basic health information and services, which is related to the behaviour of obtaining and using health information on the Web (Cashen et al, 2004). Furthermore, the consumers' interest in health information is not dependent on the individual's health status but more related to their general information profile and their attitude towards healthcare (Ginman, 2000). Therefore, consumers with low literacy are unlikely to use the Internet or Web for information to promote their conditions.

Funding

Despite the huge potential benefits for consumers of health informatics, computerisation and technology do not come cheap. One of the important factors that may enhance or prevent health informatics applications in the patient education area is the financial status of the country in general and the budget of the health sector in particular. The use of information Technology in health care systems costs millions and billions of Dollars. For example, in the UK the official cost for the NHS National Program For IT (NPFIT) introduction is around £6 billion, but nursing informatics experts in IT suggest the true cost will be closer to £30 billion when hardware, software, training and staff replacement costs are taken into consideration (Parish, 2006). In the USA, President George W. Bush proposed allocating $100 million for health information technology including electronic medical records. Moreover, in Australia, the NSW Department of health began prototyping the new electronic health records project, which was the first wide- scale online patient information data

– base in Australia with a fund of $ 19.4 million over five years (Doyle, 2006).

The previous examples were from some developed countries, which are rich countries and can fund information technology applications in various sectors including health care system. However, developing countries that are mainly poor economically, cannot implement the same applications. For example, in Syria, the health informatics initiatives are at the early stage of development in all sectors. The Syrian Ministry of Health started pilot projects in the fields of electronic medical records and Smart Card System. In Ghana, a large data base was set up containing the names, ages, pregnancies, births, illness, recoveries and deaths of the population in the Northern Ghana that was considered the most risky place to live during infancy period. This database was a component of the project named (Health Net Project), which aimed to improve the quality of life in Northern Ghana (Alemna & Sam, 2006). Financial funding is pivotal for any information technology project or application in health care system and other sectors.

Security Issues

The privacy, confidentiality and security of patients' health records and information are serious issues in health informatics applications. Privacy includes the right to secrecy of information, to determine the extent of information shared, to protection against misuse of information and freedom from intrusion. However, confidentiality is concerned with the respect of privacy of the information received and the ethical treatment of the information (Malloy, 2003). On the other hand, security is an ethical imperative to ensure the respect for human rights and freedoms of the individual, particularly the confidentiality of the information in the health informatics systems (Mommens, 1999). It is one of the fundamental rights that the patient's health information is private and it is the responsibility of the health care providers who deals with this information to protect this right. Then a relationship of trust between the patient and the nurse or physician- for example- can be built to share complete information that will further improve the quality of health care. By using technologies and electronic forms of health records, patients' information can be easily accessed to improve care, clinical decision-making, and communication between patients and health care providers. Furthermore, these data can be accessed and utilized for a wide array of non- clinical and indirect clinical purposes, such as billing, insurance transactions, and research. Therefore, legislations of security to protect the privacy requirements of the patients have been formulated and issued. Data protection legislation and a wealth of and laws for data protection are found in developed countries; however, most developing countries do not have such legislations, which represents a huge challenge to implement health informatics.

Rural Population

Rural, remote populations are another challenge for the application of health informatics. The majority of rural people have limited access to health care settings. Thus telehealth can help to provide health services to rural populations and reduce the environmental stressors associated with providing health care services in rural areas, which influences the productivity of health care providers. These stressors are heavy workloads, isolation, limited access to technologies, the diversity of skills needed, lack of flexibility in staffing patterns, lower and compressed salary scales, and lack of career opportunities (Hicks et al, 2000).

Although telehealth has many advantages for both the health care team and for the consumers, there are important problems that may prevent its application. The three main problems that complicate the use of telehealth (telenursing) are: firstly, technological problems: a lack of a communal data standard is slowing down the implementation of telehealth. Secondly, the resistance from nurses thinking that they are delegating tasks to machines. Thirdly, legislation and policies regarding licensure and reimbursement need to be fully prepared and applied (who will pay for telehealth) (Peck, 2005). These problems are modifiable and can be solved in order to involve telehealth more in patient care and thus to enhance the quality of care. This situation may be present in the developed countries, where systems that use technology have been established, but in developing countries the barriers to implement telehealth are more numerous than the three problems mentioned previously. The absence of qualified IT nurses, of infrastructure technology and of security regulations, as well as financial barriers are the main barriers in developing countries to implement telehealth. The balance between the cost of telecare and the improvements of health it can provide will be measured before taking a judgment. Telecare has its economic benefits, but to start projects of telecare from zero with out any financial help in developing countries will cost more than the benefits later.

Summary

Health education and promotion programs using health informatics during the perinatal period have not been studied widely in the literature. There is a gap of knowledge related to this topic on the Internet and Web. Furthermore, there is a lack of reliable, valid educational resources for women, although the number of health consumers (women) in the perinatal period is large. In addition the perinatal period has a wide range of events through three phases of the reproductive cycle, which can be included in the educational materials. Such uses of health informatics in health education in the area of women's health can reduce perinatal, maternal and newborn mortality and morbidity.

FUTURE RESEARCH DIRECTIONS

Although the sheer volume of information available on the web is impressive, finding the right information at the right time remains a challenge. The enormous importance of web search, and the relatively small numbers of commercial search engines means that workers in this area may see the best approach as a combination of education and add-ons to these engines. Wikipedia's success emphasizes the power of so-called user generated or web 2.0 content. It has shown that by moving from a model of "review then publish", to "publish then correct", building up a broad, if not guaranteed, knowledge base is rapidly performed by large groups of individuals. Collaborative tagging systems such as digg and dellicious may be seen to perform a similar role for referencing, and it is interesting to speculate on the degree to which communities of interest – for example patient groups or professionals with an interest in this area will use such tools.

Information is being presented in many rich formats, and libraries of videos, interactive educational simulations and even games may be preferred avenues of information distribution. The next generation of young women are likely to be even more connected than their forebears and expect information presented in the format of their choice. However professionals need to provide that information with the same care and accuracy whatever the medium.

REFERENCES

AED (Academy for Educational Development), the Manoff Group, & USAID (2005). Maternal survival: improving access to skilled care- a behavior approach, *The CHANGE Maternal Survival Toolkit*, [online]. Available from: http://www.changeproject.org [Accessed 15th August, 2006].

Alemna, A. A., & Sam, J. (2006). Critical issues in information and communication technologies for rural development in Ghana. *Information Development, 22*(4), 236-241.

American Nurses' Association (ANA). (2001). *Scope and standards of nursing informatics practice*. Washington, D.C.: American Nurses Publishing.

Arunachalam, S. (2002). Reaching the unreached: How can we use information and communication technologies to empower the rural poor in the developing world through enhanced access to relevant information? *Journal of Information Science, 28*(6), 513-522.

Barton, A. J. (2005). Cultivating informatics: competencies in a community of practice. *Nurs Admin Q, 29*(4), 323-328.

Bhutta, Z. A., Darmstadt, G. L. & Ranson, E. I. (2003). *Using evidence to save newborn lives: Policy perspectives on newborn health*. Population Reference Bureau, Save the Children, Washington, USA.

Burgio, G. R., Paganelli, A., Sampaolo, P., & Gancia, P. (2006). Ethics in perinatology. *Minerva Pediatrica, 58*(1), 77-89.

Crandall, C., Zitzelberger, T., Rosenberg, M., Winner, C., & Holaday, L. (2001). Information technology and the national centers of excellence in women's health. *Journal of Women's Health & Gender-Based Medicine, 10*, 49-55.

Cashen, M. S., Dykes, P., & Gerber, B. (2004). E-Health technology and Internet resources: Barriers vulnerable populations. *Journal of Cardiovascular Nursing, 19*(3), 209-214.

Doyle, M. (2006). Home study program: promoting standardized nursing language using an electronic medical record system. *AORN Journal, 83*(6), 1335-1348.

Dye, T., Wojtowycz, M., Applegate, M., & Aubry, R. (2002). Women's willingness to share information and participation in prenatal care systems. *American Journal of Epidemiology, 156*(3), 286-291.

Eysenbach, G. (2000). Recent advances: Consumer health informatics. *BMJ, 320,* 1713-1716

Fox, S. (2005). *Health information online,* Washington, DC: Pew Internet and American Life Project

Ginman, M. (2000). Health information and quality of life. *Health Informatics Journal, 6*(4), 181-188.

Habjanic, A., Kokol, P., Zorman, M., & Slajmer-Japelj, M. (1999). CArE: A software package for computer-aided nurse education. *Health Informatics Journal, 5*(3), 119-123.

Hardiker, N. R., Hoy, D., & Casey, A. (2000). Standards for nursing terminology. *Journal of the American Medical Informatics Association, 7*(6), 523-528.

Hicks, L. L., Boles, K. E., Hudson, S. T., Koenig, S., Madsen, R., Kling, B., et al. (2000). An evaluation of satisfaction with telemedicine among healthcare professionals. *Journal of Telemedicine and Telecare, 6*(4), 209-215.

Hobbs, S. D. (2002). Measuring nurses' computer competency: an analysis of published instruments. *CIN: Computer, Informatics, Nursing, 20*(2), 63-73.

Jenkins, M. L., Hewitt, C., & Bakken, S. (2006). Women's health nursing in the context of the national health information infrastructure. *JOGNN: Journal of Obstetric, Gynecologic, & Neonatal Nursing, 35*(1), 141-150.

Kreuter, M. W., Black, W. J., Friend, L., Booker, A. C., Klump, P., Bobra, S., et al. (2006). Use of computer kiosks for breast cancer education in five community settings. *Health Education & Behavior, 33*(5), 625-642.

Lieberman, M. A., & Goldstein, B. A. (2005). Self-help on-line: An outcome evaluation of breast cancer bulletin boards. *Journal of Health Psychology, 10*(6), 855-862.

Malloy, N. P. (2003). The informatics nurse specialist as privacy officer. *Journal of Healthcare Information Management, 17*(3), 54-58.

McCartney, P. R. (2006). Using technology to promote perinatal patient safety. *Journal of Obstetric, Gynecologic, & Neonatal Nursing, 35*(3), 424-431.

Meadows, G. (2002). Nursing informatics: An evolving specialty. *Nursing Economics, 20*(6), 300-301.

Ministry of Health in Nairobi, University of Nairobi & Population Council (2005). *Safe motherhood: repositioning postpartum care in Kenya,* Safe motherhood policy alerts.

Mommens, P. (1999). Ethical issues of healthcare in the information society. *Health Informatics Journal, 5,* 233-239.

Mullner, R. M., & Chung, K. (2006). Current issues in healthcare informatics. *J Med Sys, 30*(1), 1-2.

Norris, A. C. (2002). Current trends and challenges in health informatics. *Health Informatics Journal, 8*(4), 205-213.

North American Nursing Diagnosis Association. (2003). NANDA, NIC, NOC 2002: Developing, linking and integrating nursing language and informatics. *NANDA, NIC and NOC (Joint Meeting),* Chicago, IL.

National Women's Health Resource Center (NWHRC) (2001). Women's health & the Internet. *Nursing, 32,* 17.

Parish, C. (2006). Edging towards a brave new IT world. *Nursing Standard, 20*(27), 15-16.

Park, E. (2006). Telehealth technology in case/disease management. *Lippincott's Case Management, 11*(3), 175-182.

Peck, A. (2005). Changing the face of standard nursing practice through telehealth and telenursing. *Nurs Admin Q, 29*(4), 339-343.

Pérez-López, F. R. (2004). An evaluation of the contents and quality of menopause information on the World Wide Web. *Maturitas, 49,* 276-282.

Shaw, B., Gustafson, D. H., Hawkins, R., McTavish, F., McDowell, H., Pingree, S., et al. (2006). How underserved breast cancer patients use and benefit from eHealth programs: Implications for closing the digital divide. *American Behavioral Scientist, 49*(6), 823-834.

Smedley, A. (2005). The importance of informatics competencies in nursing. *CIN: Computer, Informatics, Nursing, 23*(2), 106-110.

Tsu, V. D. (2005). Appropriate technology to prevent maternal mortality: Current research requirements. *BJOG: An International Journal of Obstetrics and Gynaecology, 112*(9), 1213-1218.

VanBiervliet, A., & Edwards-Schafer, P. (2004). Consumer health information on the web: trends, issues, and strategies. *Dermatology Nursing, 16*(6), 519-523.

WHO (1998). Postpartum care of the mother and newborn: A practical guide, [online]. Available from: http://www.who.int/reproductivehealth/publications/MSM_98_3/msm_98_3_3.html [Accessed 5th May, 2007]

WHO (2004). *Reproductive health strategy: to accelerate progress towards the attainment of international development goals and targets,* WHO, Geneva.

WHO/ Department of Reproductive Health and Research (2006). *Sexual and reproductive health-laying the foundation for a more just world through research and action: biennial report 2004- 2005,* WHO, Geneva.

Wootton, J. C. (1999). World wide web resources for perinatal nursing. *Journal of Perinatal & Neonatal Nursing, 12*(4), 15-25.

Wyatt, J. C. & Liu, J. L. Y. (2002). Basic concepts in medical informatics. *J Epidemiol Community Health, 56,* 808-812.

Zeitlin, J., Wildman, K., Breart, G., Alexander, S., Barros, H., Blondel, B., et al. (2003). PERISTAT: Indicators for monitoring and evaluating perinatal health in Europe. *The European Journal of Public Health, 13*(suppl_1), 29-37.

ADDITIONAL READING

Tapscott, D., & Williams, A. (2008). *Wikinomics: How Mass Collaboration Changes Everything.*

Wikipedia www.wikipedia.org

The health on the net foundation www.hon.ch

Donaldson, forewords by Sue, K. & Gerdin, U. (2000). *Nursing informatics : where caring and technology meet,* 3rd ed., Springer, New York ; London.

Kirshbaum, M. N. (2004). Are we ready for the Electronic Patient Record? Attitudes and perceptions of staff from two NHS trust hospitals. *Health Informatics Journal, 10*(4), 265-276.

Martin, P., & Kauser, A. (2001). An informaticist working in primary care: A descriptive study. *Health Informatics Journal, 7*(2), 66-70.

Norris, A. C., & Brittain, J. M. (2000). Education, training and the development of healthcare informatics. *Health Informatics Journal, 6*(4), 189-195.

Oliver, K. B., & Roderer, N. K. (2006). Working towards the informationist. *Health Informatics Journal, 12*(1), 41-48.

Penn, D. L., Burns, J. R., Georgiou, A., Davies, P. G. P., & Harris, M. F. (2004). Evolution of a register recall system to enable the delivery of better quality of care in general practice. *Health Informatics Journal, 10*(3), 165-176.

Roberts, C. (1998). Quality assurance in primary care with information management and technology. *Health Informatics Journal, 4*(2), 101-105.

See Tai, S., Donegan, C., & Nazareth, I. (2000). Computers in general practice and the consultation: the health professionals' view. *Health Informatics Journal, 6*(1), 27-31.

Thede, L. Q. (2003). *Informatics and nursing: Opportunities & challenges,* 2nd ed., Lippincott Williams & Wilkins, Philadelphia ; London.

Ward, R., & Scrivener, R. (2002). The development of NMAP - the UK's gateway to high quality Internet resources in nursing, midwifery and allied health. *Health Informatics Journal, 8*(3), 122-126.

Chapter XIV
Electronic Information Sources for Women's Health Knowledge for Professionals

Shona Kirtley
University of Oxford, UK

ABSTRACT

In an age where health professionals lead very busy working lives, electronic information sources provide ease of access to vast amounts of health information on an unprecedented scale. Health professionals have the ability to access the information they require from a location convenient to them and can do so at any time, day or night. This convenience has resulted in an increasing reliance upon electronic sources of information amongst women's health professionals. As technologies develop, both the importance placed on the electronic dissemination of information by women's health professionals and the use of such resources will increase dramatically. This chapter outlines the different sources of electronic information available to women's health professionals, the constantly evolving online accessibility issues, the importance of critical appraisal when assessing the validity of online resources, and the role of the information specialist in the health sector. As this topic is currently under-researched a number of future research directions are also proposed.

INTRODUCTION/BACKGROUND

Electronic information sources can be defined as sources of information that are held in a digital or electronic format that can be accessed, searched or retrieved either by an electronic network or by an electronic data processing application. These sources can take the form of, for example, a search engine, a bibliographic database, a downloadable PDF file, an electronic journal, an e-book or a podcast.

With health professionals leading very busy working lives electronic information sources provide ease of access to vast amounts of health information on an unprecedented scale. Health professionals have the ability to access the information they require from a location convenient to them without the need to visit the library or a professional organisation in person. Electronic information can be sought and delivered to health professionals quickly and at any time, day or night. The convenience of electronic information provision therefore has encouraged health professionals to utilise this method of obtaining health information and has resulted in an increasing reliance on electronic sources of information amongst women's health professionals. As technologies develop and electronic dissemination of information increases the importance placed on the electronic delivery of information to busy women's health professionals will increase dramatically.

A comprehensive literature search carried out to identify other research in this area has revealed that in fact very little has been written specifically about electronic sources of information for women's health professionals. In this context this chapter will discuss the different sources of electronic information available to women's health professionals, online accessibility issues, the importance of critical appraisal and the role of the information specialist in the health sector.

ELECTRONIC INFORMATION SOURCES FOR WOMEN'S HEALTH KNOWLEDGE FOR PROFESSIONALS

The development of the internet can be said to have revolutionised the way in which health information is delivered to clinicians around the world. As both access to and use of the internet continues to increase, the availability of internet-based knowledge sources for health professionals has soared. The development of the internet has allowed access to information on an unprecedented scale. Information on a vast array of health topics is available on the internet and delivered to the

user very quickly, easily and most importantly on a 24/7 basis. Accessed at a location convenient to the user and at a time that is suitable, the internet is an increasingly popular platform for the delivery of health information resources.

With the explosion in the use of the internet, many organisations providing health information resources to professionals identified the need to provide their resources also on the internet and to expand the services they provided where internet technology would allow them to offer additional services that they may not have traditionally been able to provide. In particular, the field of women's health has witnessed an enormous growth in the availability of electronic resources covering all aspects of women's health and aimed at all practitioners involved in the care of women. The wide variety of different health professionals working in women's health has allowed for different knowledge sources to be developed or expanded ensuring that all professionals including, for example, consultant obstetricians, consultant gynecologists, midwives, general practitioners and gynecological nurses, have access to the information they require to make health-related decisions.

The format of on-line information resources available to women's health professionals varies enormously. Women's health electronic information is available from web-based libraries, from e-journals and even through blogs and podcasts. The wide ranging formats used to provide information to women's health professionals ensure that information covering every aspect of the health of women is available and is in a format that is desirable and useful to most professionals. However, the range of electronic information sources available also raises a problem regarding the varying quality of sources of women's health information. It is important to recognise that not all electronic resources available on the internet are from a reliable, evidence-based source. It is vital therefore to ensure that the electronic information being accessed by women's health professionals is from a trusted, reliable source and is of a good quality. This section will examine the different types or formats of sources of electronic information available to women's health professionals and provide examples of electronic resources in this field.

On-Line Libraries/Databases

A number of electronic or web-based libraries have been established to serve the needs of women's health professionals. These on-line libraries generally provide access to a range of resources to health professionals including, for example, clinical guidelines, evidence-based resources such as Cochrane Reviews or evidence-based summaries, reference resources or patient information resources. On-line libraries exist in a variety of different formats utilising different internet technologies but all aim to provide reliable electronic health information to specialists in women's health.

The National Library for Health (NLH) has been developed by the UK National Health Service (NHS) to provide an information and library service to all health professionals on a 24/7 basis. The NLH is composed of a number of individual specialist libraries, one of which is a library devoted to women's health (Table 1). The women's health library aims to bring together trusted, authoritative, up-to-date information

resources in one place, providing seamless access to the best available evidence required on a daily basis by health care professionals to make health-related decisions wherever, and whenever, it is needed. The library brings together resources such as guidelines, systematic reviews, reports, drug alerts and patient information. All resources are appraised before being added to the library therefore ensuring that the information that is accessed through the library is of a good quality and searches are carried out regularly to ensure that the library is as up-to-date as possible.

The National Library of Medicine (Table 1) based at the National Institutes of Health in the US have developed an online library and a range of online health information resources. Whilst not exclusively aimed at women's health professionals the online library provides access to resources such as Pubmed (Table 1) providing a valuable source of references to journal articles relevant to women's health and access is also provided to MedlinePlus (Table 1) which contains comprehensive patient information which can be accessed by members of the public or by health professionals who can use it to help explain conditions or treatments to their patients.

The World Health Organisation (WHO) has also developed a library accessible both over the internet and on CD-ROM. The Reproductive Health Library (Table 1) is aimed at practitioners in developing countries and covers all aspects of

Table 1.

On-line libraries/databases	URL
NLH Women's Health Specialist Library	www.library.nhs.uk/womenshealth
National Library of Medicine	www.nlm.nih.gov
Pubmed	http://www.ncbi.nlm.nih.gov/pubmed
MedlinePlus	http://medlineplus.gov/
Reproductive Health Library	www.rhlibrary.com
New Zealand Guidelines Group	http://www.nzgg.org.nz

reproductive health. The library brings together the best evidence, provides information on implications for practice and provides online videos and training resources.

The New Zealand Guidelines Group (Table 1) also provides access to a library of up-to-date women's health guidelines amongst other guidelines in other specialties. The guidelines are listed by category and relevant women's health guidelines are listed under the gynecology and obstetrics, infertility, sexual health and women's health topic headings.

On-line libraries and databases have become increasingly popular amongst health professionals for both identifying and locating the references that they require, especially where links to the full-text are provided. The examples discussed above are just a small sample of the ever expanding range of on-line libraries and databases available to health proferssionals.

On-line Continuing Professional Development (CPD)/Continuing Medical Education (CME) Courses

Health professionals generally lead very busy working lives and often find it difficult to allocate time to their CPD requirements. The advent of the internet has allowed for a transformation in the way that health care training courses can be delivered. Many organisations around the world can now deliver some of their training courses over the internet allowing women's health professionals to keep up-to-date with their continuing professional development without having to travel long distances and/or take time off from work to do so. Different types of organisations provide on-line CME courses to health professionals from official colleges for obstetrics and gynaecology to commercial organisations. Most professional colleges or associations provide, amongst a range of different services, specialist training programmes for health professionals to enable them to train as consultant obstetricians and gynaecologists and

therefore many offer CME courses as an extension to this professional training which is required for college membership.

On-line CPD courses offered by organisations differ greatly in format, content and presentation with many courses utilising the latest advances in internet technology. CME on-line courses are generally designed as a series of short units allowing health professionals to complete their CME requirements over a period of time. As a result courses are often designed to cover one particular topic area and generally consist of a review of best evidence in the specific area outlined with a set of questions at the end. Courses can be made available on the internet as html pages, as downloadable PDFs or can involve multimedia presentations or webcasts. Health professionals, on completion of each course, are awarded CPD/CME points that count towards their overall CPD requirements. Access to CPD courses varies widely as some courses are restricted to members of the organisations that provide them while others are freely available over the internet.

The Faculty of Sexual and Reproductive Healthcare (FSRH) based in the UK has designed a range of on-line continuing professional development courses that can be completed whenever and wherever health professionals wish (Table 2). Courses cover topics related to sexual and reproductive healthcare and consist of a topic review with a series of short self-test questions. Health professionals earn 1 CPD point on completion of each course.

The American College of Obstetricians and Gynecologists (ACOG) has designed a set of continuing medical education courses that are available online (Table 2). The courses are designed on a pay-per-view basis and course topics cover both obstetrics and gynecology. The format of each course is a webcast and CME points are awarded on completion of courses.

The Society of Obstetricians and Gynaecologists of Canada (SOGOC) also provide a very comprehensive set of on-line CME courses (Table

2). These courses have fixed start and end dates and questions answered at the beginning of the course allow participants to test their knowledge base against other course attendees. Completion of each course contributes towards the CME programme in Canada.

The Royal Australian and New Zealand College of Obstetricians and Gynaecologists (RANZCOG) provide access to their online flexible learning programme to health professionals who wish to update their knowledge (Table 2). Designed as a training programme for trainees, this programme is also open to members of the college allowing professionals to work through a large number of course modules and accumulate self-education points upon completion.

The NHS Women's Health Specialist Library provides access to an online learning package for Group B Streptococcus (GBS) in Pregnancy (Table 2). This learning package developed with the UK National Screening Committee provides antenatal, intrapartum and postnatal management information for health professionals and provides a self-test quiz, FAQs and links to further information about GBS.

Commercial companies also offer CME courses designed for health professionals working in women's health. One such company is freeCME.

com (Table 2) which provides free access to CME courses covering a wide range of women's health topics. When considering following any CME course provided by a commercial company it is important to investigate the background of the company, funding details and any accreditations advertised on the website as the information provided in the individual courses may have been open to bias, may not be evidence-based or the content may not reflect official guidelines recommended by the government in different countries.

The above examples of on-line continuing professional development courses are just a small sample of the vast array of courses available worldwide. On-line CPD courses provide a valuable resource for busy women's health professionals and as use of the internet increases are expected to become more frequently utilised.

Professional Societies/Associations

Professional organisations for women's health clinicians perform a vital role. These organisations exist around the world to educate and support health professionals working in all areas of women's health including midwifery, general practice, obstetrics, gynecology and nursing.

Table 2.

On-line Continuing Professional Development (CPD)/ Continuing Medical Education (CME) courses	URL
Faculty of Sexual and Reproductive Healthcare, UK	http://www.fsrh.org/Default2.asp?Section=Publications&SubSection=FACTS
American College of Obstetricians and Gynecologists	http://www.acog.org/postgrad/index.cfm
Society of Obstetricians and Gynaecologists of Canada	(http://www.sogc.org/cme/online_e.asp
Royal Australian and New Zealand College of Obstetricians and Gynaecologists	http://www.ranzcog.edu.au/flp/index.shtml
NHS Women's Health Specialist Library	http://www.whsl.org.uk/gbs/
freeCME.com	http://www.freecme.com/gcourses1.php?specialty_id=41&specialty_name=OB/GYN

Women's health professional organisations around the world include: the Royal Australian and New Zealand College of Obstetricians and Gynaecologists (RANZOG - Table 3), the UK Royal College of Nursing (RCN - Table 3), the American College of Obstetricians and Gynecologists (ACOG - Table 3), the UK Royal College of Obstetricians and Gynaecologists (RCOG - Table 3), the Canadian Association of Midwives (CAM - Table 3), the UK Royal College of Midwives (RCM - Table 3), the American College of Nurse Midwives (ACNM - Table 3), the Hong Kong College of Obstetricians and Gynaecologists (HKCOG - Table 3) and the Australian College of Midwives (ACM - Table 3). There are, however, professional associations for women's health professionals in almost every country in the world. The vast majority of professional associations serving the field of women's health now use the internet to provide a range of services to their members including access to important electronic information resources. Most health professionals rely on their professional organisation for advice and guidance on their clinical practice and therefore access to up-to-date resources such as guidelines, consensus statements, reports, clinical governance and clinical standards documents, patient information and ethics and consent information is a vital service provided by each organisation. The information resources produced by professional organisations can now be provided in a full-text format easily over the internet for clinicians to access whenever and wherever they require them and as the information resources are held electronically they can be kept up-to-date. For their members, many organisations also provide on-line access to their library collections, clinical question and answering services and as the availability of and remote access to electronic journal and e-books collections increases organisations can increasingly provide electronic access to important journal and book titles that they subscribe to. Remote access to such information resources is important for clinicians in order for them to keep up-to-date with advances within their field and to help them manage individual patients.

In addition to information provision most professional organisations also have an important role in educating and training health professionals to gain their professional qualification. Increasingly, some aspects of this education and training can be delivered over the internet and organisations also provide electronic access to for example course packs and application forms for downloading. Calendars of events are also often compiled by professional organisations and made available

Table 3.

Professional societies/associations	URL
Royal Australian and New Zealand College of Obstetricians and Gynaecologists (RANZCOG)	http://www.ranzcog.edu.au/
Royal College of Nursing (RCN)	http://www.rcn.org.uk/
American College of Obstetricians and Gynecologists (ACOG)	http://www.acog.org
Royal College of Obstetricians and Gynaecologists (RCOG)	http://www.rcog.org.uk/
Canadian Association of Midwives (CAM)	http://www.canadianmidwives.org/
Royal College of Midwives (RCM)	http://www.rcm.org.uk/
American College of Nurse Midwives (ACNM)	http://www.midwife.org/
Hong Kong College of Obstetricians and Gynaecologists (HKCOG)	http://www.hkcog.org.hk/
Australian College of Midwives (ACM)	http://www.acmi.org.au/

to members, providing health professionals with information regarding important conferences, meetings and training sessions.

Professional organisations therefore are vitally important in ensuring that all women's health professionals are properly supported in their work, in their continuing education and that they are kept up-to-date with advances in their field.

Government

All health professionals are required to practise within the laws of the country in which they work. Health professionals must be kept informed of standards of practice, ethical and legal issues and overall government targets and goals for health care provision.

Most governments have separate departments that deal with all health policy issues and increasingly each department has its own website. In the UK, the Department of Health (Table 4) provides health policy information to women's health professionals as does the US Department of Health and Human Services (Table 4), Health Canada (Table 4) and the Australian Department for Health and Ageing (Table 4) for example.

Increasingly, health policy documents are being made available electronically and most government departments around the world now publish policy documents on their websites. In most cases these policy documents are made freely available on the internet in order that health professionals can access them easily and use them to guide their professional practice. The New Zealand government for example provide essential information through the National Screening Unit website regarding policy standards for cervical screening (Table 4). In the UK the Chief Nursing Officer (Table 4) provides important information through the department of health website regarding delivering the government's strategic goals. In the US the Agency for Healthcare Research and Policy provide important information for health professionals in the women's health section of their website (Table 4) and the National Health and Medical Research Council in Australia (Table 4) publish on-line government policy documents of relevance to women's health professionals working in Australia.

All government health department websites are important sources of electronic information for health professionals providing them with

Table 4.

Government	URL
Department of Health, UK	http://www.dh.gov.uk/
Department of Health and Human Services, US	http://www.hhs.gov/index.html
Health Canada	http://www.hc-sc.gc.ca/index_e.html
Australian Department for Health and Ageing	http://www.health.gov.au/
New Zealand National Screening Unit	http://www.nsu.govt.nz/Health-Professionals/1060.asp
Chief Nursing Officer, UK	http://www.dh.gov.uk/en/Aboutus/Chiefprofessionalofficers/Chiefnursingofficer/index.htm
Agency for Healthcare Research and Policy, US	http://www.ahrq.gov/research/womenix.htm
Australian National Health and Medical Research Council	http://www.nhmrc.gov.au/publications/subjects/women.htm

access to vital clinical practice regulations for practising medicine within individual countries around the world.

International Organisations

There are many women's health related international organisations in existence around the world. These organisations vary in type and in the specific aspect of women's health that they represent. On the one hand there are organisations operating on a global level such as the World Health Organisation (Table 5), co-ordinating health policy on matters of relevance to world health and influencing research agendas. The WHO is an important source of information for women's health professionals around the world but particularly to professionals caring for women in developing countries. The WHO provides free access to information resources covering important aspects of women's health including electronic access to reports, guidelines and evidence-based health information in areas such as: Making Pregnancy Safer (Table

5); Pregnancy in the European region (Table 5); Reproductive Health and Research (Table 5) and Gender, Women and Health (Table 5) amongst many other women's health issues.

The Geneva Foundation for Medical Education and Research (GFMER - Table 5) is another international organisation providing electronic information to health professionals. The GFMER aims to help encourage research programmes and collaboration for developing countries to enable them to implement research projects that investigate health issues individual to their particular situation. Access to a comprehensive list of freely available obstetrics and gynecology journal titles (Table 5) is available from this website. In addition electronic access is provided to research in family planning, gynecologic endocrinology, gynecologic oncology, gynecologic surgery, infertility, menopause, reproductive health, obstetrics and sexual health (Table 5). The GFMER also publishes an official journal, Reproductive Health, which is an open access journal title (Table 5).

On the other hand there are many women's health international societies which often fo-

Table 5.

International organisations	URL
World Health Organisation (WHO)	http://www.who.int/en/
WHO Making Pregnancy Safer	http://www.who.int/making_pregnancy_safer/en/
WHO Pregnancy in the European region	http://www.euro.who.int/healthtopics/HT2ndLvlPage?HTCode=pregnancy
WHO Reproductive Health and Research	http://www.who.int/reproductive-health/
WHO Gender, Women and Health	http://www.who.int/gender/en/
Geneva Foundation for Medical Education and Research (GFMER)	http://www.gfmer.ch/000_Homepage_En.htm
GFMER Journal Titles List	http://www.gfmer.ch/Medical_journals/Obstetrics_gynecology_reproductive_health.htm
GFMER Research	http://www.gfmer.ch/400_Publications_En.htm
GFMER Reproductive Health open access journal	http://www.reproductive-health-journal.com/home/
International Society for the Study of Women's Sexual Health	http://www.isswsh.org/
International Society for the Study of Vulvovaginal Diseases	http://www.issvd.org/

cus upon an individual issue within women's health. The International Society for the Study of Women's Sexual Health (Table 5) for example provides a structure for professionals working in this area to communicate and share experiences. An online bulletin board allows professionals to ask questions of each other and support each other in their professional practice. The International Society for the Study of Vulvovaginal Diseases (Table 5) promotes best practice and international communication between specialists working in this area of women's health worldwide. The society provides links to information sources relating to vulvovaginal diseases and comprehensive patient information.

These are of course just an example of the many international organisations that exist in the field of women's health and that provide a truly global perspective upon the professional practice of specialists in women's health.

Academic/Research

A myriad of electronic information sources exist for women's health professionals working in academia or research. Many institutions, such as universities, provide access to a range of subscription-based electronic information sources. These are often accessed from the institutions' website using a user name and password.

An important area of electronic resources used by women's health academics and researchers are general medical databases such as Medline/Pubmed (Table 6) specialising in references in the life sciences and biomedical fields, Embase (Table 6) focusing particularly on biomedical research references, Cinahl (Cumulative Index to Nursing and Allied Health Literature - Table 6) which places emphasis particularly on nursing and allied health literature, PsychInfo (Table 6) focusing on references relating to psychology, the

Table 6.

Academic/Research	URL
Medline/Pubmed	http://www.ncbi.nlm.nih.gov/sites/entrez?db=PubMed
Embase	http://www.embase.com/
Cinahl (Cumulative Index to Nursing and Allied Health Literature)	http://www.cinahl.com/
PsychInfo	http://www.apa.org/psycinfo/
BNI (British Nursing Index)	http://www.bniplus.co.uk/
Cochrane Library	http://www.thecochranelibrary.com/
TRIP (Turning Research into Practice)	http://www.tripdatabase.com/index.html
DUETs (Database of Uncertainties about the Effects Treatments)	http://www.duets.nhs.uk/SearchResults.asp?T=5&TID=25
DARE (Database of Abstracts of Reviews of Effects)	http://www.york.ac.uk/inst/crd/crddatabases.htm#DARE
ImagesMD	http://www.images.md/
Science citation index	http://scientific.thomson.com/products/sci/
Intute medicine resources	http://www.intute.ac.uk/healthandlifesciences/medicine/
Intute nursing resources	http://www.intute.ac.uk/healthandlifesciences/nursing/
Clinical Trials.gov	http://clinicaltrials.gov/
Current Controlled Trials	http://www.controlled-trials.com/

BNI (British Nursing Index - Table 6) particularly focusing upon nursing references and the Cochrane Library (Table 6) which is a particularly useful resource for health professionals as it specialises in producing and providing access to good quality systematic reviews. The databases themselves contain millions of references and each database specialises in different areas of medicine as outlined above. Within each database bibliographic details relating to women's health literature can be identified.

The TRIP (Turning Research into Practice - Table 6) database also provides free access to a collection of high quality, best-evidence references on all aspects of health. The DUETs database (Database of Uncertainties about the Effects Treatments - Table 6) provides information regarding uncertainties about the effects of treatments in areas of women's health such as endometriosis. The DARE database (Database of Abstracts of Reviews of Effects - Table 6) contains references to quality assessed systematic reviews.

In addition to medical databases institutions often provide access to online reference works such as image databases for example ImagesMD (Table 6) and the Science citation index (Table 6) which are important information sources for women's health professionals involved in research. Intute, a directory of quality assessed resources, also provides access to for example the best web-based resources in medicine (Table 6) and nursing and midwifery (Table 6). Access to on-line information about current clinical trials is important to researchers in the field of women's health and this type of information can be found from resources such as Clinical Trials.gov (Table 6) and Current Controlled Trials (Table 6).

The range of information resources required by academics and researchers is varied and the above sources are just a sample of the extensive resources available to professionals involved in women's health research.

On-Line Journals/E-Books

The internet has allowed for the development of both on-line journals and electronic books which often, but not always, exist in parallel with their hard copy equivalents. The vast majority of journal titles available worldwide are also now available in an electronic format. Electronic books, however, are less popular and consequently only a limited number of medical e-books have been produced, although this number is increasing as uptake rises. Subscriptions are generally required to access e-journals and e-books and are arranged through the publisher, with access then being provided on the publishers' website. Most women's health professionals will normally obtain access to e-journals and e-books either through the subscriptions that their institution holds or through their own personal subscriptions. However, most journal publishers do also offer access to individual journal articles for a one-off online payment.

Sources of subscription-based e-journal and e-book resources include Blackwell Synergy E-journals (Table 7), Elsevier Science Direct (Table 7), Oxford University Press E-journals (Table 7) and Wiley InterScience (Table 7). Women's health e-journals are also published and made available to members through women's health royal colleges or associations such as the British Journal of Obstetrics and Gynaecology (BJOG - Table 7) published by the RCOG, Obstetrics and Gynecology (Table 7) published by the ACOG and the Australia and New Zealand Journal of Obstetrics and Gynaecology (Table 7) published by RANZCOG.

In addition, the increasing popularity of the open access publishing model has encouraged the publication of open access or freely available journal titles available from sources such as BioMedCentral (Table 7), Free Medical Journals (Table 7), the Directory of Open Access Journals, health sciences section (DOAJ - Table 7) and Highwire (Table 7). Journal titles relevant to women's health that are freely available include Reproductive Health (Table 7) published by GFMER, BMC Pregnancy and Childbirth (Table 7), BMC Women's Health (Table 7), Reproductive Biology and Endocrinology (Table 7) and the International Breastfeeding Journal (Table 7).

E-journal publishers often also provide a table of contents alerting service, where health professionals can sign up to receive by email the table of contents of a particular journal every time a new issue of the journal is published. This is a highly valuable service to women's health professionals and enables them to keep up-to-date with the latest research and issues in the field.

Access to journals and books has always been of great importance to health professionals. With the development of electronic access to these information sources, e-journals and e-books have become an increasingly important and heavily utilised source of electronic information for women's health professionals, ensuring that they are kept up-to-date with, for example, information on best practice, results of clinical trials and expert opinion pieces.

E-Newsletters/Blogs/Podcasts/RSS Feeds

As the internet has continued to develop new internet technologies allowing for more effective and efficient information provision have emerged and these have been increasingly utilised by providers of information resources to health professionals.

Electronic newsletters are often regarded as an effective method of information provision for health professionals and have become popular

Table 7.

On-line journals/e-books	URL
Blackwell Synergy E-journals	http://www.blackwell-synergy.com/
Elsevier Science Direct	http://www.sciencedirect.com/
Oxford University Press E-journals	http://www.oxfordjournals.org/
Wiley InterScience	http://www3.interscience.wiley.com
British Journal of Obstetrics and Gynaecology (BJOG)	http://www.rcog.org.uk/index.asp?PageID=554
Obstetrics and Gynecology	http://www.acog.org/navbar/current/greenJournalLeader.cfm
Australia and New Zealand Journal of Obstetrics and Gynaecology	http://www.ranzcog.edu.au/publications/anzjog.shtml
BioMedCentral	http://www.biomedcentral.com/
Free Medical Journals	http://freemedicaljournals.com/
DOAJ	http://www.doaj.org/doaj?func=subject&cpid=20)
Highwire	http://highwire.stanford.edu/lists/freeart.dtl
Reproductive Health	http://www.reproductive-health-journal.com
BMC Pregnancy and Childbirth	http://www.biomedcentral.com/bmcpregnancychildbirth/
BMC Women's Health	http://www.biomedcentral.com/bmcwomenshealth/
Reproductive Biology and Endocrinology	http://www.rbej.com/
International Breastfeeding Journal	http://www.internationalbreastfeedingjournal.com/

in recent years. E-newsletters aimed at women's health professionals are available on a wide range of topics and are mainly used as a form of current awareness. Many contain, for example, information about newly published resources, conference and course announcements and general women's health news or current issues. Sources of women's health e-newsletters include the NLH Women's Health Specialist Library Update (Table 8), the US Centre for Disease Control CDC/ATSDR Women's Health Update and Pathways to Women's Health (Table 8) and the ACOG Today newsletter (Table 8).

Blogs are another source of health information being utilised to impart information to health professionals. However, there are very few good quality, reliable blogs specifically aimed at women's health professionals at the present time.

Podcasts or webcasts are another very popular method of information provision for women's

health professionals. Podcasts are simply a series of digital media files made available over the internet for downloading or for users to play back, using feeds, on their own computers or personal media players. They can be delivered over the internet either live or on demand. Examples include the RCOG webcasts on maternal age and motherhood, psychiatric disease in pregnancy and fibroid embolisation (Table 8), the Society of Obstetricians and Gynaecologists of Canada (Table 8) on topics such as HPV, birth control, reproductive ageing and STIs, the Medical University of South Carolina (Table 8) who provide access to podcasts regarding cervical cancer, female urinary incontinence, hysterectomy and miscarriage amongst many other women's health topics and the British Journal of Obstetrics and Gynaecology Journal podcasts (Table 8).

RSS feeds are also an increasingly popular source of information for women's health profes-

Table 8.

E-newsletters/ blogs/podcasts/RSS feeds	URL
NLH Women's Health Specialist Library Update	http://www.library.nhs.uk/womenshealth/SearchResults.aspx?catID=10394
US Centre for Disease Control CDC/ATSDR Women's Health Update and Pathways to Women's Health	http://www.cdc.gov/women/pubs.htm
ACOG Today newsletter	http://www.acog.org/member_access/lists/newslett.cfm
RCOG Webcasts	http://rcog.mediaondemand.net/login.aspx?ReturnUrl=http%3A%2F%2Frcog%2Emediaondemand%2Enet%2Fplayer%2Easpx%3FEventID%3D325
Society of Obstetricians and Gynaecologists of Canada Podcasts	http://sogc.medical.org/media/podcasts_e.asp
Medical University of South Carolina Podcasts	http://www.muschealth.com/multimedia/Podcasts/index.aspx?type=topic&groupid=3
British Journal of Obstetrics and Gynaecology Journal Podcasts	http://www.blackwellpublishing.com/podcast/bjog.asp
Royal College of Midwives RSS	http://www.rcm.org.uk/news/rss/rss.php
NLH Women's Health Specialist Library RSS	http://www.library.nhs.uk/womenshealth/RSS/CMS.aspx?feed=56
BMC Women's Health Journal RSS	http://www.biomedcentral.com/bmcwomenshealth/rss/
WHO Reproductive Health Library Training Videos	http://www.rhlibrary.com/

sionals. RSS feeds generally provide news, current awareness and table of contents type information and are delivered direct to the subscriber. Users can subscribe to a number of feeds and have the feeds delivered regularly to their desktop. RSS feeds are therefore especially useful for busy health professionals. Organisations such as the UK Royal College of Midwives (Table 8), the NLH Women's Health Specialist Library (Table 8) and the BMC Women's Health Journal (Table 8) all currently provide an RSS feed service amongst a range of other women's health organisations and publishers across the world.

A number of organisations also provide access to online videos providing information to health professionals. The WHO Reproductive Health Library produces and provides access to training videos (Table 8) covering for example best practice in how to carry out medical procedures such as caesarean section or vacuum extraction.

The information sources and technologies discussed above are just a sample of the more recent internet-based techniques for delivering health information to women's health professionals.

As discussed, the range of different sources of electronic information for women's health professionals is vast. Important health information for professionals is still often published by and delivered from traditional sources such as professional organisations or medical libraries but with the increasing use of and availability of the internet information can now be delivered electronically by these organisations in a variety of additional ways such as through on-line libraries, e-journals, podcasts, on-line training courses and of course as downloadable electronic PDF or word documents. This has allowed for both an expansion in information services provided to women's health professionals and for a revolutionary change in the way that professionals access the information that they require. However, as internet technology advances new electronic techniques for the effective delivery of information will be developed, enhancing the methods

currently being utilised and ultimately improving access to and delivery of electronic information to women's health professionals.

ACCESSIBILITY ISSUES

The range of providers of electronic information sources for women's health is vast and very varied, ranging from individuals to large journal publishing companies. As a result of this wide variation, the level of access that each provides to their resources varies enormously. This proves confusing and time-consuming for many health professionals who simply wish to access the most appropriate resource to answer their question or interest. Most health professionals are used to the electronic resource access arrangements that their institutions provide but there are a number of different ways that access can be provided to individuals and institutions and these are outlined below.

In general access to electronic resources can be categorised into four main types: freely accessible; registration required; subscription-based and one-off payment.

Freely accessible resources are resources that anyone can access over the internet. These resources can be accessed by following links available on the website which take users to the full-text of a resource or research article or link to the full-text resource if it is freely available on another website. Some organisations provide free access to a limited range of information sources and in addition provide subscription and/or registration-only access to the rest of the content that they produce.

Increasingly, providers of electronic information resources require users to register with their website in order to be able to access full-text resources. The registration process is often free and simply involves filling out an online form which is held by the organisation providing the service. Resources are then accessible by 'signing in' every time the user visits the website. Websites requiring a form of registration can often deter health professionals from using them as it takes time to register and, of course, requires the user to remember their user name and password as they are required to be entered into the system each time the site is visited.

The vast majority of sources of electronic information for women's health professionals are subscription-based. However, there are numerous different types of subscriptions offered by providers of electronic information and these entail different terms of and means of access to the resources provided.

One example is personal subscriptions. These are subscriptions that individuals pay, for example, to professional organisations or to publishers that entitle them to access information resources published by or provided by that organisation. This could involve membership of a professional obstetrics and gynecology college that entitles the member to receive electronically the professional journal published by the organisation or a health professional may arrange to subscribe to a particular journal title through a publisher. Access to the resource is only made available to those who have subscribed and usually involves the user entering a password and user name which will be recognised by the system and the resources subscribed to will then be made available to them.

Institutions such as universities or hospitals also often take out subscriptions to electronic information sources. Subscriptions taken out by organisations usually involve a site-wide or organisation-wide subscription allowing access to the resource by all staff or health professionals associated with the organisation. These subscriptions are usually managed through the organisations' library which is responsible for administering access to the resources subscribed to. Accessing resources subscribed to in this way is similar to personal subscriptions as user names and passwords are required but in addition to this

the system often also uses IP address recognition which ensures that only people using computers within the network of the organisation that has subscribed can access the resources. For many health professionals around the world ATHENS (Table 9), an access management system for web-based resources, is the system that is used to provide users with access to the electronic resources that their organisation purchases. Organisations purchasing multiple user subscriptions to electronic resources often subscribe to a range of different resources from different information providers, such as e-journals, e-books, online learning packages, electronic reference resources and evidence-based medicine resources. These are made available to health professionals through the organisations' website, using a single log on system so that users do not have to repeatedly enter passwords and user names to access individual resources.

Lastly, access to a range of women's health information resources can also be provided by a one-off payment system. This access arrangement is most often provided by journal publishers and allows individuals who do not hold a personal subscription or whose institution does not hold an institutional license to access a particular article in a journal. The publisher advertises a price for each article it publishes and a one-off online payment is required in order for access to be provided to the user. Upon payment the user is automatically allowed to access the article which can then be downloaded. Recently, publishers have introduced a time-barred access arrangement for accessing articles. This also involves an online payment but access to the article may be provided for only one day for example and after the time limit has passed the user will no longer be able to access that particular article. This access arrangement is particularly useful for women's health professionals who require access to particular journal articles but who do not wish to hold an annual subscription.

The examples discussed above are just a few of the most common arrangements for providing

Table 9.

Accessibility issues	URL
ATHENS	www.athens.ac.uk

access to electronic sources of women's health information. Each publisher or provider has its own subscription model and these vary across the world. Ultimately, no electronic access system can be regarded as a model system as they all provide different arrangements depending upon the type of subscriber and the access arrangements that publishers/providers wish to provide to their customers, members, staff or users.

IMPORTANCE OF QUALITY ASSESSMENT

The growth in the use of and access to the internet has fuelled the development of different websites and electronic services advertising information resources for women's health. The quality of information provided by the vast array of different websites and online services varies enormously with only some providing information that is reliable and of good quality. As a result it is increasingly difficult for busy health professionals to ensure that they are accessing sources that provide good quality information. Consequently, it is important for health professionals to assess websites and electronic sources of women's health knowledge and the information that they publish in order to ensure that the information accessed by women's health professionals is evidence-based and from a reliable and trusted source.

The process used to assess information sources and resources is referred to as critical appraisal. Critical appraisal is an important part of evidence-based practice. The process of critical appraisal involves systematically examining research to determine its validity and relevance

and therefore the overall quality of the research. Over the last few years a great deal of research has been undertaken to determine the most effective critical appraisal tools.

Critical appraisal tools are checklists to guide the user through assessing the quality of a resource. Critical appraisal tools generally cover areas such as whether the research addressed a clearly focussed question; the appropriateness of the methodology used and how rigorous it is; the data collection and data analysis methods used; if the reported results of the research are valid; whether the results can be applied to local situations; whether the research could have been open to bias in any way. The tools are designed to be used alongside the reading of the research paper, website or information source and the individual checklist points in the tool applied to the resource. At the end of the appraisal the information drawn out from the resource can be used to assess the quality of the resource. Critical appraisal tools have been developed to examine different types of research such as quantitative or qualitative research and to assess different types of resources such as papers, websites and online guidelines for example.

Organisations such as CASP (the Critical Appraisal Skills Programme - Table 10) in the UK have developed and tested various different tools examining for example systematic reviews, randomised controlled trials (RCTs), qualitative studies, case control studies and economic evaluations. The CASP tools are based on guides produced by the Evidence-Based Medicine Working Group at McMaster University in Canada. The Alberta Heritage Foundation for Medical Research in Canada have developed a tool called

Standard Quality Assessment Criteria for Evaluating Primary Research Papers from a Variety of Fields (Table 10) which has been specifically developed for working with Health Technology Assessments (HTAs). In New Zealand a collaborative team based at Auckland University have established EPIQ (Effective Practice, Informatics and Quality Improvement - Table 10) and have developed the GATE (Graphic Appraisal Tool for Epidemiology) tool and a series of critical appraisal checklists covering different types of study. The AGREE (Appraisal of Guidelines Research and Evaluation) instrument has been developed by an international collaboration of experts (Table 10) and is designed to be used to assess the quality of clinical guidelines. The internet search engine SUMSearch (Table 10), developed by the University of Texas Health Science Centre, searches only for good quality, evidence-based resources available on the internet. It does this by applying certain criteria to the way it searches for the terms entered into search box and it applies filters to ensure that the results retrieved are likely to be well conducted, evidence-based research studies or resources produced by professionals.

In general, critical appraisal tools have been developed to assess the quality of RCTs, systematic reviews, guidelines and other research studies. Effective tools to assess for example websites, newsletters and blogs containing health information have not been studied in depth and very little is available for assessing this type of information resource. The DISCERN tool (Table 10), mainly aimed at consumers and patients, is a checklist of 16 questions that can be used to evaluate health information websites. Another tool that can be used to assess website quality is the Health Information Quality Assessment Tool (Table 10). This is an automated tool that allows users to work through a set of evaluation questions while viewing the website to be assessed and then when finished the tool will calculate whether it 'passes' or 'fails' the evaluation and

list comments on the strengths and weaknesses of the website. In Geneva, the Health on the Net Foundation (Table 10) provides and promotes the use of a code that website developers can sign up to to ensure that the information provided by them meets certain quality criteria.

In addition to the development of tools to help health professionals critically appraise resources themselves a number of organisations have also begun to provide access to their own critical appraisals of resources, known as CATs (critically appraised topics). CATs are brief summaries of the evidence from a research paper or resource. The College of Family Physicians of Canada (Table 10), the University of Michigan Department of Pediatrics (Table 10) and EPIQ (Table 10) in New Zealand all provide free access to their own CATs. The organisations select research papers or resources to appraise and then make the results of the appraisal available on their websites for professionals to access. Another way of creating CATs is to use the CATmaker (Table 10), developed by the Centre for Evidence-based Medicine. The CATmaker is a software tool that can be downloaded and used to create CATs for different types of research.

As the quantity of electronic resources available to health professionals increases, the need for applying a quality check to these information resources becomes more and more important and critical appraisal is regarded as being the most robust way of assessing quality. Increasingly, the ability to be able to critically appraise resources is regarded as a highly valuable skill for health professionals to acquire and as a result many institutions run courses on critical appraisal for their staff. Journal clubs are also gaining popularity around the world as a way to encourage health professionals to regularly practise their critical appraisal skills. Ultimately, there are no definitive answers as to the best methods for critically appraising resources but the fact that it is regarded as an increasingly important skill and that it is

Table 10.

Importance of quality assessment	URL
CASP (the Critical Appraisal Skills Programme)	http://www.phru.nhs.uk/Pages/PHD/CASP.htm
Alberta Heritage Foundation for Medical Research in Canada, Standard Quality Assessment Criteria for Evaluating Primary Research Papers from a Variety of Fields	http://www.ihe.ca/documents/hta/HTA-FR13.pdf
Auckland University, EPIQ (Effective Practice, Informatics and Quality Improvement)	http://www.health.auckland.ac.nz/population-health/epidemiology-biostats/epiq/index.html
AGREE (Appraisal of Guidelines Research and Evaluation)	www.agreecollaboration.org/pdf/agreeinstrumentfinal.pdf
SUMSearch	http://sumsearch.uthscsa.edu/
DISCERN	www.discern.org.uk
Health Information Quality Assessment Tool	http://hitiweb.mitretek.org/iq/
Health on the Net Foundation	www.hon.ch
College of Family Physicians of Canada CATs	http://www.cfpc.ca/English/cfpc/clfm/critical/
University of Michigan Department of Pediatrics CATs	http://www.med.umich.edu/pediatrics/ebm/Cat.htm
EPIQ CATs	http://www.health.auckland.ac.nz/population-health/epidemiology-biostats/epiq/index.html
CATmaker	http://www.cebm.net/index.aspx?o=1216

being promoted to health professionals worldwide attests to its importance in strengthening the practice of evidence-based medicine.

ROLE OF THE INFORMATION SPECIALIST

The job title 'information specialist' is an increasingly popular term within the library and information field, particularly within the area of health librarianship. The title itself is a relatively new one becoming increasingly more popular as the role of libraries and information centres has changed with the increasing use and availability of the internet and the electronic delivery of resources. The expansion in services provided by libraries as a result of this revolutionary shift in the way that information is provided to users has consequently resulted in a change and expansion of roles within the library and information field,

and the emergence of information specialists is just one of these new and highly varied roles.

Information specialists have differing roles depending upon the sector in which they work. This section will concentrate particularly on the role of information specialists within the health sector.

Essentially the role of the health information specialist is to identify, access, evaluate, make sense of and disseminate health information to health professionals. Information specialists can be viewed as gatekeepers, allowing access to relevant information and filtering out resources that are not appropriate. Health information specialists fundamentally are mediators between the mass of health information that exists worldwide and the specific information that is sought by a particular health professional. Health information specialists often work in designated fields within medicine (such as women's health) and over time build up an in-depth knowledge of the information resources and research available within their field, allowing for a more effective service to be provided to health professionals. Health information specialists can be found in a variety of institutions such as hospital libraries, university libraries, hospital departments, charities, university departments, government departments, pharmaceutical companies and in the local community.

In order to correctly and efficiently identify all relevant resources on a particular topic information specialists have to be highly trained in how to search for information and resources. Search skills are vitally important and involve an in-depth knowledge of how different databases work and the availability of web-based resources relevant to the search topic. The information specialist has the ability to design highly comprehensive search strategies by combining free-text search terms, controlled vocabularies in databases and relevant search filters and ensure that these are combined in a way that they search specifically for the type and subject area of the resources desired. The results of these searches can then be merged together in a bibliographic database and made available to health professionals.

Information specialists increasingly also have a role in filtering information resources or research to weed out poor quality resources. Filtering could be applied to the results of a complex search or a new website or information source. The filtering process involves the use of critical appraisal and can be done in various ways depending upon the type of research or resource that requires appraising. Once the health information specialist has filtered out the inappropriate resources, a list of relevant and good quality resources can be made available. The availability of lists of pre-appraised resources and research is of great benefit to busy health professionals who often seek resources that they know have gone through some quality appraisal process already due to their tight work schedules.

The ability of information specialists therefore to compile and carry out complex searches, manage the resultant bibliographic references and re-package these into user-friendly documents is of great benefit to busy health professionals.

Signposting is one of the main roles of the health information specialist. This involves the information specialist directing or alerting health professionals to good quality information resources. As a result of the continued development of, increasing use of and availability of the internet information specialists are increasingly able to do this using web-based techniques. The information specialist's role therefore involves the signposting to and delivery of information on a number of different platforms, both traditional and electronic, to health professionals. Information specialists often use their searching and critical appraisal skills to make available on the web collections of links to good quality resources in health care. They also increasingly produce email newsletters or RSS feeds alerting health professionals to new research, guidelines or resources and information specialists often set up alerting services for health topics that professionals can sign up to to receive the latest evidence from within their particular field. Web-based developments such as blogs and podcasts are also increasingly being used by information specialists as a way of disseminating important information to busy health professionals. Information specialists aim to keep up-to-date not only with new information resources in their field but also with new technology that will allow them to utilise all available platforms to disseminate relevant and important health information to health professionals who require it. Providing the right information at the right time in a convenient location is the ultimate aim.

In addition, information specialists are also increasingly involved in teaching health professionals how to search effectively, use bibliographic databases, critically appraise resources and also how to access different electronic resources. These skills are all essential in ensuring that health professionals locate evidence-based research/resources to make health-related decisions. In recent years the importance of these skills to health professionals has been recognised and often this now forms a part of the medical curriculum in medical schools across the world.

The role of an information specialist in the health sector therefore is a very broad one. Information specialists essentially manage information: identifying information sources, filtering out poor quality information, re-packaging it into useable and user-friendly formats and disseminating this information in formats relevant to health professionals. Information specialists keep abreast of new research and developments in particular fields so that busy health professionals do not have to.

CONCLUSION

Utilising electronic information resources is now an essential part of the information seeking patterns of women's health professionals. The range of resources available electronically and the differing levels of access arrangements ensure that most women's health professionals have access to the resources that they require in order to make health related decisions. The round-the-clock availability of electronic resources has greatly benefited health professionals enabling them to access evidence-based information at a time and place convenient to them. Recognition of and education about the importance of critical appraisal has enabled many health professionals to ensure that they assess the quality of the information resources that they use, this being even more important with regard to electronic information sources. Health professionals are also increasingly turning to information specialists to help them with their literature searches as information specialists can mediate between the vast array of health information available worldwide and the specific information sought by a clinician,

ultimately making sense of and signposting the clinician to the best-quality information available in their specific research area.

The ease of access that the electronic provision of information has enabled has had a hugely beneficial effect on the working lives of busy health professionals. This explosion in electronic sources of information has however also introduced new problems, as not only do women's health professionals have to keep up-to-date with new research or medical advances in their field, they also have to keep abreast of the ever-increasing sources of electronic women's health information available worldwide and the technologies used to deliver them. Internet technologies look set to continue to develop rapidly. In the years to come, therefore, we will not only continue to witness an ever-increasing range of women's health information sources but also the development of new delivery techniques and platforms that will need to be utilised to ensure that information continues to be disseminated to women's health professionals wherever and whenever it is needed.

FUTURE RESEARCH DIRECTIONS

As discussed earlier, a comprehensive literature search has revealed that very little research has actually been conducted in the specific area of electronic information sources for women's health professionals. The lack of an evidence base regarding the current information-seeking patterns of women's health professionals contributes to the problems experienced by information specialists in designing useful and relevant information resources and services for women's health professionals.

It is therefore crucial to encourage research to be conducted to assess: firstly the different publication types, such as guidelines, bottom-line summaries, systematic reviews etc., that women's health professionals feel are important to be delivered in an electronic format; secondly the frequency with which women's health professionals wish to both search for and receive this information such as daily, monthly, or only when they seek to find a particular resource; thirdly the method by which women's health professionals wish the information to be delivered to them for example as text files, email updates, websites, RSS feeds, pdf attachments etc.; lastly what the most appropriate methods of information skills training would be for women's health professionals, such as online tutorials, classroom-based teaching or one-to-one teaching in their place of work.

As technologies continue to develop and electronic dissemination of information increases, the importance placed on the electronic delivery of information to busy women's health professionals looks likely to continue to escalate. Only by conducting user research will information specialists be able to be confident that they are fulfilling the information needs of all women's health professionals.

REFERENCES

Agency for Healthcare Research and Policy, US. (n.d.). Retrieved September 13, 2007 from Agency for Healthcare Research and Policy, US.

Agree Collaboration (n.d.). Retrieved September 8, 2007, from http://www.agreecollaboration.org/pdf/agreeinstrumentfinal.pdf

AHC Media LLC, freeCME.com (n.d.). Retrieved September 13, 2007 from http://www.freecme.com/gcourses1.php?specialty_id=41&specialty_name=OB/GYN

Heritage Foundation for Medical Research Alberta (n.d.). Retrieved September 8, 2007, from http://www.ihe.ca/documents/hta/HTA-FR13.pdf

American College of Nurse Midwives (n.d.). Retrieved September 13, 2007 from http://www.midwife.org

American College of Obstetricians and Gynecology, Today newsletter (n.d.). Retrieved September 15, 2007 from http://www.acog.org/member_access/lists/newslett.cfm

American College Obstetricians and Gynecology, Obstetrics and Gynecology Journal (n.d.). Retrieved September 14, 2007 from http://www.acog.org/navbar/current/greenJournalLeader.cfm

American College of Obstetricians and Gynecologists (n.d.). Retrieved August 17, 2007 from http://www.acog.org/postgrad/index.cfm

ATHENS (n.d.). Retrieved September 13, 2007 from http://www.athens.ac.uk

Australian College of Midwives (n.d.). Retrieved September 14, 2007 from http://www.acmi.org.au/

Australian Department for Health and Ageing (n.d.). Retrieved September 14, 2007 from http://www.health.gov.au/

BioMedCentral (n.d.). Retrieved September 14, 2007 from http://www.biomedcentral.com/

Blackwell Synergy E-journals Retrieved September 14, 2007 from http://www.blackwell-synergy.com/

BMC Pregnancy and Childbirth (n.d.). Retrieved September 14, 2007 from http://www.biomedcentral.com/bmcpregnancychildbirth/

BMC Women's Health (n.d.). Retrieved September 14, 2007 from http://www.biomedcentral.com/bmcwomenshealth/

BMC Women's Health Journal RSS (n.d.). Retrieved September 15, 2007 from http://www.biomedcentral.com/bmcwomenshealth/rss/

BNI (British Nursing Index) (n.d.). Retrieved September 13, 2007 from http://www.bniplus.co.uk/

British Journal of Obstetrics and Gynaecology Journal, podcasts (n.d.). Retrieved September 15, 2007 from http://www.blackwellpublishing.com/podcast/bjog.asp

Canadian Association of Midwives (n.d.). Retrieved September 14, 2007 from http://www.canadianmidwives.org/

CASP (n.d.). Retrieved September 6, 2007 from http://www.phru.nhs.uk/Pages/PHD/CASP.htm

CATmaker, Centre for Evidence-based Medicine (n.d.). Retrieved September 8, 2007 from http://www.cebm.net/index.aspx?o=1216

Centre for Disease Control CDC/ATSDR, US (n.d.). Retrieved September 15, 2007 from http://www.cdc.gov/women/pubs.htm

Chief Nursing Officer, UK (n.d.). Retrieved September 13, 2007 from http://www.dh.gov.uk/en/Aboutus/Chiefprofessionalofficers/Chief-nursingofficer/index.htm

Cinahl (Cumulative Index to Nursing and Allied Health Literature) (n.d.). Retrieved September 14, 2007 from http://www.cinahl.com/

Clinical Trilas.gov (n.d.). Retrieved September 14, 2007 from http://clinicaltrials.gov/

Cochrane Library (n.d.). Retrieved September 13, 2007 from http://www.thecochranelibrary.com/

College of Family Physicians of Canada (n.d.). Retrieved September 15, 2007 from http://www.cfpc.ca/English/cfpc/clfm/critical/

Critical appraisal and using the literature (n.d.). Retrieved September 7, 2007 from www.shef.ac.uk/scharr/ir/units/critapp/websites

Current Controlled Trials (n.d.). Retrieved September 14, 2007 from http://www.controlled-trials.com/

DARE database (Database of Abstracts of Reviews of Effects) (n.d.). Retrieved September 13, 2007 from http://www.york.ac.uk/inst/crd/crd-databases.htm#DARE

Department of Health, UK (n.d.). Retrieved September 13, 2007 from http://www.dh.gov.uk/

Department of Health and Human Services, US (n.d.). Retrieved September 13, 2007 from http://www.hhs.gov/index.html

Directory of Open Access Journals, health sciences section (n.d.). Retrieved September 14, 2007 from http://www.doaj.org/doaj?func=subject&cpid=20

DISCERN (n.d.). Retrieved September 6, 2007 from www.discern.org.uk

DUETs database (Database of Uncertainties about the Effects Treatments) (n.d.). Retrieved September 13, 2007 from http://www.duets.nhs.uk/SearchResults.asp?T=5&TID=25

Elsevier Science Direct (n.d.). Retrieved September 14, 2007 from http://www.sciencedirect.com/

Embase (n.d.). Retrieved September 13, 2007 from http://www.embase.com/

EPIQ (n.d.). Retrieved September 8, 2007 from http://www.health.auckland.ac.nz/population-health/epidemiology-biostats/epiq/index.html

Evidence-based medicine.co.uk, What is critical appraisal? (n.d.). Retrieved September 6, 2007 from www.evidence-based-medicine.co.uk

Faculty of Sexual and Reproductive Healthcare, UK (n.d.). Retrieved August 17, 2007 from

http://www.fsrh.org/Default2.asp?Section=Publications&SubSection=FACTS

Free Medical Journals (n.d.). Retrieved September 14, 2007 from http://freemedicaljournals.com/

Geneva Foundation for Medical Education and Research (GFMER) (n.d.). Retrieved September 14, 2007 from http://www.gfmer.ch/000_Homepage_En.htm

Geneva Foundation for Medical Education and Research, Journal list (n.d.). Retrieved September 14, 2007 http://www.gfmer.ch/Medical_journals/Obstetrics_gynecology_reproductive_health.htm

Geneva Foundation for Medical Education and Research, Research resources (n.d.). Retrieved September 14, 2007 from http://www.gfmer.ch/400_Publications_En.htm

Geneva Foundation for Medical Education and Research, Reproductive Health Journal (n.d.). Retrieved September 14, 2007 from http://www.reproductive-health-journal.com/home/

Health Canada (n.d.). Retrieved September 13, 2007 from http://www.hc-sc.gc.ca/index_e.html

Health Information Quality Assessment Tool (n.d.). Retrieved September 8, 2007 from http://hitiweb.mitretek.org/iq/

Health on the Net Foundation (n.d.). Retrieved September 7, 2007 from www.hon.ch

Highwire (n.d.). Retrieved September 14, 2007 from http://highwire.stanford.edu/lists/freeart.dtl

Hong Kong College of Obstetricians and Gynaecologists (n.d.). Retrieved September 14, 2007 from http://www.hkcog.org.hk/

ImagesMD (n.d.). Retrieved September 14, 2007 from http://www.images.md/

International Breastfeeding Journal (n.d.). Retrieved September 14, 2007 from http://www.internationalbreastfeedingjournal.com/

International Society for the Study of Vulvovaginal Diseases (n.d.). Retrieved September 14, 2007 from http://www.issvd.org/

International Society for the Study of Women's Sexual Health (n.d.). Retrieved September 14, 2007 from http://www.isswsh.org/

Intute, medicine section (n.d.). Retrieved September 14, 2007 from http://www.intute.ac.uk/healthandlifesciences/medicine/

Intute, nursing and midwifery section (n.d.). Retrieved September 14, 2007 from http://www.intute.ac.uk/healthandlifesciences/nursing/

Medical University of South Carolina, podcasts (n.d.). Retrieved September 15, 2007 from http://www.muschealth.com/multimedia/Podcasts/index.aspx?type=topic&groupid=3

Medline/Pubmed (n.d.). Retrieved September 13, 2007 from http://www.ncbi.nlm.nih.gov/sites/entrez?db=PubMed

National Library of Medicine, US (n.d.). Retrieved September 13, 2007 from www.nlm.nih.gov

National Health and Medical Research Council, Australia (n.d.). Retrieved September 13, 2007 from http://www.nhmrc.gov.au/publications/subjects/women.htm

National Screening Unit, New Zealand (n.d.). Retrieved September 13, 2007 from

http://www.nsu.govt.nz/Health-Professionals/1060.asp

New Zealand Guidelines Group (n.d.). Retrieved August 18, 2007 from http://www.nzgg.org.nz

Oxford University Press E-journals (n.d.). Retrieved September 14, 2007 from http://www.oxfordjournals.org/

PsychInfo (n.d.). Retrieved September 14, 2007 from http://www.apa.org/psycinfo/

Reproductive Biology and Endocrinology (n.d.). Retrieved September 14, 2007 from http://www.rbej.com/

Royal Australia and New Zealand College of Obstetricians and Gynaecologists, Australia and New Zealand Journal of Obstetrics and Gynaecology (n.d.). Retrieved September 14, 2007 from http://www.ranzcog.edu.au/publications/anzjog. shtml

Royal Australia and New Zealand College of Obstetricians and Gynaecologists (n.d.). Retrieved August 18, 2007 from http://www.ranzcog.edu. au/flp/index.shtml

Royal College of Midwives, UK (n.d.). Retrieved September 14, 2007 from http://www.rcm.org. uk/

Royal College of Midwives, RSS (n.d.). Retrieved September 15, 2007 from http://www.rcm.org. uk/news/rss/rss.php

Royal College of Obstetricians and Gynaecologists, UK (n.d.). Retrieved September 14, 2007 from http://www.rcog.org.uk/

Royal College of Obstetricians and Gynaecologists, UK, British Journal of Obstetrics and Gynaecology (n.d.). Retrieved September 14, 2007 from http://www.rcog.org.uk/index.asp?PageID=554

Royal College of Obstetricians and Gynaecologists, UK, webcasts (n.d.). Retrieved September 15, 2007 from http://rcog.mediaondemand.net/ login.aspx?ReturnUrl=http%3A%2F%2Frcog% 2Emediaondemand%2Enet%2Fplayer%2Easpx %3FEventID%3D325

Science citation index (n.d.). Retrieved September 14, 2007 from http://scientific.thomson. com/products/sci/

Society of Obstetricians and Gynaecologists of Canada (n.d.). Retrieved August 18, 2007 from http://www.sogc.org/cme/online_e.asp

Society of Obstetricians and Gynaecologists of Canada, podcasts (n.d.). Retrieved September 15, 2007 from http://sogc.medical.org/media/pod-casts_e.asp

SUMSearch (n.d.). Retrieved September 9, 2007 from http://sumsearch.uthscsa.edu/

TRIP (Turning Research into Practice) (n.d.). Retrieved September 14, 2007 from http://www. tripdatabase.com/index.html

University of Michigan, Department of Pediatrics (n.d.). Retrieved September 8, 2007 from http:// www.med.umich.edu/pediatrics/ebm/Cat.htm

Wiley InterScience (n.d.). Retrieved September 14, 2007 from http://www3.interscience.wiley.com/

Women's Health Specialist Library, UK (n.d.). Retrieved August 18, 2007 from www.library. nhs.uk/womenshealth

Women's health Specialist library GBS Teaching Package, UK (n.d.). Retrieved August 17, 2007 from http://www.whsl.org.uk/gbs/

Women's Health Specialist Library Update, RSS (n.d.). Retrieved September 15, 2007 from http://www.library.nhs.uk/womenshealth/ SearchResults.aspx?catID=10394

World Health Organisation (n.d.). Retrieved September 13, 2007 from http://www.who.int/en/

World Health Organisation, Making Pregnancy Safer (n.d.). Retrieved September 13, 2007 from http://www.who.int/making_pregnancy_safer/ en/

World Health Organisation, Pregnancy in the European region (n.d.). Retrieved September 13, 2007 from http://www.euro.who.int/healthtop-ics/HT2ndLvlPage?HTCode=pregnancy

World Health Organisation, Reproductive Health and Research (n.d.). Retrieved September 13, 2007 from http://www.who.int/reproductive-health/

World Health Organisation, Gender, Women and Health (n.d.). Retrieved September 13, 2007 from http://www.who.int/gender/en/

World Health Organisation, Reproductive Health Library (n.d.). Retrieved August 17, 2007 from www.rhlibrary.com

ADDITIONAL READING

Centre for Health Evidence User Guides - http://www.cche.net/usersguides/main.asp

NLH Women's Health Specialist Library - www.library.nhs.uk/womenshealth

Reproductive Health Library - www.rhlibrary.com

Geneva Foundation for Medical Education and Research (GFMER) http://www.gfmer.ch/000_Homepage_En.htm

WHO Reproductive Health and Research - http://www.who.int/reproductive-health/

CASP (the Critical Appraisal Skills Programme) - http://www.phru.nhs.uk/Pages/PHD/CASP.htm

Agree Collaboration - http://www.agreecollaboration.org/

Centre for Evidence-Based Medicine http://www.cebm.net/

Chapter XV
Computerised Decision Support for Women's Health Informatics

David Parry
Auckland University of Technology, New Zealand

ABSTRACT

Decision analysis techniques attempt to utilize mathematical data about outcomes and preferences to help people make optimal decisions. The increasing uses of computerized records and powerful computers have made these techniques much more accessible and usable. The partnership between women and clinicians can be enhanced by sharing information, knowledge, and the decision making process in this way. Other techniques for assisting with decision making, such as learning from data via neural networks or other machine learning approaches may offer increased value. Rules learned from such approaches may allow the development of expert systems that actually take over some of the decision making role, although such systems are not yet in widespread use.

INTRODUCTION

Decision analysis involves formally identifying the important aspects of making decisions in terms of the required information, the process followed, and the outcomes expected. Of course, people make decisions all the time without going through this process, so decision analysis is often reserved for situations where the decisions are particularly difficult because there is no good precedent or the decision maker is uncertain, the consequences of making the wrong decision are

serious or because the decision making process needs to be particularly explicit and verifiable. As with all informatics activities, computer support is helpful, but not a complete replacement for clinical judgement, or a remedy for poor knowledge of the area.

Computational intelligence involves the use of computers to make decisions themselves, in conjunction with humans, or independently.

Formalising decision making processes allows for a reflection on the decision-making process, and the sharing of this process with others such

Figure 1. The audit cycle

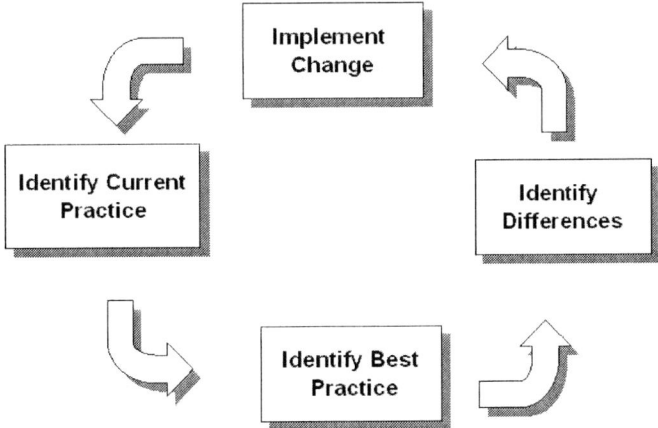

as colleagues, patients or researchers. The audit of behaviour is linked to the use of evidence–based practice (Rosenberg & Donald, 1995). As part of evidence based practice, clinicians are seen to need to justify their actions in the light of scientific research. Briefly, evidence based practice requires the following stages:

- Identification of a clinical problem
- A systematic search for evidence
- Assessment of the evidence in a structured way
- Synthesis of the evidence
- Decision on what is "best practice"

The best practice thus identified becomes the second part of the audit cycle (Figure 1). Decision analysis involves the incorporation of data from good sources of evidence, such as clinical trials in order to identify best practice. This best practice may involve a quite complex process of decision making that depends on many factors, and it may be that decisions need to be segmented in terms of whether they apply to individual cases, groups of patients or whole populations.

CLINICAL DECISION MAKING

Decision analysis is intended to both model and improve decision-making. The techniques used have a number of similarities but the importance of different aspects of the decision changes with the size of the group being affected. In general, as the groups affected get larger, the distribution of values for parameters are easier to predict , while as groups get smaller then the variation between individuals becomes more important. Dowie made an important point in a 1996 paper (Dowie, 1996) that the decision making process needs to incorporate evidence, cost effectiveness and preferences of the people involved. The use of evidence of clinical benefit, although it is necessary for the choice of action, is not always sufficient to make the decision obvious.

Decision Making for One Patient

Classically, clinical decision making concerns the actions taken to improve the health of one patient. This is at the heart of the clinicians role and has been expressed in the form of the Hippocratic Oath *"To practice and prescribe to the best of my ability for the good of my patients, and to try to avoid harming them.* "(Anonymous, 2007). In the case of decisions affecting a single patient, it is obviously important to know what the patient herself regards as an acceptable outcome. The acceptability or otherwise of an outcome is known as its "utility" in decision analysis terms. It is important to realise that these utilities can vary to quite a large degree. For example work described in (J. Thornton & R. Lilford, 1989; J. G. Thornton & R. J. Lilford, 1989) has shown that there is a very wide variation in the risk that women are prepared to accept, and that this is not simply a matter of lack of information, or an immediate emotional response. Thus, blanket policies for decision making may not reflect the patient's wishes, and reflects back on the importance of patient preference. This is not surprising if one accepts that healthcare is another part of life where autonomy and personal choice are important, just as for example the choice of whether to have a baby in the first place !

This problem cannot be solved simply by providing information – what is an acceptable risk to one person may not be to another. Indeed even within the professional body, there are wide variations in what the professional would perceive to be the best approach to a particular situation. Studies examining obstetricians attitude to decision –making in childbirth- for example whether a caesarean section is appropriate have show wide variations in preference. (Land, Parry, Rane, & Wilson, 2001).

A practical issue arises in that individuals react differently to therapy and have unique combinations of pre-existing conditions, genetic makeup and physiological response.

Decision Making for a Group of Patients

Complexity arises in treating pregnant women where there is more than one individual involved

in the outcome. A detailed discussion of the ethics involved is out of the scope of this chapter but one should realise that there may be potential conflicts between the optimum outcomes for mothers, babies, twins and even siblings in the case of "saviour" embryos (Brownsword, 2004).

Decision Making for Population Health

When the focus changes to the population, then the emphasis changes from individual benefits and utilities, to the wider common good. However, strict utilitarian approaches are not acceptable in most cases, so individual rights, and general principles such as equity need to be taken into consideration. On the positive side, variation between individuals will tend to become less important when deciding on policies for populations, although the identification of subgroups may be important. Example of this sort of decision making may include screening for cervical cancer, and provision of HPV vaccination within a population(Jones et al., 2007)

DECISION ANALYSIS

Pubmed defines decision analysis as : "Mathematical or statistical procedures used as aids in making a decision. They are frequently used in medical decision-making."

Decision analysis techniques attempt to bridge the gap between knowledge and information – that is by somehow representing the knowledge that is available, they allow information to be used to inform decision making. In terms of the use of computers, the continuum ranges from an effectively paper-based approach, such as clinical algorithms, to computer –supported decision making, as may be seen in a decision analysis spreadsheet, to a fully automatic artificial intelligence system.

Sources of Information for Decision Making

Some decisions are relatively easy to support with even limited information. For example, early trials of penicillin-based antibiotics for peritonitis in the 1940's showed that only those patients given the drug survived. Fortunately, most decisions are not as stark as this, but in order to make use of decision analysis techniques, there are some important parameters to consider. Firstly, the information must be reliable and apply to this particular patient group. Thus it is important to have correct reference data for predicted growth charts depending on the ethnic background of the patient, such statistics are described in chapter 14. It is also very important to have the best possible evidence, and this has been made easier by the growth of evidence-based medicine (Rosenberg & Donald, 1995), and in particular the availability of systematic reviews. The Cochrane Collaboration Database on pregnancy and childbirth was one of the earliest libraries of systematic reviews available (Cochrane Collaboration, 1997), and has continued to grow as part of the wider Cochrane library. For many of the techniques such as statistical decision analysis and Bayesian methods, data on the prevalence or likelihood of certain conditions are important and these can be discovered form some of the sources described in the statistical measures chapter. For knowledge discovery techniques, comprehensive databases, which may be derived from electronic health records (see the chapter on the electronic health record), may be needed, these are particularly useful when multiple factors are included in the outcome calculation, or to gain an understanding of the expected outcome in local conditions.

When people make decisions without any decision support tools, it is also helpful if the available evidence and information is collated and available, and electronic sources such as the web are increasingly valuable for this purpose (see Chapter XIII). This can be especially useful in the case of rare conditions or unusual combinations of factors, where there may be no compelling evidence from good clinical trials.

Bayesian Methods

The reverend Thomas Bayes had his essay on probability published posthumously (Bayes, 1764). Bayesian methods involve trying to quantify the likelihood of a particular event occurring given what has happened before. This differs from classical statistics which deals with the frequency of observed events. In simple terms a Bayesian approach allows you to suggest how likely a diagnosis is given data about how often the diagnosis occurs in the population you are studying and the results of any diagnostic tests, given the sensitivity and specificity of them.

In addition, modern Bayesian approaches often include the use of utility values. In order to select a recommended course of action, the chance of something happening and the desirability of that outcome are combined. This is a very common human activity, and usually a simple multiplication is performed to produce a utility score (desirability*likelihood). It is important to note that the desirability of an outcome may vary hugely between and within populations, which supports the work of Dowie (Dowie, 1996). There has been extensive debate about the validity of Bayesian approaches to decision-making, with a number of authors making the point that the prior odds of an event may not be widely available, and that the different means of reporting trials of diagnostic tests can lead to confusion and incorrect estimates (Cooper, 1992; Harris, 1981)

One of the most important things that Bayesian approaches make plain is the importance of the prior likelihood of any condition. This is particularly helpful in the situation where

If A is an event that you are trying to detect and B is the result of a test. P(A) represents the prior probability of a particular event, and P(B) the prior probability of getting the result then:

$$P(A \mid B) = \frac{P(B \mid A)P(A)}{P(B)}$$

Where P(B|A) is the probability of getting the result B given the condition A, and P(A|B) is the probability that the patient has the condition A given the result B. This allows the accuracy of the test, in terms of true positive and false positive, of the test to be included in the calculation, along with the general prevalence. So for example, imagine the situation where there is a test such as Foetal Fibronectin (FF) for preterm labor. Assuming that the probability of having preterm labor in this population is .1, and the probability of getting a true positive result is 0.99 and the probability of a false positive result is .01 then the probability of a positive result when the patient actually has preterm labour is given by (0.99*0.1)/((0.99*0.1)+(0.01*0.9))=0.917.so that around 92 % of the time, a positive test means that the patient is having preterm labor. Note that this calculation is sensitive to the base rate, or prior probability of having preterm labor, if this was halved (ie it was .05)then the calculation would be:

(0.99*0.05)/((0.99*0.05)+(0.01*0.95))=0.84 or 84%. Effectively Bayes theorem says in this case that the less common the condition, the less likely a positive result is likely to be true.

Bayesian networks (Heckerman & Wellman, 1995) are extensions of the Bayesian approach where the prior probability of a certain node being in a certain state is dependent on the posterior probability of nodes that lead to that state – a chain of causation.

Decision Trees

Decision trees are useful for mapping the data recorded in studies into potential outcomes. They have been used for deciding on the management of ectopic pregnancies (J. Elson et al., 2004). They can also be derived from data and may allow easier understanding of the processes involved. While they can be derived as part of the Knowledge Discovery process (see the section below) they can also be created by people directly from observations.

The fictional example shown below (Figure 2) concerns a hypothetical patient who is at 36

Figure 2. Decision tree

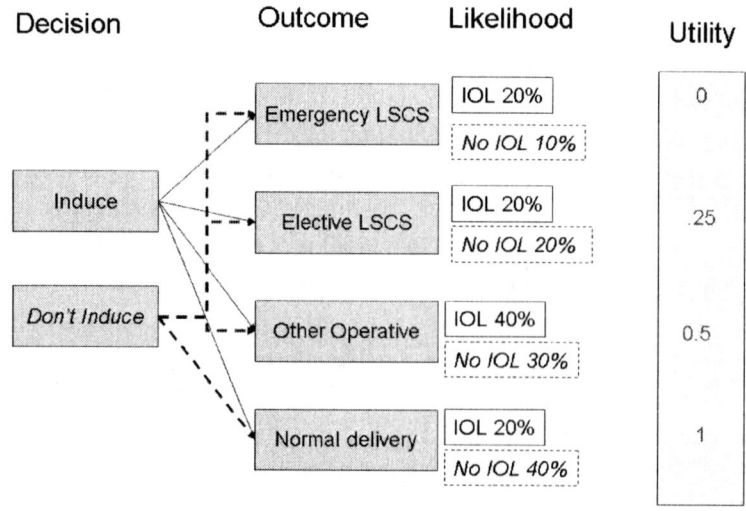

weeks gestation with pre-eclampsia. Induction of Labour (IOL) is suggested as being helpful, in this circumstance, but it may cause an increase in the chance of less- desired outcomes, such as emergency Lower segment caesarean section (LSCS). Utility values for different outcomes can be included in order to try to make the "best decision". In the example the utility value for each outcome is multiplied by the probability of each outcome. The overall result is that IOL has a utility of :

$$(0.1*0+0.2*0.25+0.3*0.5+0.2*1)=0.4,$$

but not inducing has a utility of

$$(0.2*0+0.2*0.25+0.3*0.5+0.4*1)=0.6,$$

so the non-IOL approach is preferred.

Sensitivity analysis can also be performed on these models, with the probability of each outcome being changed. More complex multi-stage trees can also be devised.

Decision Support Systems

Decision support systems (DSS), also known as decision aids, cover a wide range of approaches, as their name suggests the emphasis is on helping to make decisions, rather than removing the decision making process from the control of clinicians and patients.

A recent study (Montgomery et al., 2007) used a decision analysis tool to assist pregnant women in making a decision in the context of vaginal birth after caesarean section (VBAC). VBAC is a particularly interesting area of study because there is no universally accepted approach, and the consequences of a simple decision rule –"all women who have had a caesarean section will have another one" leads to unwanted consequences for the healthcare system – a rise in the caesarean section rate and consequent costs– and harm to the women – the morbidity associated with a

caesarean section. In VBAC there are essentially 3 possible outcomes –

1.   Vaginal birth – lowest risk of morbidity to mother, but some possibility of requirement to go to 3.
2.   Planned caesarean-
3.   Emergency caesarean – highest risk of morbidity for mother

The tool used was effectively a decision tree, each women was asked how much she preferred each outcome on a scale of 0-100. After she had done this the program combined this information with the prior odds of each outcome to produce a decision tree, which was then printed out.. This study showed a small but significant increase in vaginal birth in the group that used the tool. Interestingly this effect was not seen when comparing patients who were given information only to help them make the decision. The degree of uncertainty in decision making measured by a decision conflict scale among the women also decreased when they used the DSS tool. However this level was even lower amongst the "information only" group. An accompanying editorial (Lauer & Betran, 2007) makes the point that this DSS is designed to allow the preferences to be made before the possible outcomes are known. It also acknowledges that this approach may be more successful than exhortation in reducing Caesarean section rates.

ARTIFICIAL INTELLIGENCE AND DECISION SUPPORT

Artificial Intelligence (AI) has been defined as "The study and implementation of techniques and methods for designing computer systems to perform functions normally associated with human intelligence, such as understanding language, learning, reasoning, problem solving," (U.S. National Library of Medicine, 2001). Some authors detect a difference between artificial intelligence as a way of mimicking human decisions, and as a way of studying them. More succinctly it can be thought of way of using computers to turn data into decisions.

Different techniques are covered by the use of the term AI – some involve discovering knowledge and some involve using existing or derived knowledge for decision-making.

KNOWLEDGE DISCOVERY FROM DATABASES (KDD)

KDD is also known as machine learning and involves the use of data that has been collected to understand the causes and outcomes of events. There are some broad categories of knowledge discovery (Fayyad, Piatetsky-Shapiro, & Smyth, 1996); classification, regression, clustering, summarisation, dependency modelling and change and deviation. The conversion from data to knowledge is at the heart of intelligence, and hence artificial intelligence. The interested reader is encouraged to experiment with freely available machine learning tools – one of the most well known is "WEKA" (Witten & Frank, 2005) available from the University of Waikato New Zealand (http://www.cs.waikato.ac.nz/ml/weka/). One particularly well known method of knowledge discovery is the use of artificial neural networks, but decision trees and Bayesian networks as well as more traditional statistical methods have their place.

Neural Network Techniques

Artificial Neural networks (ANN) attempt to model decision making on the processes existing in the brain of humans or animals. They have a perhaps surprisingly long history of development and use with early work beginning in the 1950's and 1960's. An excellent review of the history can be found in (Widrow, Widrow, & Lehr, 1990).

Simply, ANN use one or more layers of "neurons" represented in a computer with connections between them (Figure 3). When a neuron is activated – i.e. the input values correspond to a particular value or range of values, then it "fires". The next layer then examines the input from the connections – which are assigned different weights -and this may then cause another layer to be stimulated, or an output to be produced. ANN are often used for learning the relationship between inputs and outputs, and can represent very complex relationships, more so than linear regression etc. They are also able to "learn" behaviour. This can be done in a number of ways, but essentially, it involves using a "training set" of data, where both the inputs and desired outputs are known, as each set of inputs as placed into the system the weights of the connections, number of connections and sometimes number of neurons are adjusted in order to create the desired outputs, using some appropriate adjustment scheme. The success of this process is then measured by using a "testing set" of data where the desired output is known but the network is not changed.

Various approaches such as accuracy of classification, a confusion matrix, sensitivity and/or specificity are then calculated. One of the issues to consider when training such a network is the danger of "overtraining" that is the situation where the network becomes extremely good at modelling the dataset used for training, but this dataset is not representative of the general case.

Classifiers – these are systems that use data about a person or condition to make a decision as to which class they belong – e.g. their diagnosis. These are usually learning systems that should get better as examples are presented to them.

If the classes are unknown – for example the outcome of the patients is not yet determined then similar techniques called *clustering* algorithms are used. Examples of classifiers are neural networks, decision trees such as C4.5and statistical methods.

Figure 3. Example of a neural network

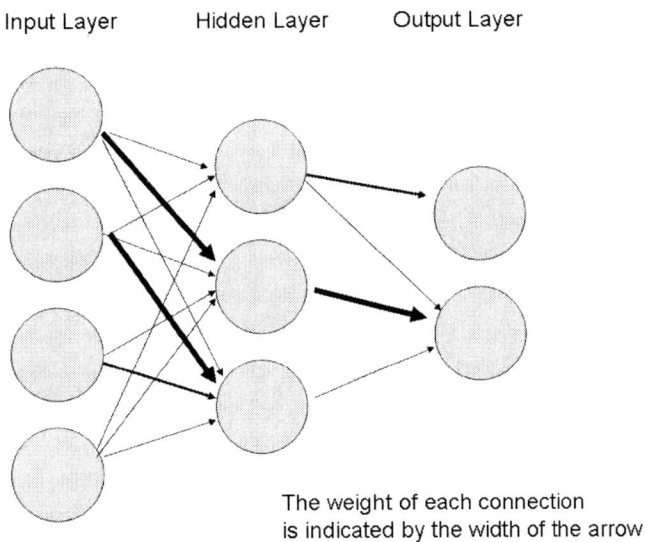

Input Layer   Hidden Layer   Output Layer

The weight of each connection
is indicated by the width of the arrow

Evolutionary computation methods such as genetic algorithms (Pena-Reyes & Sipper, 2000) and particle swarm optimisation (Kennedy, Kennedy, & Eberhart, 1995) can be thought of as systems that attempt to model different solutions to the problem of linking input to output and choose the one that is best. In technical terms this is called traversing the solution space; essentially these techniques use different methods to find functions that best give the expected outputs from the known inputs.

Generally KDD systems act on data to produce knowledge, that is they induce rules. The opposite approach, using existing knowledge to deduce outcomes is also used, in particular in the form of the expert system.

EXPERT SYSTEMS AND KNOWLEDGE BASED APPROACHES

These systems attempt to encode expert knowledge about an area as a set of rules in a knowledge base. An Expert System is: 'a computer program that represents and reasons with knowledge of some specialist subject with a view to solving problems or giving advice' (Chard & Schreiner, 1990) (p. 185). Expert Systems have had chequered history in medicine, with work starting in the early 1960's. A number of systems such as MYCIN (a system for selecting anti microbial drugs) and INTERNIST (a general internal medicine diagnosis program) were produced in the 1970's and work has continued using this and similar models. Work up to the mid '80s was reviewed by Shortliffe (Shortliffe, 1997) and de Vries (de Vries & Robbe, P.F., 1985). Medicine is an attractive target for expert systems because there is a great deal of information available on how clinicians make decisions, and it seems reasonable to view diagnosis and treatment as the application of rules. Clinical expertise is expensive, the consequences of mistakes are serious and there are many situations where such expertise is not readily available in human form. Examples of the latter include systems developed for diagnosing the acute abdomen for use on ships (Grigorenko, Zaiats, Kleshchev, Lifshits, & Samsonov, 1989). However, because of the potential risks and the complexities of the problems involved most medical expert systems have been used as decision support rather than decision making systems e.g. (Sittig, Gardner, Pace, Morris, & Beck, 1989). In fact the practical systems have mostly been advisory, and linked to databases of medical records such as the HELP system (Haug, Gardner, & Tate, 1994) to flag unusual or undesirable events. The only major systems that have 'closed the loop' i.e. act autonomously, are those in electronic pacemakers and especially implantable defibrillators which decide on very simple rules whether to attempt to cardiovert the patient, but this is really more in the domain of signal processing than artificial intelligence (Reid et al., 1983). An explanation of why expert systems are not in general use is given in (Shortliffe, 1997) and (Berg, 1994) and many other authors. Because it is rare for systems in the medical domain to be given complete authority for decision making, the term *intelligent decision support systems* has been introduced. Although many evaluations have been performed, very few of these have had the rigour expected for the assessment of other medical developments. Interestingly, the study by Johnston (Johnston, Langton, Haynes, & Mathieu, 1994) found that the well-conducted studies they collected showed that decision support systems did generally provide benefits in terms of patient outcome.

Applications in Women's Health

Women's Health Informatics is a particularly interesting area for the application of AI techniques for the following reasons:

- Large amounts of data are routinely collected, particularly in the Maternity domain, and there is some agreement about what is collected and what outcomes are important, so that data can be compared over long series and between centres.
- Screening programmes – especially cervical cancer screening- have been in place for a long time and audit of these programmes has produced a large amount of data, along with the requirement to examine large numbers of images(see chapter 11).
- In maternity, decisions are often made under uncertainty – so support for decision making from AI techniques is attractive (see chapter 10)

However, there remain formidable obstacles to use, including the fact that each woman is different, and many variables are open to interpretation, such as severity of pre-eclampsia.

SYSTEMS IN ACTION

Decision Support for Obstetrical Interventions

Induction of Labour can be a difficult decision to make, because of the lack of definitive evidence of the best course of action in a particular case. It is difficult to study because:

- Indications are formulated in a vague way (i.e. severe pre-eclampsia, rather than blood pressure (BP)>140/90)
- Published indications may not reflect actual practice.
- The indications for IOL are not completely agreed between experts - or even consistently applied by individual experts. For example, Figure 2 shows the rate at which 3 clinicians perform IOL for post-dates at 40, 41 or 42 weeks. In theory, if each clinician was consistent and the number of weeks gestation was the only criteria being considered, all post-dates induction would be performed at the same gestation.

IOL decision making is also important because of the potential risk and cost of the procedure. IOL has been associated with higher rates of other interventions and with greater reported pain during delivery and use of analgesia (E. C. Parry, Parry, & Pattison, 1999). There is no doubt that IOL is a valuable procedure that can improve outcomes for mother and baby in the correct circumstances as systematic reviews by (The Cochrane Collaboration, 1997) have shown. It is of concern if it is under used as well as over-used. With rates of IOL rising to over 25% in some centres, small changes in the IOL rate affect large numbers of women. A more philosophical problem is that pregnancy and birth are a natural process and are being reclaimed from "medicalization" by women. If unnecessary IOL's are being performed, or even if the reasons cannot be clearly explained then women will not tolerate it.

IOL is an interesting problem to study because the problem is similar to a lot of medical decisions made under uncertainty. However it has the advantage over many medical decision-making problems that the parameters involved are generally agreed, the domain is relatively small, and there has been a large amount of work done to study the effect of different decision making schemes

Finally, the greatest problem confronting the study of the decision making process in IOL is the fact that each mother and baby is different, and the outcome if the other course of action was followed will never be known. Happily, the rate of foetal deaths and complications is very low and the safety of IOL is very high so it is impossible to tell from epidemiological, retrospective or even reasonably-sized prospective study such as reported by Hannah (Hannah et al., 1996) evidence whether the correct number of IOL's is being performed. In essence, any IOL strategy used in current 1st world practice is as good as any other for preventing bad outcomes. The title of a paper "Induction of Labour, not how but why" (O'Connor, 1994), sums up this paradox. In a similar context, it has been calculated (Grant, 1994) that 200 unnecessary Caesarean sections are performed for every life-saving one. Similarly, the

IOL debate is not about reducing bad outcomes; it is about reducing the rate of unnecessary IOL's.

There has been a fair amount of work to try and simulate the decision making process in Obstetrics. This can be seen as the first step in trying to support or even automate the decisions. Neural networks have been used to try and model the decision making process using historical data (MacDowell et al., 2001) and simulated patients have been presented to obstetricians in order to try an ascertain what information they use (D. T. Parry, Yeap, & Pattison, 1998). Machine learning tools have been used to try and predict the likelihood of preterm birth (Woolery & Grzymala-Busse, 1995).

Machine learning and other types of knowledge discovery require large datasets, and future electronic records and datasets may begin to provide this sort of resource.

REMINDER SYSTEMS

There is another category of decision support tools that fall between the fully automatic, and the fully manual. Reminder or alert systems sit within an electronic health record and allow deviations from expected practice, or failure to follow protocols to be highlighted. Systems such as PRODIGY and other guideline-based approaches can integrate with the clinical record and alert clinicians during clinical episodes(Peleg, Tu, Bury, Ciccarese, & al., 2003).

DISCUSSION

There has been relatively little use of Artificial intelligence in clinical practise in women's health. This reflects the generally small impact that Artificial intelligence techniques have had in supporting the general decision making in medicine. However the picture is not all gloom for a number of reasons. Special purpose datainterpretion systems such as CTG expert systems and Cervical smear analysis tools (see chapters 10 and 11) have become more popular and effective, and embedded into diagnostic systems. However, general models designed to predict outcome or support decision-making are not widely used. This is partly because of their dependency on exact figures that may pot be available, (Harris, 1981), and partly because of their dependence on data being available in computerised form.

However a recent review (Kawamoto, Houlihan, Balas, & Lobach, 2005), has demonstrated that systems that fit into clinical workflow, are available in clinical settings, give recommendations and require justification for non-compliance with their recommendations, are likely to produce an improvement in clinical outcomes.

The increasing development of appropriate protocols, and the implementation of them within clinical systems is likely to assist in this process. With the rise of internet-based tools it is likely that such protocols may become increasingly easy to produce and maintain(D. T. Parry, Parry, Chebi, Dorji, & Stone, 2008 (in press)), especially in an open-source environment. The central relationship between clinician and woman must, however, be preserved and these developments represent an aid, rather than a replacement for clinical judgement.

FUTURE RESEARCH DIRECTIONS

Decision-making remains a key task for health professionals and it is unreasonable to expect them to meekly hand it over to machines. However, decision analysis and intelligent decision support tools offer a wide range of potential benefits to professionals and patients. Undoubtedly this area has suffered from a perception that it is dry and mathematical, and too hard to understand. It is heartening to see more efforts made to make such systems usable, and useful. Many of the most used systems are effectively hidden from the

user, embedded within electronic health record or measurement systems. This follows a trend that has seen decision support tools incorporated into commercial database management systems, and particularly placed on the web.

This area is a potentially very rewarding one for clinical workers as they can help improve the care of many future patients by allowing their knowledge and experience to be reused.

REFERENCES

Anonymous. (2007, 3rd October 2007). *Wikipedia - Hippocratic Oath*. Retrieved 16th October 2007, 2007, from http://en.wikipedia.org/wiki/Hippocratic_Oath

Bayes, T. (1764). Essay Towards Solving a Problem in the Doctrine of Chances *Philosophical Transactions of the Royal Society of London*.

Berg, M. (1994). Modeling Medical Work: On some Problems of Expert Systems in Medicine. *SIGBIO Newsletter of the ACM*, 2-6.

Brownsword, R. (2004). Reproductive Opportunities and Regulatory Challenges. *Modern Law Review, 67*(2), 304-321.

Chard, T., & Schreiner, A. (1990). Expert systems in obstetrics and gynaecology. Review. *Baillieres.Clinical.Obstetrics.&.Gynaecology., 4*, 815-840.

Cochrane Collaboration. (1997). Cochrane Pregnancy and Childbirth Database (Version III) [CD-Rom]. Oxford,UK: Update Software.

Cooper, M. (1992). Should Physicians be Bayesian Agents? *Theoretical Medicine, 13*, 349-361.

de Vries, P. H., & Robbe, P.F. (1985). An Overview of Medical Expert Systems. *Methods of Information in Medicine, 24*, 57-64.

Dowie, J. (1996). 'Evidence-based', 'cost-effective' and 'preference-driven' medicine: decision analysis based medical decision making is the pre-requisite. *Journal of Health Services Research and Policy, 1*(2), 104-113.

Elson, J., Tailor, A., Banerjee, S., Salim, R., Hillaby, K., & Jurkovic, D. (2004). Expectant management of tubal ectopic pregnancy: prediction of successful outcome using decision tree analysis. *Ultrasound in Obstetrics and Gynecology, 23*(6), 552-556.

Fayyad, U., Piatetsky-Shapiro, G., & Smyth, P. (1996). From Data Mining to Knowledge Discovery in Databases. *AI Magazine* (Fall), 37-53.

Grant, J. M. (1994). Induction of labour confers benefits in prolonged pregnancy. *Br. J. Obstet. Gynaecol., 101*(2), 99-102.

Grigorenko, G. F., Zaiats, G. A., Kleshchev, A. S., Lifshits, A., & Samsonov, V. V. (1989). The outlook for introducing the Konsul'tant-2 expert medical system on board ships. *Voen Med Zh*(2), 49-50.

Hannah, M. E., Ohlsson, A., Farine, D., Hewson, S. A., Hodnett, E. D., Myhr, T. L., et al. (1996). Induction of labor compared with expectant management for prelabor rupture of the membranes at term. *N. Eng. Med. J., 334*(16), 1005-1010.

Harris, J. M. (1981). The hazards of bedside Bayes. *Journal of the American Medical Association, 246*(22), 2602-2605.

Haug, P. J., Gardner, R. M., & Tate, K. E. (1994). Decision Support in Medicine: Examples from the HELP System. *Computers & Biomedical Research, 27*, 396-418.

Heckerman, D., & Wellman, M. P. (1995). Bayesian Networks. *Communications of the ACM, 38*(3), 27-30.

Johnston, M. E., Langton, K. B., Haynes, R. B., & Mathieu, A. (1994). Effects of computer-based clinical decision support systems on clinician performance and patient outcome. A critical appraisal of research. *Ann Intern Med, 120(2)*, 135-142.

Jones, R. W., Coughlan, E., Reid, J. S., Sykes, P., Watson, P. D., & Cook, C. (2007). Human papilloma virus vaccines and their role in cancer prevention. *Journal of the New Zealand Medical Association, 120*(1266), U2829.

Kawamoto, K., Houlihan, C. A., Balas, E. A., & Lobach, D. F. (2005). Improving clinical practice using clinical decision support systems: A systematic review of trials to identify features critical to success. *BMJ, 330*(7494), 765-.

Kennedy, J., Kennedy, J., & Eberhart, R. (1995). *Particle swarm optimization*

Particle swarm optimization. Paper presented at the Neural Networks, 1995. Proceedings IEEE International Conference

Land, R., Parry, E., Rane, A., & Wilson, D. (2001). Personal preferences of obstetricians towards childbirth. *Aust N Z J Obstet Gynaecol, 41*(3), 249-252.

Lauer, J. A., & Betran, A. P. (2007). Decision aids for women with a previous caesarean section. *BMJ, 334*(7607), 1281-1282.

MacDowell, M., Somoza, E., Rothe, K., Frye, R., Brady, K., & Bocklet, A. (2001). Understanding Birthing Mode Decision Making Using Artificial Neural Networks. *Med Decis Making, 21*(6), 433-443.

Montgomery, A. A., Emmett, C. L., Fahey, T., Jones, C., Ricketts, I., Patel, R. R., et al. (2007). Two decision aids for mode of delivery among women with previous caesarean section: randomised controlled trial. *BMJ, 334*(7607), 1305-.

O'Connor, R. A. (1994). Induction of labour - not how but why? *British. Journal. of. Hospital. Medicine., 52*(11), 559-563.

Parry, D. T., Parry, E. C., Chebi, A., Dorji, P., & Stone, P. (2008 (in press). Open source software – a key component of E-Health in Developing nations. *International Journal of Health Information Systems and Informatics.*

Parry, D. T., Yeap, W. K., & Pattison, N. (1998). Using Rough Sets to study expert behaviour in induction of labour. *Australian Journal of Intelligent Information Processing Systems, 5*(3), 219-225.

Parry, E. C., Parry, D. T., & Pattison, N. (1999). Induction of labour for post-term pregnancy: an observational study. *Australian and New Zealand Journal of Obstetrics and Gynaecology, 38*(3), 275-279.

Peleg, M., Tu, S., Bury, J., Ciccarese, P., & al., e. (2003). Comparing computer-interpretable guideline models: A case-study approach. Journal of the American Medical Informatics Association 52. *Journal of the American Medical Informatics Association,, 10*(1), 52-69.

Pena-Reyes, C. A., & Sipper, M. (2000). Evolutionary computation in medicine: An overview. *Artificial Intelligence in Medicine, 19*(1), 1-23.

Reid, P. R., Mirowski, M., Mower, M. M., Platia, E. V., Griffith, L. S., Watkins, L., Jr., et al. (1983). Clinical evaluation of the internal automatic cardioverter- defibrillator in survivors of sudden cardiac death. *Am J Cardiol, 51*(10), 1608-1613.

Rosenberg, W., & Donald, A. (1995). Evidence based medicine: an approach to clinical problem-solving. *British Medical Journal, 310,* 1122-1126.

Shortliffe, E. H. (1997). Computer Programs to Support Clinical Decision Making. *Journal of the American Medical Association, 258*(1), 61-66.

Sittig, D. F., Gardner, R. M., Pace, N. L., Morris, A. H., & Beck, E. (1989). Computerized management of patient care in a complex, controlled clinical trial in the intensive care unit. *Comput Methods Programs Biomed, 30*(2-3), 77-84.

The Cochrane Collaboration. (1997). Cochrane Pregnancy and Childbirth Database (Version III) [CD-Rom]. Oxford,UK: Update Software.

Thornton, J., & Lilford, R. (1989). The caesarean section decision: patients' choices are not determined by immediate emotional reactions. *J.Obs. Gyn., 9,* 283-288.

Thornton, J. G., & Lilford, R. J. (1989). Basic reference gambles recommended for utility assessment. *Am.J.Obstet.Gynecol., 161*(1), 256-257.

U.S. National Library of Medicine. (2001, 15 November 2001). *Medical Subject* Headings. Retrieved 11 January, 2002, from http://www.nlm.nih.gov/mesh/

Widrow, B., Widrow, B., & Lehr, M. A. (1990). 30 years of adaptive neural networks: perceptron, Madaline, and backpropagation

30 years of adaptive neural networks: perceptron, Madaline, and backpropagation. *Proceedings of the IEEE, 78*(9), 1415-1442.

Witten, I., & Frank, E. (2005). *Data Mining: Practical machine learning tools and techniques* (2 ed.). San Francisco: Morgan Kaufmann.

Woolery, L. K., & Grzymala-Busse, J. (1995). Machine learning for development of an expert system to predict premature birth. *Biomedical. Sciences.Instrumentation., 31,* 29-34.

ADDITIONAL READING

Shortliffe, E., & Cimino, J. (Eds.). (2006). *Biomedical Informatics: Computer Applications in Health Care and Biomedicine (Health Informatics)* (Third ed.): Springer.

Journal - Artificial Intelligence in Medicine

Chapter XVI
Organizational Factors:
Their Role in Health Informatics Implementation

Michelle Brear
University of New South Wales, Australia

INTRODUCTION

The influence of organizational factors on the success of informatics interventions in healthcare has been clearly demonstrated. This health specific research, informed by a larger body of evidence emerging from interdisciplinary organizational, psychological and sociological research, has confirmed the view that organizational factors can be the decisive factor in the success of an intervention (Lorenzi *et al*, 1997).

However it remains rare for organizational factors to be explicitly addressed in the implementation process. As such their contribution to the success or failure of informatics applications is not properly understood. This has implications for future interventions. Applications which were not utilized or did not perform adequately in a particular setting may be dismissed, while other, less appropriate systems may be adopted because organizational factors influenced their success. Explicit study of the role of organizational factors on the implementation of health informatics interventions is necessary to develop an understanding of their influence in the healthcare context.

Healthcare organizations tend to be highly task oriented, labor intensive and dependent on interdisciplinary teamwork, so the influence of organizational factors within them may differ considerably from the business settings in which they have traditionally been studied (Chau, 2001). Health organisations are also increasingly under-resourced due to the global downturn in government social spending, health sector privatization and aging populations. It is these characteristics which necessitate rapid uptake of informatics applications, capable of automating aspects of healthcare provision and reducing labor intensity (Coiera, 2004).

From a technical perspective, rapid and fundamental transformation of the healthcare sector through informatics is achievable. However, without a clear understanding of, and ability to manage organizational factors it is unlikely that informatics applications will realize their potential in the health sector. This short review provides an overview of the key organizational factors influencing the success of informatics interventions. It begins by positioning informatics interventions in the broader context of organizational change, before discussing the current understanding of selected factors.

INFORMATICS IMPLEMENTATION AS ORGANIZATIONAL CHANGE

Implementing informatics applications is essentially "a politically textured process of organizational change" (Berg, 1999, p87), aimed at achieving user acceptance and utilization of informatics applications. Organizational change requires people to be aware of a need for change, identify a particular course through which the change can occur and take actions to make it happen (Lorenzi, 2004). Resistance to change occurs if users are not aware of the need for change, not convinced of the course of action set out or unable to carry out the necessary action. It is the users, not the technology that should be the centre of the change process, as the decision to utilise the system is ultimately theirs (Berg, 1999).

Even the best-designed and well-intentioned informatics interventions are likely to lead to productivity losses in the early stages and create major changes (Lorenzi, 2004). Timely and effective training of users can reduce the disruption, however is not enough to ensure success as even a correctly used system can have far reaching effects. Informaticians taking a 'socio-technical' approach, view the application as one component of a complex system, the health organisation, whose introduction will disrupt other components of the system (e.g. patients and clinicians). They advocate design approaches which aim to create technology which 'fits' within the complex system (Kaplan, 2001).

The multi-disciplinary nature of health sector organisations makes finding the correct 'fit' challenging (Kaplan, 2001). A range of professionals with different needs, expectations and work norms, are likely to use an application and each will expect it to 'fit' with their work practice. When an application does not fit resistance will increase. This is often due to valid concerns about increased workload or ability to care for patients (Timmons, 2003). When systems do not 'fit', the best way to overcome resistance is to change them. However when they are essentially effective, resistance can be overcome by changing people's opinions or work norms. Organizational culture and social networks, from which many of these norms and opinions arise, need to be understood and managed.

ORGANIZATIONAL CULTURE

Organizational culture is the set of shared norms and values and tacit rules within which members of an organisation function (Lorenzi & Riley, 2000). "Every culture supports a political and social values system" (Lorenzi, 1997, p85) which will influence the reaction to an informatics application. Healthcare settings often involve a professional hierarchy between doctors and nurses, are characterized by high levels of informal and disruptive communication and place value on clinician/patient relationships and patient care.

It is necessary to identify and target the aspects of organizational culture presenting opportunities for and barriers to success when changing the organisation through an informatics intervention. Managing change requires mediating the influence of culture on events, rather than necessarily aiming to change it (Demeester, 1999). Where organizational culture and informatics applications appear incompatible, adaptation of the application should be considered.

If it is not possible to modify the system, success is dependent on changing the organizational culture to make it compatible. Cultural change directly targeted at the strongly held values of users, may only increase resistance. If the organisational culture supports a belief that informatics applications undermine good clinician/patient relationships, attempting to convince clinicians that good relationships with their patients are not important is unlikely to be a successful strategy for winning acceptance of the application. However it may be possible, through an educational process, to convince clinicians that informatics applications do not necessarily undermine good relationships and in the right conditions can even enhance them. Users may already be convinced of the need to change some aspects of organizational culture which do not threaten the values they are most passionate about. The structure of an organisation and work patterns and roles of individuals within it are influential and may be appropriate areas to encourage change.

Organizational Structure

The structure of an organisation will affect the way in which decisions are made, the type of leadership which emerges and the way resistance is dealt with in the implementation process. 'Flatter' organizational structures tend to encourage the sharing of ideas, emergence of innovation and broader involvement in decision-making (Leonard *et al*, 2004). In these types of organisations management tends to adopt a collaborative approach, working alongside, listening to and involving those working on the ground, rather than making decisions on their behalf and communicating orders. Management is supportive, approachable and accountable and shows dedication to continuous learning (Zimmerman, 1993). These types of organisations are more likely to include practicing clinicians in formal decision-making bodies such as management committees. They are also more likely to recognize, encourage and legitimize the role of grass roots leaders with clinical credibility and presence and have

a commitment to involving informatics users in the implementation process.

User involvement throughout the process "leads to increased user acceptance and use by encouraging realistic expectations, facilitating the user's system ownership, decreasing resistance to change, and committing users to the system" (Lorenzi, 1997, p86). It also allows better definition of problems and solutions, from the user's perspective and develops a better understanding amongst users of the application (Lorenzi, 1997). Involving users in the design and implementation of a system is more likely to result in applications suited to the current work patterns of the intended users.

Work Patterns and Roles of Clinicians

Any informatics application must be compatible with the current work practices and values of the organisation (Greenhalgh, 2004; Kaplan, 2001; Lorenzi & Riley, 2000). Compatibility will differ between organisations and cultures so applications require the capacity to be tailored to the needs of individual organisations. Take an electronic prescribing system for example. In one hospital it may be used to enter prescription orders during ward rounds via a laptop computer however a different hospital (or even another ward within that hospital) may find it more appropriate to install the system on a computer terminal at the nurses stations so that orders can be entered retrospectively. Bearing in mind the necessity to consider the unique context of individual organisations, it is possible to make some generalizations regarding the work patterns and roles of clinicians to broadly inform the design of informatics interventions.

Doctors have traditionally worked with a high degree of professional autonomy and status (Gagnon, 2003). Applications perceived to undermine their autonomy and status as professionals or "subvert the art of medical practice" (Kaplan, 2001, p4) are more likely to meet with resistance.

In a qualitative study examining factors influencing adoption of a CDSS involving automatic clinical reminders, Rousseau et al (2004) found clinicians favored on-demand evidence systems to automatically generated reminders. The latter were perceived to be intrusive, often inapplicable and not particularly useful for making patient management decisions.

Clinicians tend to be patient focused, require an ability to maintain control of patient care and make decisions specific to individuals which computers are not capable of. They must be convinced that applications will not jeopardize their ability to care for patients (Timmons, 2003). Overly prescriptive systems, or those which attempt to take on the uniquely human quality of thinking, are unlikely to be successful. Rouseau et al (2004) noted inapplicable reminders were a barrier to effective use and found that practitioners formed a habit of ignoring all reminders. In a study of adherence to electronic HIV treatment reminders, Patterson *et al* (2004) found the inapplicability of reminders to many patients' specific situations, and the time taken to document why the reminders were not adhered to, were significant barriers to effective system use.

All applications will create some change to normal work patterns and roles. That is essentially what their implementation is intended to do (Berg & Toussaint, 2003). Users need to be realistically informed of and prepared for changes to normal work practice. It is inevitable that users will expect some future benefit from adapting their behaviors and realistic communication of the likely benefits, particularly if they are indirect or not clearly visible, should form an integral part of the communication strategy.

Communication

Communication binds individuals together and is integral to the implementation process. Without effective communication it is impossible to lead, learn, make decisions, prepare individuals for an intervention or use it effectively (Zimmerman, 1993). Lack of communication, or ineffective communication which lacks trust, can negatively influence the uptake of a technology (Ash, 1997). There is no 'magic formula' for effective communication, however there are some key principles which should be applied to enhance the effectiveness of communication.

Communication must be timely. People require time to digest information and prepare for changes (Tilley & Chambers, 2004). However they also forget. Users who are trained to use a system months before its implementation may not remember how to use it when it finally arrives. Information must also be communicated at an appropriate time. Disrupting a lunch break or patient care, may not be the most appropriate way to inform users about a new application.

Communication must be sincere and truthful. Users must be offered an honest and realistic assessment of the potential negative consequences and expected benefits of an application. For example if an electronic medical record application is introduced, it may be realistic to expect its use to be more time consuming in the initial stages while users master the system. However in time, its ability to provide comprehensive patient information at the click of a button may save time and provide better quality information. It is also important to acknowledge unexpected benefits and problems if they occur.

Sources of communication have an immense impact on the perceived message, its credibility and influence (Kaplan, 2001). A manufacturer's leaflet declaring the new system easy to use is unlikely to carry much weight with users, however a respected clinical peer conveying this information may be quite influential.

It is essential the communication be recognized as multi-dimensional, rather than a one-way channel from management to users. Mechanisms for receiving feedback must be created and where it is not forthcoming, should be actively elicited from users. Magrabi *et al* (2004) incorporated two mechanisms for feedback into an online DSS. Users could volunteer feedback at any time, however it was also actively elicited by randomly prompting users. Once received, feedback should be acted upon to adapt the application to meet user needs (Greenhalgh, 2004). For example, in response to clinician feedback, the patterns of automatically generated reminders in a clinical decision support system (CDSS) was altered to limit the number of reminders perceived by clinicians to be inapplicable. Communication through informal structures (e.g. gossiping in the tea room) is inevitable and ability to manage it directly, limited. However the less effective formal communication mechanisms are, the more likely it is that communication will take place through informal channels in the social network.

SOCIAL NETWORKS

A social network consists of the individuals, groups and organizations with whom, and patterns of communication by which individuals in an organisation interact. It is through social networks that organizational culture and behaviors are reinforced and adapted (Lorenzi, 1997). The culture represented within a social network can be influential. For example, Gagnon *et al* (2003) found that physicians who perceived social and professional responsibility to adopt telemedicine applications [from others in their social network] had a stronger intention to do so. The culture represented in each individual's social network will differ, and each individual within will interact and be influenced differently.

To properly understand a social network it is necessary to examine the interactions, not the individuals. Frequency of interaction is important but should not be viewed in isolation from the style of communication (e.g. formal or informal), type of communication (e.g. synchronous or asynchronous) the strength of ties between the participants in an interaction and power relations

involved (Katz et al, 2004). When implementing an informatics application, interactions which occur in clinical teams and with respected opinion leaders, are particularly influential in relation to individuals decisions to utilise applications.

Effective Teamwork

The clinical team has been identified as the organizational unit most influential in the diffusion of innovation (Gosling *et al*, 2003). Well functioning teams facilitate effective communication, encourage continuous learning and offer a trusting environment in which ideas and issues can be raised. Through these interactions, teams develop shared visions and common goals which support the introduction of new innovations to fulfill these goals. As work in health organisations is highly dependent on teamwork and it is teams, not individuals, which must adopt informatics applications, well functioning teams are a pre-requisite for successful informatics implementation (Goldstein *et al*, 2004).

In organisations where well functioning teams do not exist, an informatics intervention may be an opportunity to develop teams, by uniting individuals around a shared vision and common goals which the application can fulfill. Doctors and nurses take on different roles and responsibilities in the process of caring for patients so a shared vision may not be immediately apparent. However both groups ultimately work towards the goal of providing optimal patient care, so incorporating an application into a vision of improved patient care may be a way to unite users.

Consideration should also be given to the size and composition of teams. Teams of more than 15 tend to fragment into sub-teams, while very small teams have a tendency to become cliquish, so ideally they should consist of 10-15 members (Gosling *et al*, 2003). The work environment may largely dictate a team's composition. In healthcare settings teams are usually multidisciplinary. Individuals however, are more likely to create ties with those they perceive to be similar, so identifying similarities amongst multidisciplinary teams is pertinent (Katz *et al*, 2004). Identifying and utilizing the influence of respected clinicians within the team can also be useful.

Clinical Champions and Opinion Leaders

Respected clinicians with influence amongst their peers, who support the intervention play an important role in convincing others of an application's worth, as do those who oppose the intervention. They are commonly referred to as clinical champions or opinion leaders. As the name 'champions' tends to imply a positive influence and does not necessarily imply the champion has influence amongst peers (Lolock *et al*, 2001), 'opinion leader' will be used in this paper.

Opinion leaders are individuals with the ability to influence others in the social network, who make a major personal commitment to diffusing information about an informatics application (Lorenzi & Riley, 2000). Such diffusion may have a negative or positive influence, and can discourage or encourage the adoption of the application. For example Ash (1997) identified the presence of 'champions' as a significant factor in the diffusion of email in academic health science centres. Conversely Timmons (2003) discusses a "strong and articulate" ward sister whose resistance to using an electronic system in the ward was successful in preventing its implementation. It is not unusual to have both negative and positive opinion leaders within a network.

Whatever their persuasion they tend to be charismatic individuals with good interpersonal relationships based on trust and understanding. They act through clinical conviction, generally outside of the formal structures, and give applications credibility at a local level. Their role is essentially informal, and, on the proviso their colleagues respect them, they tend to be self-appointed (Lolock, 2001). The role is largely

dependent on personal motivation and conviction and therefore difficult to formalize. The potential alienating effect of being an opinion leader means that those without sufficient commitment are likely to be reluctant to take on such a role (Lolock, 2001)

Despite a general consensus that successful interventions are more likely when champions are present, there is a lack of understanding about exactly what it is they do, the circumstances in which they will be influential and how best to describe them. As with each of the factors mentioned here, opinion leaders are one small component of a large and complex system (the health organisation) and it is difficult to isolate their effect. There is also considerable evidence to suggest that other factors, in particular the suitability of the application, influence the emergence of opinion leaders. As with all the factors mentioned here, further research is needed to identify how opinion leaders influence and how the 'champions' amongst them can be encouraged.

CONCLUSION

There is a general recognition that numerous organizational factors will influence the success of an informatics intervention. This is supported by a body of evidence from multi-disciplinary and health specific research. In particular research has noted the influence of: organizational culture and social networks. Organisational culture, the shared norms and values within which members of an organisation function influences the organization's structure and patterns of communication. Social networks, the individuals and groups with whom one interacts and the interactions which occur between them, are the social space in which teams are formed and work and individuals are influenced, particularly by those individuals known as opinion leaders or clinical champions. Organizational factors are highly inter-related and the exact nature and contribution of each to the success of an intervention is not clear. A health specific understanding and recognition of these factors is necessary if informatics applications are to reach their potential in healthcare settings.

REFERENCES

Berg, M. (1999). Patient care information systems and health care work: a sociotechnical approach. International Journal of Medical Informatics 55, 87-101.

Berg M. & Toussaint, P. (2003). The Mantra of Modeling and the Forgotten Powers of Paper: A Sociotechnical View on the Development of Process-oriented ICT in Health Care. International Journal of Medical Informatics, 69, 223-234.

Chau, P.Y.K. & Hu, P.J.-H. (2002). Investigating Healthcare Professionals' Decisions to Accept Telemedicine Technology: an Empirical Test of Competing Theories. Information and Management, 39, 297-311.

Coiera, E. (2004). Four Rules for the Reinvention of Healthcare. British Medical Journal, 328, 1197-1199.

Demeester, M. (1999). Cultural Aspects of Information Technology Implementation. International Journal of Medical Informatics, 56, 25-41.

Gagnon, M.-P. Godin, G. Gagne, C. Fortin, J.-P. Lamothe, L. Reinharz, D. & Cloutier, A. (2003). An Adaption of the Theory of interpersonal Behaviour to the Study fo Telemedicine Adoption by Physicians. International Journal of Medical Informatics, 71, 103-115.

Goldstein, M.K. Coleman, R.W. Tu, S.W. Shankar, R.D. O'Connor, M.J. Musen, M.A. Martins, S.B. Lavori, P.W. Shilipak, M.G. Oddone, E. Advani, A. A. Gholami, P. & Hoffman, B.B. (2004). Translating Research into Practice: Organisational Issues in Implementing Automated Decision Support for Hypertension in Three Medical Centers. Journal of the American Medical Informatics Association, 11(5), 368-376.

Gosling, A.S. Westbrook, J.I. & Braithwaite, J. (2003). Clinical Team Functioning and IT Innovation: A Study of the Diffusion of a Point-of Care Online Evidence System. Journal of the American Medical Informatics Association, 10(3), 244-251.

Greenhalgh, T. Robert, G. MacFarlane, F. Bate, P. & Kyriakidou, O. (2004). Diffusion of Innovations in Service Organisations: Systematic Review and Recommendations. The Millbank Quarterly, 82(4), 581-629.

Kaplan, B. (2001). Evaluating informatics applications- some alternative approaches: theory, social interactionism, and call for methodological pluralism. International Journal of Medical Informatics 64, 39-56.

Katz, N. Lazer, D. Arrow, H. & Contractor, N. (2004). Network Theory and Small Groups. Small Group Research, 35(3), 307-332.

Leonard, M. Graham, S. Bonacum, D. (2004). The Human Factor: The Critical Importance of Effective Teamwork and Communication in Providing Safe Care, Quality and Saftey in Health Care, 13(Suppl 1), i85-i90.

Lolock, L. Dopson, S. Chambers, D. & Gabbay, J. (2001). Understanding the role of opinion leaders in improving clinical effectiveness. Social Science and Medicine, 53, 745-757.

Lorenzi, N.M. Riley, R.T. Blythe, A.J.C. Southon, G. & Dixon, B.J., (1997). Antecedents of the People and Organizational Aspects of Medical Informatics: Review of the Literature. Journal of the American Medical Informatics Association, 4(2), 79-93.

Lorenzi, N.M. (2004). Beyond the Gadgets: Non-technological barriers to information systems need to be overcome. British Medical Journal 328, 1146-1147.

Lorenzi, N.M. & Riley, R.T. (2000). Managing Change: An Overview. Journal of the American Medical Informatics Association, 7(2), 116-124.

Magrabi, F. Westbrook, J.I. Coiera, E. W. & Gosling, A.S. (2004). Clinicians' Assessments of the Usefulness of Online Evidence to Answer Clinical Questions. Proceedings of the 11th World Congress on Medical Informatics, 297-300.

Patterson, E.S. Nguyen, A.D. Halloran, J.P. & Asch, S.M. (2004). Human Factors Barriers to the Effective Use of Ten HIV Clinical Reminders. Journal of the American Informatics Association, 11(1), 50-59

Rousseau, N. McColl, E. Newton, J. Grimshaw, J. & Eccles, M. (2003). Practice-based, Longitudinal, Qualitative Interview Study of Computerised Evidence Based Guidelines in Primary Care. British Medical Journal, 326, 314-321.

Tilley, S. & Chambers, M. (2004). The process of implementing evidence-based practice- the curates egg. Journal of Psychiatric and Mental Health Nursing, 11, 117-119.

Timmons, S. 2003, Nurses Resisting Information Technology. Nursing Inquiry, 10(4), 257-269.

Zimmerman, J.E. Shortell, S.M. Rousseau, D.M. Duffy, J. Gillies, R.R. Knaus, W.A. Devers, K. Wagner, D.P. & Draper, E.A. (1993). Improving Intensive Care: Observations based on organisational case studies in nine intensive care units: A prospective multicenter study. Critical Care Medicine, 21(10), 1143-1451.

KEY TERMS

Clinical Champion: Clinical Champions are opinion leaders who 'champion' or encourage the uptake of an application.

Opinion Leader: An opinion leaders is an individual, respected amongst their peers who acts out of clinical conviction to influence the opinions of others vis-à-vis an informatics application.

Organisational Culture: Organisational culture is the set of shared norms and values and tacit rules within which members of an organisation function.

Organisational Factors: In an informatics context, organisational factors are factors relating to the culture and functioning of an organisation which, negatively or positively, influence its ability to adapt to an informatics intervention.

Social Network: A social network consists of the individuals, groups and organisations with whom an individual interacts, and the interactions which take place between the individual and other components of their social network.

Socio-technical Approach: A socio-technical approach is one which views informatics applications as part of the broader social and political context within which they are implemented.

Teamwork: The co-operative effort of a small group to achieve a specified outcome.

Chapter XVII
Standardization in Health and Medical Informatics

Josipa Kern
Zagreb University Medical School, Croatia

INTRODUCTION

When things go well then often it is because they conform to standards (ISO, 2005). According to the Oxford Dictionary of Modern English, there is a lot of explanation of what standard means, but, in context of the first sentence, the best meaning is «standard is a thing or quality or specification by which something may be tested or measured». Personal computer is a standardized computer. It means that any of its components is made according to strictly defined specification. Consequently, it does not matter who produces components and where they are produced.

Industry put the first demand for standards. Especially standardization is extremely important for electronics, for information and communication technology (ICT), and its application in different areas. Nowadays developing of standards is organized on global, international level, but it exists also on national level, well harmonized with international one.

Developers of standards are organizations and groups working on this matter. The leading standard developer in the world is International Standards Organization (ISO). ISO is a non-governmental organization established on 23 February 1947. Its mission is to promote the development of standardization and related activities in the world with a view to facilitating the international exchange of goods and services, and to developing cooperation in the spheres of intellectual, scientific, technological and economic activity (ISO, 2005). ISO collaborates with its partners in international standardization, the International Electrotechnical Commission (IEC), a non-governmental body, whose scope of activities complements ISO's. The ISO and the IEC cooperate on a joint basis with the International Telecommunication Union (ITU), part of the United Nations Organization and its members are governments. The ISO standard can be recognized by the ISO logo, ISO prefix and the designation, "International Standard".

European developer of standards is the European Committee for Standardisation (Comité Européen de Normalisation – CEN). It was founded in 1961 by the national standards bodies in the European Economic Community and EFTA countries. CEN promotes voluntary technical harmonization in Europe in conjunction with worldwide bodies and its partners in Europe and the conformity assessment of products and their certification (CEN, 2005). CEN cooperates with the European Committee for Electrotechnical Standardization (CENELEC), and the European Telecommunications Standards Institute (ETSI). Product of this cooperation is the European standard which can be recognized by the prefix EN. Any added prefix to the existing one, for both ISO and CEN standard, means that this standard is result of cooperation with other standardization group or organization. The prefix ENV in European standardization means that this standard is not yet a full standard (it is under development by CEN).

ISO and CEN have Technical Committees working in the specific areas. ISO/TC215, established in 1998, and CEN/TC251, established in 1991, are corresponding technical committees working on standardization in health and medical informatics in ISO and CEN. Both standardization bodies, the ISO and CEN cooperate, and they mutually exchange their standards.

There are also a variety of organizations and groups developing standards, cooperating with ISO and CEN or acting as administer and coordinator in standardization. For example, there are Health Level 7 (HL7), Digital Imaging and Communications in Medicine (DICOM), American National Standards Institute (ANSI), non-profit organization that administers and coordinates the U.S. voluntary standardization and conformity assessment system, etc.

BACKGROUND

Definition: A standard is a set of rules and definitions that specify how to carry out a process or produce a product, or more precisely standard is a document established by consensus, and approved by a recognized body, that provides, for common and repeated use, guidelines or char-

acteristics for activities or their results, aimed at the achievement of the optimum degree of order in a given context.

The main role of standard is in raising levels of quality, safety, reliability, efficiency and interchangeability, and consequently in lower cost (ISO, 2005).

Standard creation process: There are several *phases* in the process of standardization: The first phase of this process is characterized by demand for standard. There must be someone who needs standard. Most standards are prepared at the request of industry. The European Commission can also request the standards bodies to prepare standards in order to implement European legislation. This standardization is 'mandated' by the Commission, through the Standing Committee of the Directive, in support of the legislation. Group of users can also ask for standard in the field of their interest. The second phase of standardization means developing of standards by following specification based on needs defined in the first phase. Experts of specific field are working on related standards. After the standard has been approved by standardization body, it becomes prototype which goes to testing and evaluation. Positive test results imply dissemination of standards and they start to live. It should be highlighted that standard is dynamic category and it changes time after time. Most standards require periodic revision. Several factors combine to render a standard out of date: technological evolution, new methods and materials, new quality and safety requirements. To take account of these factors, the general rule has been established that all standards should be reviewed at intervals of not more than several, predefined time period. On occasion, it is necessary to revise a standard earlier (Hammond and Cimino, 2001).

Standardization in health and medical informatics - why and what: Standardization has been a major factor in the company's financial and clinical success, enabling faster implementation, greater quality control and significant cost-savings (Ball et al., 2004). The contribution of the standardization process in healthcare terminology initiated by CEN/TC251 and supported now by the work of CEN/TC215/WG3 to this new approach can be summarized as the practical realization of ontology (Rodrigues et al., 2002). The standard CEN ENV 12924 contains a security categorization model for information systems in healthcare, distinguishing six categories, plus some refinements. For each category it specifies the required protection measures (Louwerse, 2002). Standards support interoperability and electronic health record (EHR) communication. It supports co-operative work among health agents, and it is necessary to share healthcare information about patients in a meaningful way. Examples of requirements to EHR are provided in four themes: EHR functional requirements; Ethical, legal, and security requirements; Clinical requirements; Technical requirements. The main logical building blocks of an EHR use the terminology of CEN TC251 ENV13606. (Marley, 2002; Maldonado et al., 2004; Lloyd and Kalra, 2003). Many specific medical records, like medical records of patients suffering from beta-thalassaemia which are inevitably complex and grow in size very fast, are based also on ENV 13606 (Deftereos et al., 2001). The wider electronic exchange of clinical information between heterogeneous information systems in the delivery of diabetes care demands a common structure in the form of a message standard, and close co-operation with CEN/TC 251 (Vaughan et al., 2000).

CURRENT STATUS OF STANDARDIZATION IN HEALTH AND MEDICAL INFORMATICS

All the standards developers work through their working technical committees in health and medical informatics, and a number of working groups specialized in a specific area.

What are Specific Areas of Work and Results of the ISO/TC215?

Table 1 shows working groups acting in the ISO/TC215. Table 2 shows list of standards given by this Technical Committee.

What are Specific Areas of Work and Results of the CEN/TC251?

The work is carried out by the Working Groups mentioned in the Table 3.

CEN TC251 has been operating for 10 years. By October 2004, it had created 10 full standards, or EN (Table 4).

FUTURE TRENDS IN STANDARDIZATION IN HEALTH AND MEDICAL INFORMATICS

There is no doubt that candidate for standardization in medical informatics will be core data sets for healthcare speciality groups, decision-support

Table 1. Working groups of ISO/TC215

ISO/TC215 WG 1 Health records and modelling coordination
ISO/TC215 WG 2 Messaging and communication
ISO/TC215 WG 3 Health concept representation
ISO/TC215 WG 4 Security
ISO/TC215 WG 5 Health cards
ISO/TC215 WG 6 Pharmacy and medicines business

Table 2. Standards in health and medical informatics given by ISO/TC215

ISO/IEEE 11073-10101:2004	Health informatics -- Point-of-care medical device communication -- Part 10101: Nomenclature
ISO/IEEE 11073-10201:2004	Health informatics -- Point-of-care medical device communication -- Part 10201: Domain information model
ISO/IEEE 11073-20101:2004	Health informatics -- Point-of-care medical device communication -- Part 20101: Application profiles -- Base standard
ISO/IEEE 11073-30200:2004	Health informatics -- Point-of-care medical device communication -- Part 30200: Transport profile -- Cable connected
ISO/IEEE 11073-30300:2004	Health informatics -- Point-of-care medical device communication -- Part 30300: Transport profile -- Infrared wireless
ISO/TR 16056-1:2004	Health informatics -- Interoperability of telehealth systems and networks -- Part 1: Introduction and definitions
ISO/TR 16056-2:2004	Health informatics -- Interoperability of telehealth systems and networks -- Part 2: Real-time systems
ISO/TS 16058:2004	Health informatics -- Interoperability of telelearning systems
ISO/TS 17090-1:2002	Health informatics -- Public key infrastructure -- Part 1: Framework and overview
ISO/TS 17090-2:2002	Health informatics -- Public key infrastructure -- Part 2: Certificate profile
ISO/TS 17090-3:2002	Health informatics -- Public key infrastructure -- Part 3: Policy management of certification authority
ISO/TS 17117:2002	Health informatics -- Controlled health terminology -- Structure and high-level indicators
ISO/TR 17119:2005	Health informatics - Health informatics profiling framework
ISO/TS 17120:2004	Health informatics -- Country identifier standards
ISO 17432:2004	Health informatics -- Messages and communication -- Web access to DICOM persistent objects
ISO 18104:2003	Health informatics -- Integration of a reference terminology model for nursing
ISO/TR 18307:2001	Health informatics -- Interoperability and compatibility in messaging and communication standards -- Key characteristics
ISO/TS 18308:2004	Health informatics -- Requirements for an electronic health record architecture
ISO 18812:2003	Health informatics -- Clinical analyser interfaces to laboratory information systems -- Use profiles
ISO/TR 21089:2004	Health informatics -- Trusted end-to-end information flows
ISO 21549-1:2004	Health informatics -- Patient healthcard data -- Part 1: General structure
ISO 21549-2:2004	Health informatics -- Patient healthcard data -- Part 2: Common objects
ISO 21549-3:2004	Health informatics -- Patient healthcard data -- Part 3: Limited clinical data
ISO/TS 21667:2004	Health informatics -- Health indicators conceptual framework
ISO/TR 21730:2005	Health informatics -- Use of mobile wireless communication and computing technology in healthcare facilities -- Recommendations for the management of unintentional electromagnetic interference with medical devices
ISO 22857:2004	Health informatics -- Guidelines on data protection to facilitate trans-border flows of personal health information

ISO/TS is normative document representing the technical consensus within an ISO committee
ISO/TR is an informative document containing information of a different kind from that normally published in a normative document (Beolchi, 2003).
IEEE is Institute of Electrical and Electronic Engineers, USA

Table 3. CEN/TC251 working groups

CEN/TC251 WG1 Communications: information models, messaging and smart cards
CEN/TC251 WG2 Terminology
CEN/TC251 WG3 Security, safety and quality
CEN/TC251 WG4 Technology for interoperability (Devices)

Table 4. Standards in health and medical informatics given by CEN/TC251

EN 14484:2003	International transfer of personal health data covered by the EU data protection directive - High level security policy
EN 14485:2003	Guidance for handling personal health data in international applications in the context of the EU data protection directive
EN 1828:2002	Categorial structure for classifications and coding systems of surgical procedures
EN ISO 18104:2003	Integration of a reference terminology model for nursing (ISO 18104:2003)
EN ISO 18812:2003	Clinical analyser interfaces to laboratry information systems – Use profiles (ISO 18812:2003)
EN ISO 21549-1:2004	Patient healthcard data - Part 1: General structure (ISO 21549-1:2004)
EN ISO 21549-2:2004	Patient healthcard data - Part 2: Common objects (ISO 21549-2:2004)
EN ISO 21549-3:2004	Patient healthcard data - Part 3: Limited clinical data (ISO 21549-3:2004)
EN 12251:2004	Secure user identification for healthcare - Identification and authentication by passwords - Management and security
EN 12252:2004	Digital imaging - Communication, workflow and data management (which endorses all of DICOM as a European Standard)

algorithms and clinical guidelines, and vocabulary. Identification of patient, content and structure of electronic patient record, and messages communicating in the health care system are also object candidates for international standards. Standard formats need to be defined for special kinds of data like images, signals and waveforms, sound and voice, and video, including motion video. Data security, security of objects and communication channels, data archiving, especially in case of catastrophe of any kind, should be standardized. Some of these standards exist or have been under way, but standardization is a continuous process, depending on development of information and communication technology, and therefore all of them need to be improved and adapted to new technology coming day after day.

CONCLUSION

Standards in health and medical informatics are means enabling the better health care. Health care is supposed to be better if health care providers can access data in patient health record, can read it or add some new data relevant for other health care providers taking care about patient. Information technology used in diagnostics produces data about patient as images, signals or waves, as well as classic alphanumeric data. Format of such data should be standardized, usable and readable, at any instrument of this kind, wherever in the world. Medical language should be standardized, coding systems universal. Transfer of medical data should be secure as well as data storage and communication. Some of patient data should be portable by health cards, especially for patient suffered of chronic diseases. Bad medical informatics can kill patient, and standardization in the field can help that this not happen.

REFERENCES

Ball, M.J., Cortes-Comerer, N., Costin, M., Hudson, K. and Augustine B. (2004). HCA Inc.: standardization in action, *Journal of Healthcare Information Management*, 18(2),59-63.

Beolchi, Luciano (ed.) (2003). European Telemedicine Glossary of Concepts, Technologies, Standards and Users, 5th Edition, Brussels: European Commission.

CEN, http://www.cenorm.be/cenorm/index.htm , accessed on February, 11 2005.

Deftereos, S., Lambrinoudakis, C., Andriopoulos, P., Farmakis, D., Aessopos, A. (2001). A Java-based electronic healthcare record software for beta-thalassaemia. Journal of Medical Internet Research, 3(4):E33.

Hammond, W.E. and Cimino, J.J. (2001). Standards in Medical Informatics, *Medical Informatics – Computer Applications in Health Care and Biomedicine*, Edward H. Shortliffe and Leslie E. Perreault (eds.), New York: Springer, 212-255.

ISO, Why standards matter? http://www.iso. org/iso/en/aboutiso/introduction/index.html#one, accessed on February, 11 2005.

Lloyd, D., Kalra, D. (2003). EHR requirements. *Studies in Health Technology and Informatics*, 96, 231-237.

Louwerse, K. (2002). Demonstration results for the standard ENV 12924. *Studies in Health Technology and Informatics*, 69,111-139; discussion 229-237.

Maldonado, J.A., Crespo, P., Sanchis, A., Robles, M. (2004). Pangea: a mediator for the integration of distributed electronic healthcare records. *Medinfo 2004*, (CD),1738.

Marley, T. (2002). Standards supporting interoperability and EHCR communication--a CEN TC251 perspective. *Studies in Health Technology and Informatics*, 87,72-77.

Rodrigues, J.M., Trombert Paviot, B., Martin, C., Vercherin. P., Samuel, O. (2002). Co-ordination between clinical coding systems and pragmatic clinical terminologies based on a core open system: the role of ISO/TC215/WG3 and CEN/TC2511/WG2 standardisation?, *Studies in Health Technology and Informatics*, 90,401-405.

Vaughan, N.J., Cashman, S.J., Cavan, D.A., Gallego, M.R., Kohner, E., Benedetti, M.M., Sando, S.H., Sonksen, P.H., Storms, G.E., Vermeij, D. (2000). A detailed examination of the clinical terms and concepts required for communication by electronic messages in diabetes care. Diabetes, Nutrition and Metabolism, 13(4), 201-209.

KEY TERMS

Standard: A set of rules and definitions that specify how to carry out a process or produce a product

Standardisation: Process of producing of standards

International Standardisation: Activity of the world authority for standards

ISO (International Standard Organization): World authority for standards

ISO/TC 215 – ISO Technical Committee for standardisation in health and medical informatics

European Standardisation: Activity of the European authority for standards

CEN (Comité Européen de Normalisation: European Committee for Standardisation) – the European authority for standards

CEN/TC 251: CEN Technical Committee for standardisation in health and medical informatics

ANSI (American National Standards Institute): A private, nonprofit membership organization responsible for approving official American National Standards

EN: European standard made by CEN

ISO: International standard made by ISO

This work was previously published in Handbook of Research on Informatics in Healthcare and Biomedicine, edited by A. Lazakidou, pp. 44-50, copyright 2006 by Information Science Reference, formerly known as Idea Group Reference (an imprint of IGI Global).

Chapter XVIII
Evaluation of Health Information Systems:
Challenges and Approaches

Elske Ammenwerth
University for Health Sciences, Medical Informatics and Technology (UMIT), Austria

Stefan Gräber
University Hospital of Saarland, Germany

Thomas Bürkle
University of Münster, Germany

Carola Iller
University of Heidelberg, Germany

ABSTRACT

This chapter summarizes the problems and challenges which occur when health information systems are evaluated. The main problem areas presented are the complexity of the evaluation object, the complexity of an evaluation project, and the motivation for evaluation. Based on the analysis of those problem areas, the chapter then presents recommendations how to address them. In particularly, it discusses in more detail what benefits can be obtained from applying triangulation in evaluation studies. Based on the example of the evaluation of a nursing documentation system, it shows how both the validation of results and the completeness of results can be supported by triangulation. The authors hope to contribute to a better understanding of the peculiarities of evaluation.

INTRODUCTION

It is hard to imagine health care without modern information and communication technology (ICT). It is evident that the use of modern information technology offers tremendous opportunities to reduce clinical errors, to support health care professionals and to increase the efficiency of care, and even to improve the quality of patient care (Institute of Medicine, 2001).

However, there are also hazards associated with ICT in health care: modern information systems are costly, their failures may cause negative effects on patients and staff, and possibly, when inappropriately designed, they may result in spending more time with the computer than with the patient. This all could have a negative impact on the efficiency of patient care. Therefore, a rigorous evaluation of IT in health care is recommended (Rigby, 2001) and of great importance for decision makers and users (Kaplan & Shaw, 2002). Evaluation can be defined as the decisive assessment of defined objects, based on a set of criteria, to solve a given problem (Ammenwerth et al., 2004).

The term ICT refers to technologies as such. Whether the use of these technologies is successful depends not only on the quality of the technological artefacts but also on the actors, i.e. the people involved in information processing and the organisational environment in which they are employed. ICT embedded in the environment, including the actors, is often referred to as an Information System (IS) in a sociotechnical sense. (Winter et al., 2001), (Berg, Aarts, & van der Lei, 2003).

Many different questions can lead the evaluation of information technology. Within evaluation research, two main (and often rather distinct) traditions can be found: the objectivist (positivistic) and the subjectivistic tradition (Friedman & Wyatt, 1997), which are related to the dominant use of either quantitative or qualitative methods (for details, see chapter 13).

Despite a large amount of published evaluation studies – e.g., (van der Loo, 1995) found over 1.500 citations on evaluation of healthcare IT between 1967 and 1995, and (Ammenwerth & de Keizer, 2004) found 1.035 studies between 1982 and 2002 - many authors report problems during evaluation. One of the main problems frequently discussed is the adequate choice of evaluation methods. While objectivistic researchers tend to concentrate on quantitative methods, subjectivistic researchers mainly rely on qualitative methods. Sometimes, a mixture of methods is applied. For example, qualitative methods are used to prepare quantitative studies, or quantitative measurements are used to support qualitative argumentation. However, there is still usually one tradition which dominates typical evaluation studies, leading to a focus either on quantitative or qualitative methods.

Many researchers point to the fact that this domination of one method or tradition may not be useful, but that a real integration of various methods from both traditions can be much more helpful to get comprehensive answers to given research questions. The integration of the complementary methods (and even beyond this, of data sources, theories and investigators), is discussed under the term "triangulation".

In this paper, we first want to review some of the underlying reasons which make evaluation of health care IT so difficult. We will structure the problems into three main problem areas: the complexity of the object of evaluation, the complexity of the evaluation project, and the motivation to perform evaluation. We will discuss means how to overcome the discussed problems.

As one more detailed example, we then discuss what benefits can be obtained from applying triangulation in an evaluation study. Based on the example of the evaluation of a nursing documentation system, we show how both the validation of results and the completeness of results can be supported by triangulation.

TYPICAL PROBLEMS IN EVALUATION OF IT IN HEALTH CARE

First Problem Area: Complexity of the Evaluation Object

When understanding IT as part of the information system of an organization, it is clear that evaluation requires not only an understanding of computer technology, but also of the social and behavioral processes that affect and are affected by the technology. This complexity of the evaluation objects has some important consequences. First, the **introduction of IT takes time**. It is not enough to implement the technology and then to immediately measure the effects. Users and workflow need a lot of time to get used to new tools and to completely exploit the new possibilities (Palvia, Sharma, & Conrath, 2001). Thus, evaluation results can develop and change during this first period of use. Then, even after an introduction period, the **evaluation object may steadily change** (Moehr, 2002) (moving evaluation target). For example, the use of information technology may be affected by changes in work organization, or in staff. It is nearly impossible to reach a stable situation in a flexible health care environment which makes evaluation results dependant of the point in time where the evaluation took place. In addition, each information system in our definition is quite **unique**. While the information technology may be similar in various departments, workflow, users and used functionality may be different. In addition, the organization of its introduction as well as the overall user motivation may differ. Thus, even when the same information technology is introduced, its effects may be varying (Kaplan & Shaw, 2002). The influence of such factors on the results of an evaluation study is often hard to disentangle (Wyatt, 1994), posing the problem of **external validity** (Moehr, 2002): Many evaluation studies may be valid only for the particular institutions with their specific information system.

The complexity of the evaluation object is an inherent attribute in health care IT evaluation and cannot be reduced. However, there are some ways to handle this problem in evaluation studies. To address the problem of external validity, the information technology and its environment which is going to be evaluated should be **defined in detail** before the beginning of the study. Not only the software and hardware which is used should be described, but also the number of users and their experience and motivation, the way information technology is introduced and used, the general technical infrastructure (e.g. networks) and any further aspects which may influence the usage of an information technology and its effects. Of special importance should also be the functionality and the way it is really used. Only this information may allow interpretation of the study results and comparison of different locations. Then, to address the problem of the moving evaluation target, **all changes in the information technology** and its interaction with the users should be carefully documented during the study. For example, changes in workflow, in staffing, or in hardware or software should be documented with reference to the ongoing evaluation. This permits the explanation of changes and differences in effects measured during the study period. Another approach to address the problem of the moving evaluation target may be to define smaller **evaluation modules**. This would allow the evaluation design or evaluation questions to be adapted to changes in the environment. Each module answered a question related to a defined phase of the introduction of the information technology. In addition, an evaluation must be planned in a **long-term perspective** in order to allow the users and the environment to integrate the new information technology. Hence enough resources for long-term evaluation (e.g. over several months or even years) should be available.

Second Problem Area: Complexity of the Evaluation Project

Evaluation of information technology is performed in the real and complex health care environment, with its different professional groups, and its high dependency on external influences such as legislation, economic constraints, or patient clientele. This poses problems to the evaluation projects, meaning the planning, executing and analyzing of an IT evaluation study. For example, the different stakeholders often have different conceptions and views of successful information technology (Palvia et al., 2001). The different stakeholder requirements can serve as a frame of reference for evaluation during the early phases of the IT life cycle, but also guide evaluations during later phases. In each case, multiple stakeholder view may lead to a multitude of (possibly conflicting) evaluation questions (Heathfield et al., 1999).

Depending on the point of view adopted, the evaluation will require different study designs and evaluation methods. The evaluation researcher must decide e.g. on the evaluation approach, on the adequate evaluation methods (e.g. quantitative vs. qualitative), and on the study design (e.g. RCT vs. observational study). Each has its own advantages and drawbacks (Moehr, 2002), (Frechtling, 1997), making their selection a rather challenging endeavor. This multitude of possible evaluation questions and available evaluation methods makes the planning of an evaluation study quite complex.

The complexity of the evaluation project has several consequences. First, the overall success of information technology is elusive to define (Palvia et al., 2001), and it is therefore often difficult to establish **clear-cut evaluation criteria** to be addressed in a study (Wyatt, 1994). Each stakeholder group may have individual questions, and a universal evaluation in terms of absolute or relative benefits is usually not feasible (or, from a more subjectivistic point of view, even not possible). It is also unrealistic to expect that

the information technology itself will have a direct and easy to measure effect on the outcome quality of patient care like in a drug trial (Wyatt, 1994). Thus **indirect measures** are often used such as user satisfaction or changes of clinical processes, which, however, do not give a really complete picture of the benefits of information technology. Often, **changes in the evaluation questions** may occur during the study, e.g. based on intermediate evaluation results, new insights, changes in stakeholders' opinions, or changes of the information technology (scope creep) (Dewan & Lorenzi, 2000). Changes in study questions, however, may be difficult to balance with study resources. Finally, the selection of **adequate evaluation designs and evaluation methods** is often regarded as a problem during evaluation studies. Evaluators may not be sufficiently aware of the broadness of available approaches, or be too deeply embedded in either the qualitative or the quantitative paradigm, neglecting the possible contributions of the complementary approach. Thus, inadequate methods or study designs may be chosen which may not be able to answer the original study questions.

The following suggestions may be useful in order to deal with the complexity of the evaluation project. First, it is recommended that the **general intention of the evaluation** and the starting point should be agreed early on. In principle, evaluation should start before the new information technology is implemented, in order to allow for early gathering of comparative data, and then continue during all phases of its life cycle (VATAM, 2000). Then, the **areas of evaluation should be restricted** to aspects which are of most importance to the involved stakeholders, and which can be measured with the available resources. A complete evaluation of all aspects of a system (such as economics, effectiveness, and acceptance) is usually not feasible. A balance between the resources of a study and the inclusion of the most relevant aspects has to be found. In addition, sufficient time should be invested into the definition of **relevant study questions**. All involved stakeholder groups should discuss and agree on the goals of evaluation (VATAM, 2000). The selected study questions should be relevant for decision-making with regard to introduction, operation or justification of information technology (Ammenwerth et al., 2004). Conflicting goals should be discussed and solved, as they are not only problematic for an evaluation, but for the overall management of new information technology. Fourth, when **new evaluation questions** emerge during the study, they should only be included in the study design when it is possible without creating problems. Otherwise, they should be tackled in consecutive studies. Each shift in evaluation questions must thoroughly be documented. For each study question, **adequate methods** must be chosen. A triangulation of methods may be useful to best answer the study questions (Heathfield, Pitty, & Hanka, 1998). For example, to address the effects of a nursing documentation system, both quantitative methods (time measurement, user acceptance scales, documentation quality measurement) as well as qualitative methods (focus group interviews) were used. We will discuss this example later on in more detail.

Third Problem Area: Motivation for Evaluation

An evaluation study can normally only be conducted when there is sufficient funding, and a sufficient number of participants (e.g. staff members, wards). Both these variables depend on the motivation of stakeholders (e.g. hospital management) to perform an evaluation. Sometimes, this motivation is not very high, because, for example, of fear for negative outcome, or of fear for revealing deficiencies of already implemented technology (Rigby, Forsström, Roberts, & Wyatt, 2001). In addition, the introduction of IT in an organization is a deep intervention that may have large consequences. It is thus often very difficult to organize IT evaluation in the

form of an experiment, and to easily remove the system again at the end of the study in case the evaluation was too negative.

Even with a motivated management, it may be difficult to find suitable participants. Participating in a study usually requires some effort from the involved staff. In addition, while the users have to make large efforts to learn and use a new, innovative system, the benefit of joining a pilot study is usually not obvious (the study is conducted in order to investigate possible effects), but participation may even include some risks for the involved staff such as disturbances in workflow. In summary, due to the given reasons, the hospital management, as well as involved staff members are often reluctant to participate in IT evaluation studies.

The described problem has consequences for the study. Without the support and motivation of the stakeholders to conduct an evaluation study, it will be difficult to get **sufficient resources** for an evaluation and sufficient participants willing to participate. Second, due to the given problems, the study organizer tends to recruit any participant who volunteers to participate. However, those participants may be more motivated to participate than the 'normal' user. This leads to the well-known **volunteer effect**, where results are better when participants are motivated. In addition, evaluation results are not only important for the involved units, but also for the overall organization or for similar units in other organizations. To allow transfer of results, the pilot wards or pilot users must be **sufficiently representative** for other wards or users. But, as each information technology within its environment is quite unique (see problem area 1), it is difficult to find comparable or representative participants.

To increase the number of participants, two approaches should be combined. First, the responsible management should be **informed and motivated** to support the study. The result of an evaluation study may be important to decide on new information technology, and to support its continuous improvement. Then, the possible participants could be directly addressed. It should be made clear that the study provides the opportunity to influence not only the future development of IT in health care but also the own working environment. User feedback of study results may act as an important driving force for users to participate in the study. Offering **financial compensation** or additional staff for the study period may help to gain support from participants and from management. As in clinical trials, **multi-centric studies** should be considered (Wyatt & Spiegelhalter, 1992). This would largely increase the number of available participants. This means however, that study management requires much more effort. A multi-centric study design is difficult when the environment is completely different. In addition, the variation between study participants will be bigger in multi-centric trials than in single-centre ones. This may render interpretation and comparison of results even more difficult (cp. discussion in problem area 1).

Summary of General Recommendations

The above discussed problems and approaches will now be summarized in a list of 12 general recommendations for IT evaluation in healthcare:

1. Evaluation takes time, thus take your time for thorough planning and execution.
2. Document all of your decisions and steps in a detailed study protocol. Adhere to this protocol; it is your main tool for a systematic evaluation.
3. Strive for management support, and try to organize long-term financial support.
4. Clarify the goals of the evaluation. Take into account the different stakeholder groups. Dissolve conflicting goals.
5. Reduce your evaluation questions to an appropriate number of the most important questions which you can handle within the

available time and budget. If new questions emerge during the study, which cannot easily be integrated, postpone them for a new evaluation study.
6. Clarify and thoroughly describe the information technology which is the object of your evaluation, and the environment. Take note of any changes of the information technology and its environment during the study that may affect results.
7. Select an adequate study design. Think of a stepwise study design.
8. Select adequate methods to answer your study questions. Neither objectivist nor subjectivist approaches can answer all questions. Take into account the available methods. Consider being multi-methodic and multi-disciplinary, and consider triangulation of methods, data sources, investigators, and theories. Strive for methodical (e.g. biometrics) advice.
9. Motivate a sufficient number of users to participate. Consider multi-centric trials and financial or other compensation.
10. Use validated evaluation instruments wherever possible.
11. Be open to unwanted and unexpected effects.
12. Publish your results and what you learned to allow others to learn from your work.

One of the most discussed aspects is the selection of adequate methods and tools (point 6), and here especially the adequate application of multi-methodic and multi-disciplinary approaches (Ammenwerth et al., 2004). The interdisciplinary nature of evaluation research in medical informatics includes that a broad choice of evaluation methods is available for various purposes. In section 2 and 3 of this book, several distinct quantitative and qualitative evaluation methods have been presented and discussed in detail. All of them have their particular application area. However, in many situations, the evaluator may want to combine the methods to best answer the evaluation questions at hand. Especially in more formative (constructive) studies, a combination of methods may seem necessary to get a more complete picture of a situation. To support this, the method of triangulation has been developed and will now be presented in more detail.

THE THEORY OF TRIANGULATION

The term triangulation comes from navigation and means a technique to find the exact location of a ship base on the use of various reference points. Based on this idea, triangulation in evaluation means the multiple employment of data sources, observers, methods, or theories, in investigations of the same phenomenon (Greene & McClintock, 1985). This approach has two main objectives: First, to support a finding with the help of the others (validation); second, to complement the data with new results, to find new information, to get additional pieces to the overall 'puzzle' (completeness) (Knafl & Breitmayer, 1991).

Triangulation is, based on work by (Denzin, 1970), usually divided into the following four types which can be applied at the same time:

- **Data triangulation:** Various data sources are used with regard to time, space, or persons. For example, nurses from different sites are interviewed, or questionnaires are applied at different times.
- **Investigator triangulation:** Various observers or interviewers with their own specific professional methodological background take part in the study, gathering and analyzing the data together. For example, a computer scientist and a social scientist analyze and interpret results from focus group interviews together.
- **Theory triangulation:** Data is analyzed based on various perspectives, hypotheses or theories. For example, organizational

changes are analyzed using two different change theories.
- **Methods triangulation:** Various methods for data collection and analysis are applied. Here, two types are distinguished: within-method triangulation (combining approaches from the same research tradition), and between-method triangulation (combining approaches from both quantitative and qualitative research traditions, also called across-method triangulation). For example, two different quantitative questionnaires may be applied to access user attitudes, or group interviews as well as questionnaires may be applied in parallel.

It should be noticed that the term triangulation is only used when *one* phenomenon is investigated with regard to *one* research question.

The term "triangulation" is often seen strongly related to the term "multi-method evaluation" because methods triangulation is seen as the most often used triangulation approach. However, as we want to stress, it is not limited on the combination of methods, but also describes combination of data sources, investigators, or theories.

EXAMPLE: TRIANGULATION DURING THE EVALUATION OF A NURSING DOCUMENTATION SYSTEM

Background of the Study

Nursing documentation is an important part of clinical documentation. There have been some attempts and discussions on how to support the nursing documentation using computer-based documentation systems.

In 1997, the Heidelberg University Medical Center started to introduce a computer-based nursing documentation system in order to systematically evaluate preconditions and consequences. Four different (psychiatric and somatic) wards were chosen for this study.

In the following paragraphs, we will concentrate on those parts of the study which are relevant for the triangulation aspects of the study. Please refer to other publications for more details on methods and results, such as (Ammenwerth, Mansmann, Iller, & Eichstädter, 2003b), (Ammenwerth et al., 2001).

Three of the four study wards had been selected by the nursing management for the study. On all three wards, the majority of nurses agreed to participate. Ward B volunteered by themselves to participate. The four study wards belonged to different departments. Ward A and B were psychiatric wards with 21 resp. 28 beds, ward C was a pediatric ward for children under two years with 15 beds, ward D, was a dermatological ward with 20 beds.

Our study wards were quite different with regard to nursing documentation. On wards A and B, a complete nursing documentation based on the principles of the nursing process - for details on nursing process, see (Lindsey & Hartrick, 1996) - had been established for several years. In contrast, on ward C and D, only a reduced care plan was usually documented. Documentation was mostly conducted in the ward office. Only on ward C, major parts of documentation were also conducted in the patients' room. The youngest staff could be found on ward D, the staff least experienced in computer use on ward C.

Study Design

The software PIK ("Pflegeinformations- und Kommunikationssystem", a German acronym for "nursing information and communication system") was introduced on those four wards. The functionality covered the six phases of the nursing care process. The study period was between August 1998 and October 2001. Ward A

and B started in 1998 with the introduction of the documentation system, Ward C and D joined in 2000.

The study consisted of two main parts: The objective of the more **quantitative study** was to analyze the changes in the nurses' attitudes with regard to nursing process, computers in nursing, and nursing documentation system, after the introduction of the computer-based system. Standardized, validated questionnaires were applied based on (Bowman, Thompson, & Sutton, 1983) for nurses' attitudes on the nursing process, on (Nickell & Pinto, 1986) for computer attitudes, on (Lowry, 1994) for nurses' attitudes on computers in nursing, and on (Chin, 1988) and (Ohmann, Boy, & Yang, 1997) for nurses' satisfaction with the computer-based nursing documentation system itself. We carefully translated those questionnaires into German and checked the understandability in a pre-study. We used a prospective intervention study with three time measurements: approx. 3 months before introduction ("before"); approx. 3 months after introduction ("during"); approx. 9 months after introduction ("after").

The second part of the study was a more **qualitative study**. Here, the objective was to further analyze the reasons for the different attitudes on the wards. The quantitative study exactly described these attitudes, and the qualitative study was now intended to further explain those quantitative results. The qualitative study was conducted in February 2002, after the analysis of the quantitative study was finished. In this qualitative study, open-ended focus group interviews were conducted with up to four staff members from each ward (most of them already have taken part in the quantitative study), with the three project managers from each department, and with the four ward managers from the wards. Open-ended means that the interviews were not guided by pre-defined questions. We used two general questions which started the interviews, e.g. "How are you doing with PIK?", "How was the introduction period".

The rest of the interview was mostly guided by the participants themselves, with relative little control exerted by the interviewers.

All interviews were conducted by a team of two researchers. They took about one hour each. The interviews were audio taped and analyzed using inductive, iterative content analysis based on (Mayring, 1993). This means that the transcripts were carefully and step-wise analyzed (using the software WinMaxProf98).

In the following paragraphs, only those results of the quantitative and qualitative study will be presented which are relevant for the triangulation aspects of the study. Please refer to the already mentioned study publications for more details.

Results of Quantitative Analysis of User Attitudes

All in all 119 questionnaires were returned: 23 nurses answered all three questionnaires, 17 nurses answered two, and 16 nurses answered one questionnaire. The return rates were 82% for the 1st questionnaire, 86.5% for the 2nd questionnaire, and 90.2% for the 3rd questionnaire. A quantitative analysis of the individual items of the questionnaires revealed unfavorable attitudes especially on ward C. On both wards C and D, the nurses stated that the documentation system does not "save time", and that it does not "lead to a better overview on the course of patient care". In addition, on ward C, the nurses stated that they "felt burdened in their work" by the computer-based system, and that the documentation system does not "make documentation easier". On ward A and B, the opinions with regard to those items were more positive.

The self reported daily usage of the computer-based documentation system was quite similar on all wards: about 1 – 2 hours/day during the 2nd and 3rd questionnaire, with highest values on ward B, and lowest values on ward A. The self-confidence with the system as stated by the nurses was rather high on all wards during both the 2nd

and 3rd questionnaire: the mean values were between 3 and 3.7 during the 2nd questionnaire and between 3.4 and 3.8 during the 3rd questionnaire (1 = minimum, 4 = maximum).

Statistical analysis revealed that the overall attitude on the documentation system during the 3rd questionnaire was positively correlated to the initial attitude on the nursing process, to the attitude on computers in general and to the attitude on computers in nursing. Both computer attitude scores were in turn positively correlated to the years of computer experience. For details, see (Ammenwerth et al., 2003b).

Overall, the results of quantitative analysis pointed to a positive attitude on the computer-based nursing documentation already shortly after its introduction, which significant increase on three of the four wards later on. However, on ward C, the quantitative results revealed negative reactions, showing a heavy decline in the attitude scores during the 2nd questionnaire. On ward C, the overall attitude of the computer-based system remained rather negative, even during the 3rd questionnaire. What could be the reasons? In order to answer this question, a subsequent qualitative study was conducted.

Results of Qualitative Analysis of User Attitudes

This part of the study was conducted as planned. Overall, about 100 pages of interview transcript were analyzed. Details of the interviews are published elsewhere (Ammenwerth et al., 2003a), we will now only summarize the main points.

On ward C, some distinct features came up in the interviews which seem to have leaded to low attitude scores at the beginning. For example, the nursing process had not been completely implemented before, thus the documentation efforts now were much higher. Documentation of nursing tasks covered a 24 h/day, due to the very young patients and their high need for care. Thus, the overall amount of documentation on ward C was higher. Patient fluctuation was also highest on ward C. Nurses found it time-consuming to create a complete nursing anamnesis and nursing care plan for each patient. The previous computer experience was seen as rather low on ward C, and also the number and availability of motivated key users. Then, during the introduction of the nursing documentation system, the workload was rather high on ward C due to staff shortage which increased pressure on the nurses. Finally, and most importantly, nursing documentation had previously at least partly been carried out in the patients' rooms. However, during our study, computers were only installed in the ward office. No mobile computers were available, which according to the nurses lead to time-consuming and inefficient double documentation.

Interesting differences were found between the nurses and the project management. For example, the nurses stated in the interviews to not have been sufficiently informed on the new documentation system, while the project management stated to have offered information, which had however not been used. Another example: the nurses felt that training was insufficient. In the opinion of the project management, sufficient opportunities had been offered. We will later see how this divergent information helps to complete the overall picture.

On ward D, the attitude on the documentation system was high in the interviews. The nurses saw benefits, especially in a more professional documentation, which would lead to a greater acknowledgement of nursing. Standardized care planning was seen to make care planning much easier, without reducing the individuality of the patient. Overall, the ward felt at ease while working with the new documentation system.

On ward A and B, the attitudes were also positive. The nurses stressed the better legibility of nursing documentation in the interviews. They said that time effort for nursing care planning was lower, but overall, time effort for nursing documentation was much higher than before. The

interviews showed that the introduction period had been filled with anxiety and fear about new requirements for the nurses. Now, after some time, the nurses felt self-confident with computers. An interesting discussion arose on the topic of standardization. Most nurses felt that standardized care plans reduced the individuality of the care plans, and that they did not really reflect what is going on with the patient. Finally, those wards, too, mentioned insufficient teaching and support in the first weeks.

These rather short summaries from the interviews should highlight some distinct features of the wards, showing similarities (e.g. on insufficient teaching and fears at the beginning), but also differences (e.g. on the question on standardized care plans or time effort).

Application of Triangulation in this Study

After analysis of the quantitative study and the qualitative study, we now want to see how the different results can be put together to get a broader picture of the effects and preconditions of a nursing documentation system. We thus applied all four types of triangulation as described by (Denzin, 1970):

- **Data triangulation:** Various data sources were used: Within the quantitative study, data triangulation with regard to time was used as the questionnaires were submitted three times to the same users (data triangulation with regard to time). In addition, in the interviews, not only nurses, but also project management and ward management were interviewed (data triangulation with regard to persons).
- **Investigator triangulation:** Within the qualitative study, the two interviewers had different backgrounds (one more quantitative coming from medical informatics, the other more qualitative coming from social

science). Both acted together as interviewers, analyzed the transcript together, and discussed and agreed on results and conclusions.

- **Theory triangulation:** We learned from various complementing theories to better understand the results of our studies. For example, to explain the implementation phases, we took ideas both from the book of (Lorenzi & Riley, 1995) (first-, middle- and second-order change) as well as from the change theory of (Lewin, 1947) (unfreezing, moving, refreezing phase). With regard to user evaluation, we used e.g. the Technology Acceptance Model (TAM) of (Davis, 1993), and the Task-Technology Fit model (TTF) of (Goodhue, 1995).

- **Methods triangulation:** We applied between-methods triangulation by applying both quantitative questionnaires and qualitative focus group interviews to investigate users attitudes.

As stated in the introduction, triangulation has two main objectives: To confirm results with data from other sources (validation of results), and to find new data to get a more complete picture (completeness of results). We will now shortly discuss whether triangulation helped to achieve those goals.

Validation of Results

Validation of results is obtained when results from one part of the study are confirmed by congruent (not necessarily equal) results from other parts of the study. In our example, some parts of the study showed congruent results:

First, both the questionnaire and the interviews focused on attitudes issues. In this area, both approaches lead to congruent results, showing e.g. favorable attitudes on three wards. In addition, both the questionnaires and the interviews showed

also problems with regard to the user satisfaction with the nursing documentation system on ward C. However, as the interviews were conducted later, they could better show the long-term development on the wards. Hence, both data sources thus showed congruent results.

Second, we found congruent results of the two scales "attitudes on nursing process" and "attitude on the computer-based nursing documentation system" within the standardized questionnaires. Both focus on different attitude items, both showed comparable low results on ward C and higher results on the other wards, pointing to congruent measurements.

Those two selected examples show how results of some parts of the study could be validated by congruent results from other parts of the studies.

Completeness of Results

Besides validation, triangulation can increase completeness when one part of the study presents results which have not been found in other parts of the study. By this new information, the completeness of results is increased. The new information may be complementary to other results, or it may present divergent information.

In our study, both questionnaires and interviews presented partly **complementary results**, which led to new insights. For example, impact of the computer-based documentation system on documentation processes and communication processes had not been detected by the questionnaire (this aspect had not been included in the questions). However, the documentation system seems to have influenced e.g. the way different health care professional exchanged patient-related information. This led to some discussion on this topic on all wards in the interviews and seems to have had an impact on the overall attitude. Those effects only emerged in the group interviews (and not in the questionnaires), enlarging the picture of the effects of the nursing documentation system, and helping to better understand the reactions of the different wards.

Another example is the complementarity of the results in the interviews and questionnaires on ward C. The interviews were done some time after the questionnaires. Thus, during this time, changes may have occurred. The change theory of (Lewin, 1947) states that organizational changes occur in three phases. "Unfreezing" (old patterns must be released, combined with insecurity and problems), "Moving" (new patterns are tested), and "Refreezing" (new patterns are internalized and seen as normal). The low attitude scores on ward C even at the last measurement point indicate that the ward was in the moving phase during this time. During the interviews, the stress which was articulated by the nurses seems to be less. This can be interpreted as ward C being slowly changing from the moving into the refreezing phase.

Triangulation can thus help to get a more complete picture of the object under investigation. Often, especially when applying various methods during the investigation, the results will not be congruent, but they may be divergent (e.g. contradicting). This is an important aspect of triangulation, as divergent results can especially highlight some points, present new information and lead to further investigation.

In our study, we found some **divergent results**. For example, during the group interviews, nurses from one ward stressed that they do not see a reduction in effort needed for documentation by the computer-based system. However, in the questionnaires, this ward indicated strong time reductions. This differences can lead to the questions whether e.g. time efforts are judged with regard to the situation without the nursing documentation system (where amount of documentation was much lower, and so did the time effort), or with regard to the tasks which have to be performed (the same amount of documentation can be done much quicker with the computer-based system). This discussion can help to better

understand the answers. Interesting differences of point of view could also be found between the staff and the project management of one ward in the group interviews. While the nurses of this ward claimed in the interviews that training was sub-optimal, the project management stated that sufficient offers had been made. Those apparent contradictions may point e.g. to different perceptions of the need for training by the different stakeholders. Those insights may help to better organize the teaching on other wards.

As those (selected) examples show, triangulation helped us to obtain a better picture of the reaction of the four wards. The evaluation results also led to some decision on how to improve the technical infrastructure as well as how to better organize the teaching and support on some wards. All wards are still working with the computer-based nursing documentation system.

DISCUSSION

Medical informatics is an academic discipline, and thus evaluation is an important part of any system development and implementation activity (Shahar, 2002; Talmon & Hasmann, 2002). However, many problems with regard to health care IT evaluation have been reported. (Wyatt & Spiegelhalter, 1992) as well as (Grémy & Degoulet, 1993) already discussed the complexity of the field, the motivation issue, and methodological barriers to evaluation. Examples of meta-analysis of IT evaluation studies confirm those barriers (e.g. (Johnston, Langton, Haynes, & Mathieu, 1994), (Kaplan, 2001), (Brender, 2002).

In this chapter, we elaborated a number of important problems to some more detail, and structured them into three areas: The complexity of the evaluation object, the complexity of the evaluation project with its multitude of stakeholders, and the motivation for evaluation.

A kind of framework to support evaluation studies of information systems may be useful to address the problem areas discussed in this paper. In fact, many authors have formulated the necessity for such a framework, e.g. (Shaw, 2002) or (Grant, Plante, & Leblanc, 2002). Chapter 15 will present a framework for evaluation in more detail. One important part of such a framework is the call for multi-method evaluation. While triangulation has long been discussed and applied in research (one of the first being (Campbell & Fiske, 1959), the idea of the possible advantages of multi-method approaches or triangulation in more general terms is not really reflected in medical informatics literature.

The background of multi-method approaches has been more deeply discussed in chapter 13. In general, both quantitative and qualitative methods have their areas and research questions where they can be successfully applied. By triangulation both approaches, their advantages can be combined. We found that both complementary and divergent results from the different sources gave important new information and stimulation of further discussion.

In the last years, there has been a more basic discussion whether inter-methods triangulation is possible at all. It is discussed that the epistemological underpinnings between quantitative and qualitative research paradigms may be so different that a real combination may not be possible (Greene & McClintock, 1985), (Sim & Sharp, 1998). However, this argumentation is not taking into account that a tradition of research has formed beyond subjectivistic and objectivistic paradigms. Evaluation methods are chosen accordingly to research questions and the research topic. Thus the question which methods to apply and how to combine them only can be answered with respect to the research topic and the research question and not on a general basis. Thus, as important as this discussion might be in the light of progress in research methods, evaluation researchers in medical informatics may be advised to start to select and combine methods based on their distinctive

research question. This gives evaluation researchers a broad range of possibilities to increase both completeness and validity of results independent of his or her research tradition.

CONCLUSION

Evaluation studies in health care IT take a lot of time, resources, and know-how. Clearly defined methodological guidelines which take the difficulties of information system evaluation in health care into account may help to conduct better evaluation studies. This chapter has classified some of the problems encountered in healthcare IT evaluation under the three main problem areas complexity of the evaluation object, complexity of the evaluation project and limited motivation for evaluation. We suggested a list of 12 essential recommendations to support the evaluation of information systems. A broadly accepted framework for IT evaluation in healthcare which goes more into details seems desirable, supporting the evaluator during planning and executing of an evaluation study.

Focusing on methodological aspects, we have presented some basics on triangulation and illustrated them in a case study. The correct application of triangulation requires – as other evaluation methods – training and methodological experience. Medical informatics evaluation research may profit from this well-established theory.

ACKNOWLEDGMENT

This chapter is based on two earlier publications published by Elsevier: Ammenwerth E, Gräber S, Herrmann G, Bürkle T, König J (2003). Evaluation of Health Information Systems - Problems and Challenges. International Journal of Medical Informatics; 71 (2-3): 125-35. And Ammenwerth E, Mansmann U, Iller C. Can evaluation studies benefit from a triangulation of quantitative and qualitative methods? A case study (2003). International Journal of Medical Informatics; 70 (2-3): 237-48.

REFERENCES

Ammenwerth, E., Brender, J., Nykänen, P., Prokosch, U., Rigby, M., & Talmon, J. (2004). Visions and strategies to improve evaluations of health information systems - reflections and lessons based on the HIS-EVAL workshop in Innsbruck. Int J Med Inf.

Ammenwerth, E., & de Keizer, N. (2004). An inventory of evaluation studies of information technology in health care: Trends in evaluation research 1982 - 2002. Methods Inform Med.

Ammenwerth, E., Eichstädter, R., Haux, R., Pohl, U., Rebel, S., & Ziegler, S. (2001). A Randomized Evaluation of a Computer-Based Nursing Documentation System. Methods of Information in Medicine, 40(2), 61-8.

Ammenwerth, E., Iller, C., Mahler, C., Kandert, M., Luther, G., Hoppe, B., & Eichstädter, R. (2003a). Einflussfaktoren auf die Akzeptanz und Adoption eines Pflegedokumentationssystems - Studienbericht (2/2003). Innsbruck: Private Universität für Medizinische Informatik und Technik Tirol.

Ammenwerth, E., Mansmann, U., Iller, C., & Eichstädter, R. (2003b). Factors Affecting and Affected by User Acceptance of Computer-Based Nursing Documentation: Results of a Two-Year Study. Journal of the American Medical Informatics Association., 10(1), 69-84.

Berg, M., Aarts, J., & van der Lei, J. (2003). ICT in Health Care: Sociotechnical Approaches (Editorial). Methods Inf Med, 42, 297-301.

Bowman, G., Thompson, D., & Sutton, T. (1983). Nurses' attitudes towards the nursing process. Journal of Advanced Nursing, 8(2), 125-129.

Brender, J. (2002). Methodological and Methodical Perils and Pitfalls within Assessment Studies Performed on IT-based solutions in Healthcare (ISSN 1397-9507). Aalborg: Virtual Centre for Health Informatics.

Campbell, D., & Fiske, D. (1959). Convergent and discriminant validity by the muli-trait, multi-method matrix. Psychological Bulletin, 56, 81-105.

Chin, J. (1988). Development of a tool measuring user satisfaction of the human-computer interface, Chi'88 Conf. Proceedings: Human factors in Computing (pp. 213-218). New York: Association for Computing Machinery.

Davis, F. (1993). User acceptance of information technology: System characteristics, user perceptions and behavioral impacts. International Journal of Man-Machine Studies, 38, 475-487.

Denzin, N. (1970). Strategies of multiple triangulation. In N. Denzin (Ed.), The Research Act (3rd ed., pp. 297-331). Chicago: Aldine.

Dewan, N., & Lorenzi, N. (2000). Behavioral Health Information Systems: Evaluating Readiness and User Acceptance. MD Computing, 17(4), 50-52.

Frechtling, J. (1997). User-Friendly Handbook for Mixed Method Evaluation, [Ausdruck im Eval-Ordner]. Available: http://www.ehr.nsf.gov/EHR/REC/pubs/NSF97-153/start.htm [Feb. 2003].

Friedman, C., & Wyatt, J. C. (1997). Evaluation Methods in Medical Informatics. New York: Springer.

Goodhue, D. (1995). Understanding user evaluations of information systems. Management Science, 41(12), 1827-44.

Grant, A., Plante, I., & Leblanc, F. (2002). The TEAM methodology for the evaluation of information systems in biomedicine. Comput Biol Med, 32(3), 195-207.

Greene, J., & McClintock, C. (1985). Triangulation in evaluation: Design and analysis issues. Evaluation Review, 9(5), 523-545.

Grémy, F., & Degoulet, P. (1993). Assessment of health information technology: which questions for which systems? Proposal for a taxonomy. Medical Informatics, 18(3), 185-93.

Heathfield, H., Hudson, P., Kay, S., Mackay, L., Marley, T., Nicholson, L., Peel, V., Roberts, R., & Williams, J. (1999). Issues in the multi-disciplinary assessment of healthcare information systems. Assessment of Healthcare Information Technology & People, 12(3), 253-75.

Heathfield, H., Pitty, D., & Hanka, R. (1998). Evaluating information technology in health care: barriers and challenges. British Medical Journal, 316, 1959-61.

Institute of Medicine. (2001). Crossing the Quality Chasm: A New Health System for the 21st Century. Washington: National Academy Press.

Johnston, M., Langton, K., Haynes, R., & Mathieu, A. (1994). Effects of Computer-based Clinical Decision Support Systems on Clinician Performance and Patient Outcome - A Critical Appraisal of Research. Annuals of Internal Medicine, 120, 135-42.

Kaplan, B. (2001). Evaluating informatics applications - clinical decision support systems literature review. International Journal of Medical Informatics, 64, 15-37.

Kaplan, B., & Shaw, N. (2002). People, Organizational and Social Issues: Evaluation as an exemplar. In R. Haux & C. Kulikowski (Eds.), Yearbook of Medical Informatics 2002 (pp. 91 - 102). Stuttgart: Schattauer.

Knafl, K., & Breitmayer, B. (1991). Triangulation in qualitative research: Issues of conceptual clarity and purpose. In J. Morse (Ed.), A contemporary dialogue (pp. 226-239). Newbury Park, California: Sage.

Lewin, K. (1947). Frontiers in group dynamics: concepts, methods, and reality of social sciences: Social equalization and social change. Human Relations, 1, 5-14.

Lindsey, E., & Hartrick, G. (1996). Health-promoting nursing practice: the demise of the nursing process? Journal of Advanced Nursing, 23(1), 106-112.

Lorenzi, N., & Riley, R. (1995). Organizational Aspects of Health Informatics - Managing Technological Change. New York: Springer.

Lowry, C. (1994). Nurses' attitudes toward computerised care plans in intensive care. Part 2. Intensive and Critical Care Nursing, 10, 2-11.

Mayring, M. (1993). Einführung in die qualitative Sozialforschung. Weinheim: Psychologie-Verlag-Union.

Moehr, J. R. (2002). Evaluation: salvation or nemesis of medical informatics? Comput Biol Med, 32(3), 113-25.

Nickell, G., & Pinto, J. (1986). The Computer Attitude Scale. Computers in Human Behaviour, 2, 301-306.

Ohmann, C., Boy, O., & Yang, Q. (1997). A systematic approach to the assessment of user satisfaction with health care systems: constructs, models and instruments. In C. Pappas (Ed.), Medical Informatics Europe ,97. Conference proceedings (Vol. 43 Pt B, pp. 781-5). Amsterdam: IOS Press.

Palvia, S., Sharma, R., & Conrath, D. (2001). A socio-technical framework for quality assessment of computer information systems. Industrial Management & Data Systems, 101(5), 237-251.

Rigby, M. (2001). Evaluation: 16 Powerful Reasons Why Not to Do It - And 6 Over-Riding Imperatives. In V. Patel, R. Rogers, & R. Haux (Eds.), Proceedings of the 10th World Congress on Medical Informatics (Medinfo 2001) (Vol. 84, pp. 1198-202). Amsterdam: IOS Press.

Rigby, M., Forsström, J., Roberts, R., & Wyatt, W. (2001). Verifying quality and safety in health informatics services. BMJ, 323(8 September 2001), 552-556.

Shahar, Y. (2002). Medical Informatics: Between Science and Engineering, Between Academia and Industry. Methods Inf Med, 41, 8-11.

Shaw, N. (2002). ,CHEATS': a generic information communication technology (ICT) evaluation framework. Computers in Biology and Medicine, 32, 209-200.

Sim, J., & Sharp, K. (1998). A critical appraisal of the role of triangulation in nursing research. Int J Nurs Stud, 35(1-2), 23-31.

Talmon, J., & Hasmann, A. (2002). Medical Informatics as a Discipline at the Beginning of the 21th Century. Methods Inf Med, 41, 4-7.

van der Loo, R. (1995). Overview of Published Assessment and Evaluation Studies. In E. M. S. J. van Gennip & J. S. Talmon (Eds.), Assessment and evaluation of information technologies (pp. 261-82). Amsterdam: IOS Press.

VATAM. (2000). The VATAM Websites. Validation of Health Telematics Applications (VATAM). Available: http://www-vatam.unimaas.nl/html/aboutvalidation.shtml [January 2004].

Winter, A., Ammenwerth, E., Bott, O., Brigl, B., Buchauer, A., Gräber, S., Grant, A., Häber, A., Hasselbring, W., Haux, R., Heinrich, A., Janssen, H., Kock, I., Penger, O.-S., Prokosch, H.-U., Terstappen, A., & Winter, A. (2001). Strategic Information Management Plans: The Basis for Systematic Information Management in Hospitals. International Journal of Medical Informatics, 64(2-3), 99-109.

Wyatt, J. (1994). Clinical data systems, part 3: development and evaluation. The Lancet, 344, 1682-8.

Wyatt, J., & Spiegelhalter, D. (1992). Field trials of medical decision-aids: potential problems and solutions. In P. Clayton (Ed.), 15th Annual Symposium on Computer Applications in Medical Care (pp. 3-7). New York: McGraw-Hill.

This work was previously published in E-Health Systems Diffusion and Use: The Innovation, the User and the USE IT Model, edited by T. Spil and R. Schuring, pp. 212-236, copyright 2006 by IGI Publishing, formerly known as Idea Group Publishing (an imprint of IGI Global).

Chapter XIX
eHealth Systems, Their Use and Visions for the Future

Pirkko Nykänen
Tampere University, Finland

ABSTRACT

eHealth refers to use of information and communication technologies to improve or enable health and healthcare. eHealth broadens the scope of health care delivery, citizens are in the center of services and services are offered by information systems often via the Internet. In this chapter eHealth systems are classified on the basis of their use and their functionality and the use is discussed from the viewpoints of citizens and health professionals. Citizens are increasingly using Internet and eHealth systems to search for medicine or health related information, and they become better informed and may take more responsibility of their own health. Health professionals are more reluctant to use the Internet and eHealth systems in physician-patient communication due to power and responsibility problems of decisions. In the future the socio-technical nature of eHealth should be considered and future systems developed for real use and user environment with user acceptable technology.

INTRODUCTION

In the information society it is important to develop and apply technologies in such a way that we empower citizens to play a full role in a society. An essential part of the information society are health care services, they are needed by citizens and should be provided efficiently and made accessible to all (Haglund, 2002).

With the information society a new concept, eHealth, has been introduced to refer to the use of emerging information technology to improve or enable health and health care. Silber (2003) defines eHealth as "application of information and communication technologies (ICT) across the whole range of functions that affect health" (p. 3). Eysenbach (2001) gives a broder definition for eHealth: An emerging field in the intersection of medical informatics, public health and business, referring to health services and information delivered or enhanced thorough the Internet and related technologies. Alvarez (2002) emphasises the consumer-viewpoint when he defines eHealth as a consumer-centered model of health care where stakeholders collaborate, utilising ICT and Internet technologies to manage health, arrange, deliver and account for care, and manage the health care system. All these definitions support the conception that eHealth means application of information technologies to promote health, and to support health care services delivery and use. eHealth covers all health strategies: Prevention, treatment and rehabilitation. It is essential that eHealth applications meet the needs of citizens, patients, health care professionals and policy makers. Therefore, evaluation studies are needed to assess the benefits, effects and impacts of eHealth on citizens, professionals, health care systems and health care outcomes.

eHealth conceptualization broadens the scope of health care delivery; citizens are placed at the centre of services, services are in many situations offered to be used through the Internet e.g. at home and citizens can have interaction with health professionals who look after their health needs (Silber, 2003; Wilson et al., 2004). eHealth is expected to contribute to development of new ways of delivering health services and to impact on the organisation and structure of the health care delivery system. eHealth is not only of technological improvement but it is of reengineering of health care processes, and of consideration of the socio-technical aspects of design and development of applications.

eHEALTH SYSTEMS

eHealth applications should make citizens better informed, all citizens should have access to services, use of services should be economically affordable and citizens should benefit from the use

of services. On the other hand, eHealth services should improve the quality, availability and effectiveness of health care (Grimson et al, 2000; Silber, 2003; Wilson 2004).

Types of eHealth Systems

Traditionally, three broad categories of eHealth applications can be identified: Delivery of care to patients by health care professionals, education and dissemination of health-related information and knowledge, and trading health products (Ruotsalainen et al., 2003).

The first category covers systems for delivery of care to patients by health care professionals including wide range of applications from pure administrative to those for care delivery:

- *Hospital systems,* including e.g. scheduling systems, logistics systems, management information systems, hospital and patient administration systems, laboratory information systems, radiology information systems, pharmacy systems, nursing systems and networked services such as electronic messaging between the hospital and other health care actors for communication of clinical information and administrative data, including telemedical services such as telepathology and teleconsultation for remote areas.
- *Primary care systems,* including e.g. information systems for general parctitioners, pharmacists and dentists for patient management, medical records, electronic prescribing and information exchange.
- *Home care systems,* including e.g. systems that are used to deliver care services via telecommunication or wireless to the patient at home. Examples of such systems are remote vital signs monitoring systems that enable the patient to receive targeted treatment and medication without the need to visit an out-patient clinic or occupy a hospital bed.

These kinds of systems are particularly well developed in diabetes medicine, hypertension management, asthma monitoring and home dialysis.

The second category covers systems for education and dissemination of health related information and knowledge including web-portals and specific health-related web-sites, virtual hospitals and Internet-based consultation services. These systems may be targeted for:

- *Medical consultation*, search for the second opinion, search for health, diseases or treatments related information,
- *Medical education and dissemination* of medical publications, preventive materials and public health related information.

These dissemination systems may help citizens to become informed and empowered through information and knowledge they are able to retrieve and access themselves from the Internet sources. However, the quality and validity of information can be questioned with many Internet information sources (Wilson, 2002). To promote these kinds of Internet information sources and to ensure people that they can confidently and with full understanding of known risks access and use information from the Internet, initiatives like Health on the Net, HI Ethics Program and Health Online Actions have been established to develop guidelines and quality criteria and to promote codes of ethics for health-related Websites (Spink et al., 2004; Wilson, 2002).

The third category covers systems that are developed to trade health related products. eCommerce or eTrading of medical products, health related goods, pharmaceuticals and medical devices is a growing eHealth area and current procedures enable citizens to enter Internet shopping in an easy and secure way.

eHealth applications can also be classified according to their functionality and following

this principle we may currently find the following groups of applications (Ruotsalainen et al., 2003):

- *Regional health information networks* that deploy advanced health care services at various levels of health care delivery system, including primary care, pre-hospital health emergency management and hospital care. These systems are networked and implemented using various technologies. A typical feature for these systems is the integration of existing legacy systems, imaging systems, departmental and administrative systems into one network and development of new, innovative interfaces and applications to provide comprehensive services regionally.

- *Hospital systems, clinical systems, diagnostic systems, hospital management systems* that cover hospital information systems (HIS), various departmental systems like radiology information systems (RIS), pathology information systems, laboratory information systems (LIS), diagnostic systems like decision support and knowledge based systems and hospital management systems like accounting, resource management and booking systems.

- *Telemedicine or teleconsultation systems* are used to access an expert opinion or a second opinion, or to monitor remote patient at home or in another health care organisation. These systems are especially often planned to support delivery of medical expertise for rural areas.

- *Insurance, cards or systems that present the payer view on health services.* These applications are developed to support the use of cards as means to access health services, to get information on the health insurance status and to register users that are entitled to special services or reimbursements based on their health, age or employment status.

- *Citizen-centred systems, patient-centred systems and health information portals.* These applications provide health related information for patients and health professionals, and additionally they may provide possibilities for consultation services, or for buying pharmaceuticals or other health related products.

- *Home care systems and health related fitness systems.* Home care systems are meant to monitor chronic diseases at home, to monitor elderly patients, or to teleconsult professionals from home. These systems are often based on wireless technology, e.g mobile phones or handheld computers. Home care systems are also used to help in the management of care, in preparing care plans and in coordination of actions and tasks taken by members of care teams. Health related fitness systems are those meant for healthy people that want to monitor their well-being and fitness.

We see from the typologies above for that enablers for most eHealth systems are the electronic patient records and Internet based technologies. Electronic patient records make it possible to share medical information between the care providers across the health strategies and medical disciplines and facilitate consultation between care providers on a given patient. The electronic patient records also give possibilities for further networked applications such as electronic prescribing and integrated regional health information networks (Ruotsalainen et al., 2003). However, current electronic patient records still lack a uniform infrastructure for data exchange and systems are heterogeneous and lack agreed and shared vocabularies (Safran & Goldberg, 2000). This restricts sharing of information. Today many eHealth systems are building more and more on eCommerce and eGovernment strategies and experiences on how to use Internet technologies to redesign operation of public services.

eHealth Systems use by Citizens and Health Professionals

The use of the Internet by citizens and also by health professionals is increasing worldwide (Gruen, 1999; Fallis & Fricke, 2002; Budtz & Witt, 2002; Silber, 2003; Rodrigues & Risk 2003; Wilson et al., 2004; Holliday & Tam, 2004). Internet is used to access health related information by ill-people but also by healthy people who look for advice on healthy lifestyles, diets, habits and health related products (Jones et al., 2001). Accessing health information is one of the commonest reasons for going to Internet; from 50% to 75% of the Internet users have used it to search for health related information (Powell & Clarke, 2002). In 2003 approximately 62% of American Internet users searched the Internet for health related information (Spink et al., 2004). In some cases citizens do not use tailored health-related websites but general Internet search engines to access health information. In 2003 40% of Europeans used Internet to access health care services and information (Wilson et al., 2004). A Danish study showed (Budtz & Witt, 2002) that of 93 patients in a study 20% had used the Internet to get health information. In another study Larner (2002) followed patients for six months period and found that more than 50% of them had Internet access, and 82% of them were interested in accessing websites with relevant medical information. People using the Internet for health information report that they value the convenience, anonymity and volume of online information (Powell & Clarke, 2002). The patients who search for specific information on their diseases, diagnoses and treatments report that it is beneficial to have information, advice and social support from the Internet (Potts & Wyatt, 2002).

In 2002 on average 78% of European general practitioners were online (e-Health, 2004) and 48% of them used electronic patient record systems and to some extent also other information systems to receive laboratory results and to transfer patient data to other health care organisations. Even 36% of general practitioners used telemedicine systems to home monitoring via Internet or email (Wilson et al., 2004).

When analysing the use of eHealth services and health information sources through the Internet the key findings are that the citizens want to have more information and they want better information (Wilson et al., 2004). The use of the Internet for health purposes is rising and the citizens would like to have guidance from the health professionals regarding quality websites (Silber, 2003). The major reason for the citizens to use Internet information resources is to know more, to be able to ask more precise questions from the health professionals and to understand better health and well-being. Internet health resources support citizens to become better informed and knowledgeable and through this they also may take more responsibility of their health and well-being.

However, the Internet and other new technologies will interfere with the communication between health professionals, and between them and the patient. Impacts of the Internet use do not only come from the communication but from the operational availability of information resources. In an Asian study (Holliday & Tam, 2004) more than 90% of patients had expressed their wish to communicate with their physician via email, but physicians were reluctant to do so. Physicians explained that the physician-patient confidentiality, time concerns and increased exposure for malpractice were the major reasons for their reluctance. Physicians are somewhat opposing the use of Internet especially when it interferes with their decision making activity (Gerber & Eiser, 2001; Kleiner et al., 2002). There seems to be two reasons: A question of power and a question of danger. A question of power implies that physicians want to keep the control on the medical activities, and the question of danger implies that they want to keep control on actions and decisions that are on their responsibility. Some physicians

even fear that they become technical executors of decisions taken by third parties, e.g. the Internet information sources.

Expected Benefits by eHealth Systems

Many studies (Alvarez, 2002; Ruotsalainen et al., 2003; Iliakovidis et al., 2004) identify the promises of eHealth to be in the manner and degree to which eHealth can build on the advances in ICT to support the development of the health care infrastructure. Health care services are expected to be better accessible and data available any place and any time independent on where data is stored or created.

Health care professionals expect that eHealth systems have remarkable impacts on health care routines and practices (Grimson et al., 2000; Eng 2001; Ruotsalainen et al., 2003; Wilson et al., 2004). Reliable and accurate information would be available easily and rapidly at the time and place where it would be needed. It would be possible to view information on the prior history of the patient and on diagnostic investigations to avoid redundant testing. Communication between the healthcare providers would be independent of their physical location and this results in time savings and increased accuracy of diagnosis and effectiveness of care. Health professionals would be able to update their knowledge and expertise though online training sessions and they would be able to consult international colleagues in dealing with particularly complex cases (Ruotsalainen et al., 2003).

Patients and citizens would benefit through better quality health information and services available to them (Silber, 2003; Ruotsalainen et al., 2003; Wilson et al., 2004). The possibility for home monitoring and treatment or follow-up would reduce the need for hospitalisation or travel in order to receive professional care. Patients would regulate with the consent the provision of their data to various healthcare providers. The possibility to control one's own health data would facilitate and increase the mobility of citizens and patients, particularly those suffering of chronic conditions.

eHealth systems are expected to harmonise healthcare systems thus enabling provision of seamless and continuous care (Grimson et al., 2000; Ruotsalainen et al., 2003; Wilson et al., 2004). Inter-organisational cooperation would allow sharing of data and information whenever necessary. eHealth systems are also expected to result in improved quality and cost-effectiveness of healthcare systems. The fact that healthcare processes would be better documented and thus accountable, would provide more possibilities for evaluation and quality assessment, and information could be made available to support decision making and interventions at the public health level.

Eysenbach (2001) lists the 10 e's for eHealth systems: improved efficiency in health care and decrease of costs, enhanced quality of care e.g. by comparisons of care providers, evidence-based in the sense that the effectiveness and efficiency of interventions are proved by scientific evaluations, empowerment of consumers and patients, encouragement of a new relationship between the patient and the physician, education of physicians through online resources, enabling information exchange and communication, extending the scope of health, ethics as new forms of patient-physician interaction become possible and equity to have health care more accessible to all. There is at the same time a threat that those people who do not have money, skills, computers and Internet connections cannot access eHealth services.

Despite of the availability of eHealth systems and their potential benefits eHealth systems are not yet widely used in health care practices (e-Health, 2004). Iliakovidis et al. (2004) report some example eHealth systems which are now entering the European market. However, many promises of eHealth research and development have not been fulfilled yet (Ruotsalainen et al.,

2003). The major barriers (e-Health, 2004) include among other lack of commitment by health care authorities, missing interoperability of health information systems which is mostly due to lacking conceptual models, ontologies and sharable vocabularies. Additionally, the eHealth developments by far have been rather technology-oriented and thus the developed systems are not easy to use, technology is expensive and the systems are vulnerable to changes in the environment. Maybe the most important reason for failures is that the socio-technical nature of eHealth systems have not been fully considered. Development of eHealth systems requires thorough understanding of the health care work practices where systems are to be installed. The needs of the users and the contextual aspects of the systems use should be the starting point for the development (Berg, 1999; Nykänen & Karimaa, 2004).

eHEALTH VISIONS FOR THE FUTURE

The challenges for eHealth are technical, social, economic and political. Eng (2001) pointed out that there is need for strong leadership from health policy makers and need for practical solutions for interoperable systems that are secure, respect confidentiality and promote the best possible access to health care for all citizens.

In our survey (Ruotsalainen et al., 2003) several of the respondents looked for a comprehensive e-enabled healthcare system, standardised and interoperable which meets the necessary legal and functional requirements for optimal, seamless, cross-border delivery of services. Implementation of such a system is expected to lead to more equal, accessible, holistic and human-centred healthcare.

In the future we suppose that several Internet-related and other trends will have influence on the design, content, functionality, dissemination and use of future eHealth systems. With the globalisation increasing number of eHealth resources will be developed overseas and for global audience (Eng, 2001). Thus standardisation and cross-cultural factors will become increasingly important.

The digital generation will most likely demand immediate access to information and will rely on online resources to inform health and other decisions (Eng, 2001). Wireless technologies may contribute to the growth of mobile eHealth applications for both providers and consumers. Digital television may serve in the future as a cheap and easy platform to offer eHealth systems and information for large audiences. Personalisation and tailoring of applications to specific users will put emphasis on privacy and data security issues.

There are many important questions still open with eHealth systems: Ethical and legal issues? Who will pay for the use? Who has access to eHealth systems? What are the standards, guidelines and good practices for development and use of these systems and technologies?

The basic requirements for the future eHealth applications can be derived from the current health informatics and eHealth situation. First; eHealth applications should serve the users needs, the needs of citizens, patients, health care professionals and health care organisations. Second; the applied technology should be user acceptable, cheap and not too cumbersome to use and vulnerable to changes. Third; eHealth applications should be based on the health care information systems infrastructure, they should be integrated with the environment and preferably also be interoperable. Fourth; standards should be applied on design and development and fifth; security and safety issues have to be solved within the practice and legal frameworks. And sixth, all eHealth systems and applications should be evaluated to assess the effects and impacts and to find reasons for success or failure.

REFERENCES

Alvarez RC (2002), The promise of e-health - a Canadian perspective. eHealth International 1(4), 1-8.

Berg M (1999), Patient care information systems and health care work: A socio-technical approach. Int J Medical Informatics 55, 87-101

Budtz S & Witt K (2002), Consulting the Internet before visit to general practice. Patients' use of the Internet and other sources of health information. Scan J Primary Health Care 20(3), 174-176.

e-Health - making healthcare better for European citizens: An action plan for a European e-Health area (2004), Commission of the European Communities. COM (2004) 356, Brussels.

Eng, T.R (2001), The eHealth Landscape: A Terrain Map of Emerging Information and Communication Technologies in Health and Health Care. Princeton, New Jersey, The Robert Wood Johnson Foundation, USA.

Eysenbach G (2001), What is e-health? Editorial. J Med Internet Res 1(2), e20.

Fallis D & Fricke M (2002), Indicators of accuracy of consumer health information on the Internet: a study of indicators relating to information for managing fever in children at home. JAMIA 9(1), 73-79.

Gerber BS & Eiser AR (2001), The patient-physician relationship in the Internet age: Future prospects and the research agenda. J Med Internet Res 3(2), e15.

Grimson J, Grimson W, Flahive M, Foley C, O'Moore R, Nolan J & Chadwick GA (2000), Multimedia approach to raising awareness of information and communications technology amongst health care professionals. Int J Medical Informatics 58-59, 297-305.

Gruen J (1999), The Physician and the Internet: Observer or participant? MD Comput 16(6), 46-48.

Haglund H (2002), The significance of welfare services and their electronic applications for the business activities in the future. Presentation given in the eHealth - Tomorrow's eHealth services, Tampere, November 2002, www.etampere.fi, Feb 11, 2003

Holliday I & Tam W (2004), eHealth in the East Asian tigers. Int J Medical Informatics (article in press).

Jones R, Balfour F, Gillies M, Stobo D, Cawsey AJ & Donaldson K (2001), The accessibility of computer-based health information for patients: Kiosks and the Web. Medical Information 10, 1469-73.

Iliakovidis I, Wilson P & Healy JC (2004), eHealth. Current situation and examples of implemented and beneficial e-health applications. IOS Press, Studies in Health Technology and Informatics, Amsterdam, The Netherlands.

Kleiner KD, Akers R, Burke BL & Werner EJ (2002), Parent and physician attitudes regarding electronic communication in pediatric practices. Pediatrics 109 (5), 740-744 Larner AJ (2002), Use of the Internet medical websites and NHS Direct by neurology outpatients before consultation. Int J Clin Pract 56(3), 219-221.

Nykänen P & Karimaa E (2004), Success and failure factors during development of a regional health information system - results from a constructive evaluation study. Submitted for Methods of Information in Medicine.

Potts HWW & Wyatt JC (2002), Survey of doctors' experience of patients using the Internet. J Med Internet Res 4(1), e5.

Powell J & Clarke A (2002), The WWW of the World Wide Web: Who, what and why. J Med Internet Res 18, 4(1), e4.

Rodrigues RJ & Risk A (2003), eHealth in Latin America and the Caribbean: Development and policy issues. J Med Internet Res, 5(1), e4.

Ruotsalainen P, Nykänen P, Doupi P, Cheshire P, Pohjonen H, Kinnunen J, Keskisaari-Kajaste L, Hirvonen-Kari M, Moisio I & Tripovsky T (2003), The state of eHealth in Europe. Report D1 of the MEDITRAV-project, EU IST 1999-11490, Stakes, Helsinki.

Safran C & Goldberg H (2000), Electronic patient records and the impact of the Internet. Int J Medical Informatics 60, 77-83.

Silber D (2003), The case for ehealth. European Commission, Information Society, eHealth Conference 2003, Atlanta, Belgium.

Spink A, Yang Y, Jansen J, Nykänen P, Lorence D, Ozmutlu S & Ozmutlu HC (2004), A study of medical and health queries to web search engines. Health Information and Libraries Journal 21, 44-51

Wilson P (2002), How to find the good and avoid the bad or ugly: a short guide to tools for rating quality and health information on the Internet. BMJ 9 (324), 598-602

Wilson P, Leitner C & Moussalli A (2004), Mapping the potential of eHealth. Empowering the citizen through eHealth tools and services. eHealth Conference 2004. European Institute for Public Administration. Maastricht, The Netherlands.

This work was previously published in E-Health Systems Diffusion and Use: The Innovation, the User and the USE IT Model, edited by T. Spil and R. Schuring, pp. 281-293, copyright 2006 by IGI Publishing, formerly known as Idea Group Publishing (an imprint of IGI Global).

Chapter XX
The Competitive Forces Facing E–Health

Nilmini Wickramasinghe
Stuart Graduate School of Business, USA

Santosh Misra
Cleveland State University, USA

Arnold Jenkins
Johns Hopkins Hospital, USA

Douglas R. Vogel
City University of Hong Kong, China

ABSTRACT

Superior access, quality and value of healthcare services has become a national priority for healthcare to combat the exponentially increasing costs of healthcare expenditure. E-Health in its many forms and possibilities appears to offer a panacea for facilitating the necessary transformation for healthcare. While a plethora of e-health initiatives keep mushrooming both nationally and globally, there exists to date no unified system to evaluate these respective initiatives and assess their relative strengths and deficiencies in realizing superior access, quality and value of healthcare services. Our research serves to address this void. This is done by focusing on the following three key components: 1) understanding the web of players (regulators, payers, providers, healthcare organizations, suppliers and last but not least patients) and how e-health can modify the interactions between these players as well as create added value healthcare services. 2) understand the competitive forces facing e-health organizations and the role of the Internet in modifying these forces, and 3) from analyzing the web of players combined with the competitive forces for e-health organizations we develop a framework that serves to identify the key forces facing an e-health and suggestions of how such an organization can structure itself to be e-health prepared.

INTRODUCTION

E-health is a broad term that encompasses many different activities related to the use of the Internet for the delivery of healthcare service. Healthcare professionals are extending the use of the Internet to include a source of evidence-based consumer information as well as to facilitate the research of protocols for healthcare delivery, accessing laboratory and medical records, and performing second opinion consults (Sharma and Wickramasinghe, 2004; Sharma et al., 2006). Moreover, the Internet is being used by patients to become more knowledgeable about health practices as seen from their questions to their physicians (Gargeya and Sorrell, 2004).

Although, a relatively new term and unheard of prior to 1999, e-health has now become the latest "e-buzzword," used to characterize not only "Internet medicine", but also virtually everything related to computers and medicine (Sharma et al, 2006; von Lubitz and Wickramasinghe, 2006). The scope and boundary of e-health, as well as e-heath organizations, is still evolving. However one can only imagine it will grow rapidly especially given that governments in both US and Europe, and organizations such as WHO (World Healthcare Organization) are advocating that e-health be on the top of all healthcare agendas and an integral component of any healthcare delivery initiative (von Lubitz and Wickramasinghe, 2006).

Given the growth and variety of e-health initiatives, it becomes important to examine the forces affecting these initiatives and factors leading to the success of e-health. To date, little research examines metrics of measurement pertaining to e-health initiatives or their economic value. What are the forces of competition affecting e-heath? Are the competitive forces constrained by external considerations? Is the issue of competition an appropriate concern for e-health? If so, what are the strong and weak competitive forces? We argue that analysis of these forces would lead us

to understand the long-term sustainability of any e-health initiative.

TRADITIONAL COMPETITIVE FORCES

The starting point for understanding the competitive forces facing any e-health initiative lies in understanding the fundamentals of traditional competitive forces that impact all industries and then how the Internet as a disruptive technology has impacted these forces.

The strategy of an organization has two major components (Henderson and Venkatraman, 1993). These are 1) formulation – making decisions regarding the mission, goals and objectives of the organization and 2) implementation – making decisions regarding how the organization can structure itself to realize its goal and carryout specific activites. For today's healthcare organizations the goals, mission and objectives all focus around access, quality and value and realizing this value proposition for healthcare then becomes the key (Wickramasinghe, N. et al, 2004). Essentially, the goal of strategic management is to find a "fit" between the organization and its environment that maximizes its performance (Hofer, 1975). This then describes the Market-based view of the firm and has been predominantly developed and pushed by the frameworks of Michael Porter. The first of Porter's famous frameworks is the generic strategies (Porter, 1980).

The use of technology must always enable or enhance the businesses objectives and strategies of the organization. This is particularly true for 21st Century organizations where many of their key operations and functions are so heavily reliant on technology and the demand for information and knowledge is so critical. A firms' relative competitive position i.e., its ability to perform above or below the industry average is determined by its competitive advantage. Porter (1980) identified 3

Figure 1. Porter's Competitive (Five) Forces Model

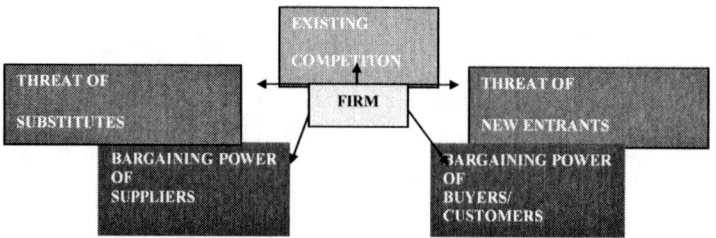

generic strategies that impact a firm's competitive advantage. These include cost, focus and differentiation. Furthermore, Porter himself notes that two and only two basic forms of competitive advantage typically exist:

1. cost leadership
2. differentiation

Firms can use these two forms of competitive advantage to either compete across a broad scope of an industry or to focus on competing in specific niches; thereby, leading to three generic strategies. Porter (ibid) notes that firms should be cautious about pursuing more than one generic strategy; namely cost, differentiation and focus. For example, if a cost leadership strategy is adopted it is unlikely that a firm can also maintain and sustain differentiation since it would not be possible to simultaneously pursue the costly capital investment or maintain high operating costs required for differentiation and thus in the long run the firm has a confused strategy which leads to failure.

In order to design and develop ones strategy an organization should first perform an industry analysis. Porters Five Forces or Competitive Forces model is most useful (Porter, 1980, 1985). Figure 1 depicts this model. Essentially, Porter has taken concepts from micro-economics and modeled them in terms of five key forces that together outline the rules of competition and at-

tractiveness of the industry.

The forces are as follows:

1. threat of new entrant: a company new to the industry that could take away market share from the incumbent firms
2. threat of substitute: an alternative means that could take market share from product/service offered by the firms in the industry
3. bargaining power of buyers: the strength of buyers or groups of buyers within the industry relative to the firms
4. bargaining power of suppliers: the strength of suppliers relative to the firms in the industry
5. rivalry of existing competition: relative position and market share of major competitors

The collective strength of these five forces determines the attractiveness of the industry and thus the potential for superior financial performance by influencing prices, costs, and the level of capital investment required (Porter, 1985). Once a thorough industry analysis has occurred it is generally easier for a firm to determine which generic strategy makes most sense for it to pursue and enables the firm to exploit most of its core competencies in its existing environment.

Table 1. The three e-opportunity domains and their components

	Components
e-operations	• Automation of administrative processes • Supply-chain reconfiguration • Reengineering of primary infrastructure • Intensive competitive procurement • Increased parenting value
e-marketing	• Enhanced selling process • Enhance customer usage experience • Enhanced customer buying experience
e-services	• Understanding of customer needs • Provision of customer service • Knowledge of all relevant providers • Negotiation of customer requirements • Construction of customer options

Table 2. The e-opportunities for healthcare organizations

	Components
e-operations	• Internet-based supply purchasing • Prescription writing, formulary checking, and interaction checking using hand-held devices
e-marketing	• Delivery of consumer health content and wellness management tools over the Internet • Use of consumer health profiles to suggest disease management and wellness programs
e-services	• Patient-provider communication and transaction applications • Web-based applications to support the clinical conversation between referring and consulting physicians
Crossing multiple domains	• Increasing the level of information content in the product • Increasing the information intensity along the supply chain • Increase in the dispersion of information

ROLE OF THE INTERNET OF THE COMPETITIVE FORCES

Feeny (2001) presents a framework that highlights the strategic opportunities afforded to organizations by using the Internet. In particular he highlights three e-opportunity domains. Table 1 details these domain and their respective components.

E-OPPORTUNITIES IN HEALTHCARE

Given the three areas of e-opportunities discussed above, Glaser (2002) identifies several key e-opportunities for healthcare. Table 2 details these.

WEB OF PLAYERS IN HEALTHCARE

Figure 2 depicts the web of healthcare players and the key elements of the any e-health architecture that serves to support the interactions between and within this web of players. In order to fully capture the flows of information it is necessary to first identify the primary producers and consumers of data and information within the healthcare system. At the center of the information flows is the HCIS (healthcare information system); i.e. the e-health network because not only does it connect the key players within the healthcare system in an efficient and effective manner but also it forms the central repository for key information such as patient medical records, billing, and treatment details. Hence the HCIS provides the foundation for supporting the information flows and decision making throughout the healthcare system. Figure 2 then represents a macro view of the inter-relationships between the key players within this system as well as the sources, destinations and flows of information between these players and the pivotal role of the HCIS.

Healthcare procedures such as medical diagnostics, treatment decisions and consequent effecting of these decisions, prevention, communication and equipment usage can be thought of as iatric in nature (Perper, 1994). Integral to these iatric procedures is the generating and processing of information (Mandke et al. 2003). The patient naturally provides key information at the time of a clinical visit or other interaction with his/her provider. Such a visit also generates other information including insurance information, medical history, and treatment protocols (if applicable) which must satisfy regulatory requirements, payer directives and, obviously, the healthcare organization's informational needs. Thus, we see that from a single intervention many forms and types of information are captured, generated and then disseminated throughout the healthcare system. All this information and its flows must satisfy some common integrity characteristics such as accuracy, consistency,

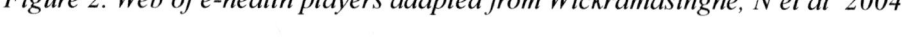

Figure 2. Web of e-health players adapted from Wickramasinghe, N et al 2004

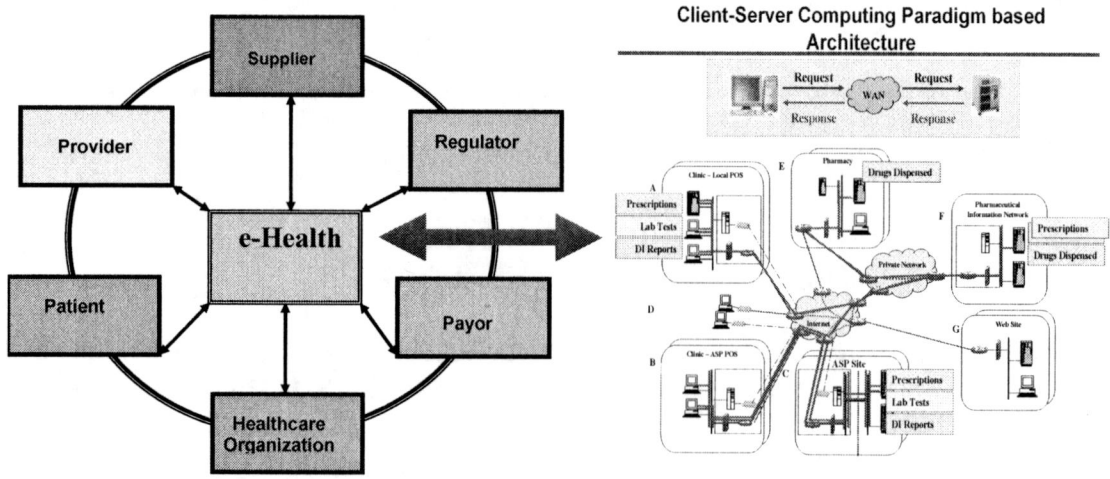

reliability, completeness, usefulness, usability and manipulability. Consequently, generating a level of trust and confidence in the information's content and processes. Since the information flows across various organizational boundaries, the challenge of ensuring information integrity is further compounded because any integrity problems will propagate with ripple effects following the same trajectory as the information itself. Given the high degree of inter-relatedness between the various players, the consequences of poor quality information (such as the cost of information integrity problems) are multiplied and far reaching. This highlights the need for robust, well designed and well managed HCIS (Applegate et al., 1986). Such a perspective should not be limited to new systems, but rather, equally and perhaps of even more importance, should be applied to existing systems as well.

MODELING THE COMPETITIVE FORCES IN E-HEALTH

In order to model e-health let us first construct a general model of the competitive forces pertaining to e-business. E-business is not simply offering traditional products and services on line. It requires broad-scale asset redeployment and process changes, which ultimately serve as the basis for a company's competitive advantage in today's Digital Economy (Rappa, 2000). For this study, the e-business model could be broken into components such as; products and services, customer value, pricing component, revenue source, the cost component and asset model as shown in figure 3.

The prime objective of business model is to make money (La Monica, 2000). The various components of business model as shown in figure 1 work together to create profit margins for the business. First of all, the electronic business model should offer products and services online.

Figure 3. Generic e-business model components

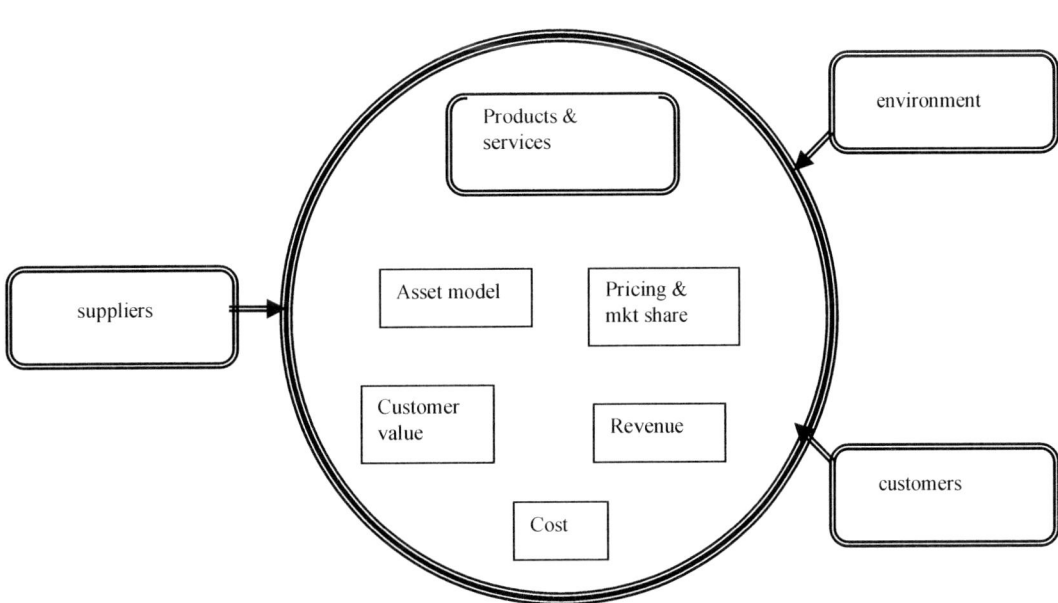

These products and services should be differentiated with competitors by low price or unique customer value. The products are differentiated if customers perceive some value in these that other products do not have. Differentiation can be done by offering different product features, timing, location, service, product mix, linkage between functions etc. (Afuah and Tucci, 2000). Customer value can be judged whether firm offering its customers something distinctive or at a lower cost than its competitors. The success of business model depends upon how does the firm price the value? An important part of profiting from the value that firms offer customers is to price it properly. For pricing, market shares and margins would be most critical. The good business model should strive for high market share and thus firm should devise strategies accordingly. Pricing of products depends upon the cost and asset model of the firm. The cost (fixed cost + variable cost) should be spread in a fashion that profit margins

remain high. The profits in electronic business model case will not only come from sales but may come from many other sources. Therefore, revenue source is another important component for business model. The sustainability of business model can be gauged based upon non-imitable nature of products and services. How can firm continue improve market share and make more money and have competitive advantage are the kind of questions needs to answers for the sustainability of business model. For example; using simple profits equation; Profits=(P-Vc)Q-Fc, firm can assess how each of the components of business model impact profitability. If a firm offers distinctive products, it can charge premium price P for it. A good business model should keep low variable cost but should have high market share for higher profitability (Afuah and Tucci, 2000). Taking these components of a business model into consideration, let us now map this to the healthcare domain (figure 4).

Figure 4. E-health business model components

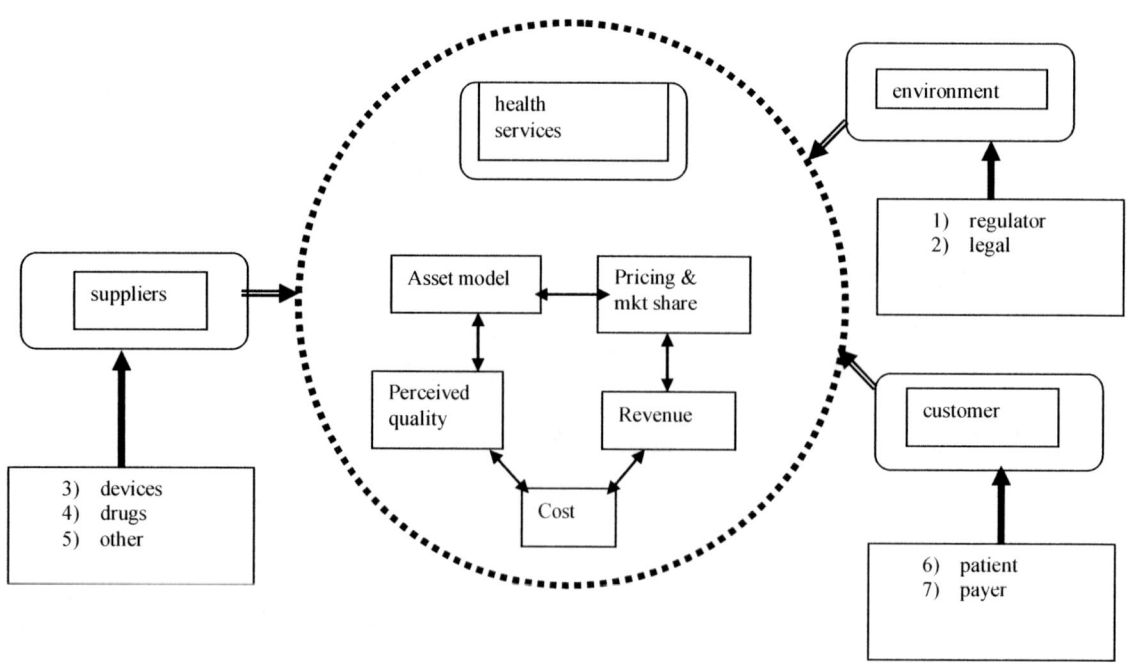

In so doing, some of the nuances pertaining to the dynamics of healthcare become apparent; such as, the receiver of services, or the patient, is not usually the principal payer. Moreover, the model serves to underscore that for e-health initiatives to truly add value and be sustainable the dynamics of a generic e-business model must be satisfied. Hence, some determination needs to be made regarding Vc, Fc, P and Q in this context.

To understand these dynamics more easily let us consider a case study example of the implementation of an electronic patient record.

Case Study

The Johns Hopkins Medicine Center for Information Services Public LAN (JPL) is a computer network designed to provide patient care providers access to clinical applications. This computer network is utilized by all types of patient care providers in both inpatient and out patient services. These providers include, but not limited to, doctors, interns, fellows, nurses, unit clerks, pharmacists, nutritionists, and admission specialists. In this paper an examination of the history of the Public LAN, the current state of the LAN, and the future of the Public LAN will be examined. Since its inception the Public LAN as been the leader in efficiency and innovation for Desktop Computing Services (DCS), a division of Information Technology @ Johns Hopkins (IT@Hopkins).

Introduction of the Public LAN

During the spring of 1996 JHMCIS and a group of doctors developed an in-house application to provide patient care. This application is called Electronic Patient Record or EPR. The application was to be used in patient areas for tracking patient record. These records can then be viewed by other clinicians throughout the hospital. A second application was introduced at the same time

to provide a graphical user interface to many of the hospital's mainframe and mid-range systems. This application is Host Interface Program or HIP. The challenge at this stage was to provide a computer system that could be used by the doctors that would allow EPR and HIP to be used to provide patient care and at the same time have a desktop system that was secure.

These desktops were to be deployed in medical exam rooms and the major problem was having a desktop that could provide these applications to the clinicians without allowing the clinicians or patients the ability to access the operating system and the computer configuration. This led to the development of the Public Desktop.

The Public desktop is a Microsoft Windows based desktop that has the clinical applications installed, as well as an Internet browser and the Microsoft Office suite. The challenge was managing these systems in areas with limited access during business hours as they were in use by clinicians providing patient care. The operating system was secured and limited access was given to the users. The users were not able to install any applications or download any programs.

The Public LAN started out will 70 desktops in three clinical areas. The Harriet Lane Clinic which is an outpatient clinic for pediatrics, the neonatal intensive care unit, and the adolescent outpatient clinic. This pilot lasted approximately six months. During the next three years the Public LAN grew to 1100 desktops.

The Growth of the Public LAN

Today the Public LAN supports over 1800 desktops and many clinical applications. During the first three years of the Public LAN the number of systems reached over 1100 systems. Included in this growth, not only the number of devices supported, but the number of applications that were supported on these desktops. The driving forces of these changes were outdated clinical applications that were being replaced with client server applications and the millennium with applications that were not year 2000 compliant.

During this time the application supported grew to include BDM, a new pharmacy application, Vision – a nutrition application and ClicTate, a pediatrics version of EPR. With the intention of more clinical applications moving from the mainframe and mid-range systems to client server applications the desktops are going to need to be able to handle these additional applications.

The process of managing these systems became a challenge as well. Since the desktops were standardized, DCS was able to implement Microsoft's System Management Server (SMS). This allowed not only the ability to manage these desktops, but also distribute software, inventory the hardware and software of a specific system, and provide remote control capabilities. SMS was included when the pilot of the Public LAN was deployed but its true value was not realized until the rapid growth of the LAN.

The Public LAN Today

The Public LAN today is well over 1800 desktops, supporting more than 30 clinical applications. Most of these applications are still accessed via HIP, however more client server applications are also supported. The additional client server applications have lead to different configurations of the desktop's application software or "flavors" of Public workstations. Currently there are currently many different configurations for the Public Workstations. These different configurations include:

- Standard configuration
- Training configuration
- Wilmer Eye Clinic configuration
- Pharmacy configuration
- Nutrition configuration
- Provider Order Entry configuration

- Operating room configuration
- DCOM image viewing configuration
- Eclypsis Point of Care configuration
- Procedure Reporting System configuration
- OB/GYN Configuration

These different configurations can be on a few as 20 desktops to as many as 600, where the standard configuration is on all of the desktops. The standard configuration is:

- Windows XP Professional
- EPR
- HIP
- Internet Explorer
- Microsoft Office Suite
- Adobe Reader
- Calculator

The additional configurations are based on adding additional clinical applications to the desktops. In addition, many of the systems have multiple clinical applications installed.

The Lessons Learned

During the growth of the Public LAN many lessons have been learned. These lessons include best practices for desktops management, application management and deployment, and reduction in the total cost of ownership of a desktop.

The current network is supported by three desktop technicians, which is an average of 600 plus desktops per technician. Desktop Computing Services needed to have a way to manage these systems not only located at the East Baltimore campus, but at other campuses within the Baltimore metropolitan area. The use of Microsoft Systems Management Software (SMS) was deployed to allow desktop management. SMS allows a technician the ability to remote control in to a desktop and perform work as if they were at the desktop. This capability also allows the support staff to view the process of the user and see the error as it happened. SMS also is used to deploy application software to the desktop.

Due to the increased number of clinical applications the number of different application software configurations increased. In order to manage this DCS used SMS for application deployment. DCS is able to determine the application software installed on the desktop and perform upgrades to the software. The upgrade to an application is preformed by using SMS to "push" and install the software on the desktop without any user intervention. Therefore, and application could be upgraded or installed without having to visit the desktop.

With the integration of SMS to manage the desktops this has reduced the total cost of ownership of supporting the Public LAN. This decrease is realized by having a ratio of one desktop technician per 600 desktops. DCS is able to remote control the desktop, this prevents the technician from have in walk across campus to help a user. In addition, the installation of applications and upgrades to applications is completed on many systems at once without having to visit each individual desktop. Also, DCS has secured the desktop to prevent the users from accessing the operating system and the hard drive. If the users were able to access the operating system and download and install applications, including spyware, this would greatly increase the support costs of the desktop.

The Future of the Public LAN

The future of the Public LAN at Johns Hopkins Hospital is ever evolving. The needs of the clinicians for resources to provide patient care are continually changing. With patients bringing medical records in on CD-ROM to access to network resources the Public LAN must evolve to meet these needs. In order to meet these needs the Public LAN support staff is required

to find clever and innovative ways to provide these resources. New hardware is being added to the Public desktops to allow viewing of clinical data on CD-ROM, the use of USB keys for file storage has been enabled and logging in with a personal account.

The ability for a clinician to login with their personal account allows them to access network resources. These resources include access to network file servers and departmental file servers. In order for a clinician to use a personal account they are required to have a timeout of their session. The timeout of the session will log the user off after a certain amount of idle time. The reason for this is to prevent others from accessing information and to prevent non Johns Hopkins employees to access data and network resources.

The future of the Public LAN is ever evolving. The Johns Hopkins Hospital is building two new clinical towers that will be state of the art. The devices that provide patient care will also need to be state of the art and provide clinicians the ability to provide patient care in a completely paperless, film-less, and wireless network. The Public LAN will be able to provide these solutions and will realize the benefits of these efforts as patients are cared for more efficiently and effectively.

Mapping the Case to the Model

The implementation of the EPR at Johns' Hopkins, represents a relatively common e-health initiative in the current healthcare environment. The EPR enables the seamless flow of patient data and thus facilitates the delivery of efficient and effective quality healthcare to the patient. This is certainly professed as a key benefit for the embracing of EPR in most instances.

The e-health sustainability model however, suggests that one must analyze the micro- and meso-dynamics more closely to actually determine the sustainability of such an initiative. Specifically, it is necessary to capture key factors including, perceived quality, fixed and variable costs, price and market share and quantity and then look at the interaction of these factors before sustainability of the initiative can be pronounced. However this is beyond the scope of this paper but will form the focus of future research.

What can be noted at this point and will be research in more detail in future work is the size or scale of the e-health initiative. Returning to the simple profit equation Profits=(P-Vc)Q-Fc, in the case scenario above fixed costs will be constant and Vc for any EPR will be marginal given the generic nature of the program and the applications of it by various providers hence we hypothesis that the sustainability of the EPR would increase with Q the quantity or size. Thus, the larger the EPR initiative the more likely it is to be sustainable. Quantitative data to support the relationship between scope and quantity and impact of ICTs in general in healthcare settings can be found in previous studies (Wickramasinghe and Silvers, 2003; Wickramasinghe and Lamb, 2002).

DISCUSSION

In mapping the John's Hopkins case to the model in figure 4 we can see that the reality of an e-health initiative involves the interactions of various groups of stakeholders. Knowledge management provides an umbrella under which we may discuss a number of opportunities and raise issues relative to components of the business model. The vision of collaboration between components of the business model recognized as stakeholders is one of great opportunity. Stakeholders in this case include suppliers, the firm, the customer and the government as a key representative of the environment. Each stakeholder brings to the table talent, resources and differentiated perspectives that, together, create a robust whole in addressing problems and projects. For example, suppliers can be a source of knowledge that can assist the firm

in delivering cost effective products and services. Customers are an additional source of knowledge in terms of personal history and preferences. The firm can manage knowledge in a form that maximizes the probability of value added products and services. The government can serve as a catalyst to create an environment conducive to knowledge exchange and management.

Unfortunately, great opportunities do not always turn into reality. Collaboration successes between suppliers, the firm and its customers much less the government can, sadly, be few and far between. In addition to strengths and distinctions, each stakeholder also brings to the table residual weaknesses and biases that can scuttle the best of collaborative intentions. For example, internal firm bureaucracy can easily drive out the best of suppler intentions and customer good will. Problems can easily be left unaddressed and efforts can easily fail as reality drives out vision. This can be exacerbated by cultural norms and historical behaviors embedded in government policies.

A case in point is the handling of SARS. Levels of suffering and unnecessary deaths were, in part, a result of lack of collaboration between stakeholders. In this case, government agencies (specifically the hospital authorities) were negligent in sharing information and allocating resources amongst hospitals. The hospitals, however, were not guilt free and were accused of withholding information to customers including patients and their families. Further, the relationship between suppliers and hospitals was insufficient to respond to the need for supplies. Shortages were evident and supplies misapplied in circumstances that could have been adverted through collaboration. The situation was further strained as lack of information sharing across governments and excessive bureaucratic delay inhibited quick action to rapidly respond to changing circumstances. In summary, stakeholder collaboration could have, arguably, avoided hardship at individual and societal levels. Unfortunately, it didn't happen and the World Health Organization (WHO) was, rightly, exasperated.

Experiences with SARS have sensitized stakeholders at all levels with respect to effectively dealing with potential pandemics e.g., H5N1-based bird flu. Over the past months, we have already seen a much higher level of information exchange and collaboration than existed in the lead-up to SARS. Governments have more readily shared information and established channels for dealing with global adversity. Hospitals have begun preparations including emergency response practice. Suppliers have opened historically propriety processes and licenses to enable extended manufacturing capability e.g., Roche with Tamiflu, as but one example. Customers have sought (and obtained) information relative to prevention and preparation for a variety of circumstances as well as acted as a source of information back to appropriate authorities regarding infectious incidences, e.g., bird flock deaths. Numerous conferences with multiple stakeholders present have provided forums for knowledge sharing, enhanced understanding leading towards the creation of action plans. In short, bird flu threats have galvanized stakeholders in a way that was unseen in the handling of SARS, in part, as a result of witnessing and experiencing hardship.

Knowledge management provides a focus that can enhance the probability of success in encouraging and sustaining broad-based stakeholder collaboration. Formalized knowledge management promotes the ultimate desire for the benefits of stakeholder collaboration to be sufficiently well developed and supported to offset inherent weaknesses. Knowledge management plays a key role in assuring that aspects of information creation, sharing and dissemination compatible with multiple stakeholder objectives can be successfully achieved (Alavi and Leidner, 2001). Problems are often beyond the scope of any particular stakeholder which encourages

cooperation in order for success to be attained (Van de Ven, 2000).

The concept of suppler, firm, customer and government collaboration is sound but operationalization is difficult and fraught with problems. This doesn't suggest that the concept should be abandoned, just managed and supported. Sadly, this situation is not unique (Lyytinen and Rose, 2003). The missing element is often cooperative knowledge creation and exchange. Each element of the collaboration needs a better understanding and focus on cooperation. Unfortunately this doesn't naturally exist and easily turns antagonistic. Cooperation is difficult to achieve even when linkages are in place. It is far too easy to say that "details can be worked out." Unfortunately, the "devil" is in the detail. Towards that end, stakeholder collaboration in achieving knowledge management objectives is paramount.

CONCLUSION

The underlying goal for healthcare is to provide cost effective quality treatment, i.e., realize its value proposition in this challenging environment. In order to do this healthcare needs to maximize its information management techniques and make prudent use of ICTs (Information Communication Technologies). In such a context e-health initiatives willl clearly play a dominant role in healthcare delivery. This has been underscored by leaders of US and the EU as well as leading bodies such as the World Healthcare Organization (WHO) that focus on global healthcare issues and policy. Moreover, Both European and US authorities define their initiatives primarily in terms of medical information technology centering on computerized patient record [CPR] or, in more acceptable parlance, the HER electronic health record as referred to by WHO. Hence e-health is here to stay. What becomes critical then is the sustainability of these e-health initiatives and their ability to bring benefits to the key actor in healthcare, the patient.

This paper has set out to delve into the abyss of e-health sustainability. A logical starting place to us seemed to identify the primary drivers in a generic e-business model and then map them into healthcare. Our e-health sustainability model then serves to identify the critical factors and important dynamics faced by any e-health initiative. In addition, we identified the importance of scale and scope economies in this process through the mapping of case study data. Finally we noted that it is necessary to incorporate the techniques and strategies of knowledge management if superior collaboration between the multiple stakeholders is to ensue. Through the example of SARS we underscored how important this aspect is not only to the sustainability of e-health but in order to realize effective healthcare delivery. Clearly this is only the beginning and we now need further investigation and research which we plan to embark upon. We close by encouraging other researchers to also delve deeper into this imperative healthcare research area.

REFERENCES

Afuah, A., and Tucci, C. L. (2000). Internet Business Models and Strategies – Text and Cases McGraw Hill Irwin.

Alavi, M. A., and Leidner, D. E. (2001). Review: Knowledge Management and Knowledge Management Systems: Conceptual Foundations and Research Issues. MIS Quarterly, 25(1), 107-136.

Feeny, D. 2001 "Making Business Sense of the e-opportunity" MIT Sloan Management Review, Winter vol. 42, no. 2 p. 42.

Gargeya, V and D. Sorrell 2004 "Moving toward an e-hospital" pp.50-64 in Wickramasinghe, N., J. Gupta and S. Sharma Eds Creating Knowledge-Based Healthcare Organizations with IdeanGroup Publishers, Hershey.

Glaser, J. 2002 The Strategic Application of Information Technology in Health Care Organizations 2nd Ed. Jossey Bass, San Francisco.

Hendersen, J and N. Venktraman 1992 "Strategic Alignment: A model for organizational transformation through information technology," in T. Kochan & M. Unseem, eds, Transforming Organisations, Oxford University Press, NY,

Hofer, C 1975 "Toward a Contingency Theory of Business Strategy" Academy of Management, vol 18, no.4 pp.784-810.

La Monica, M. (October 2000). "Building trust into e-business models," InfoWorld, 22(28): 3.

Lyytinen, K., and Rose, G. M. (2003). The Disruptive Nature of Information Technology Innovations: The Case of Internet Computing in Systems Development Organizations. MIS Quarterly, 27(4), 557-595.

Porter, M and E. Teisberg 2004 "Redefining Competition in Healthcare" Harvard Business Review pp. 65-76 June.

Porter, M. 1980 Competitive Strategy New York Free Press

Porter, M. 1985 Competitive Advantage, New York free Press.

Sharma, S. and N. Wickramasinghe, 2004 "e-health with Knowledge Management: areas for Tomorrow" pp. 110-124 in Wickramasinghe, N., J. Gupta and S. Sharma Eds Creating Knowledge-Based Healthcare Organizations with IdeanGroup Publishers, Hershey.

Sharma, S. N. Wickramasingeh, B. Xu and N. Ahmed , 2006 "Electronic Healthcare :Issues and Challenges" Int. J. Electronic Healthcare vol 2 no. 1 pp. 50-65

Van De Ven, A., Angle, H. and Poole, S. (2000). Research on the Management of Innovation, Oxford: Oxford University Press.

Von Lubitz, D and N. Wickramasinghe,. 2006 "Healthcare and Technology: The Doctrine of Networkcentric Healthcare" in press Intl. J Electronic Healthcare(IJEH).

Wickramasinghe, N. A. Fadlalla, E. Geisler, and J. Schaffer, 2005 "A Framework For Assessing E-Health Preparedness" International J. Electronic Healthcare (IJEH) vol. 1 no. 3 pp. 316-334

Wickramasinghe, N. and J. Silvers 2003 "IS/IT The Prescription To Enable Medical Group Practices To Manage Managed Care" Health Care Management Science vol. 6 no 2 pp-75-86

Wickramasinghe, N. and R. Lamb 2002 "Enterprise-wide systems enabling physicians to manage care", International Journal Healthcare Technology and Management vol 4 Nos. 3/4 pp.288-302

Compilation of References

(2000). Guidelines for referral to a gynecologic oncologist: Rationale and benefits. The Society of Gynecologic Oncologists. *Gynecologic Oncology, 78*(3 Pt 2), t-13.

(2001). ESMO minimum clinical recommendations for diagnosis, treatment and follow-up of ovarian cancer. *Annals of Oncology, 12,* 1205-7.

(2003, May, June). Determinants of success of inpatient clinical information systems: A literature review. *JAMIA: 10,3,* 235-243.

"Brown apologises for records loss." BBC 21 Nov. 2007.

"E-mails reveal data check warning." BBC 23 Nov. 2007.

30 years of adaptive neural networks: perceptron, Madaline, and backpropagation. *Proceedings of the IEEE, 78*(9), 1415-1442.

Adomat, R., & Hewison, A. (2004). Assessing patient category/dependence systems for determining the nurse/patient ratio in ICU and HDU: A review of approaches. *Journal of Nursing Management, 12*(5), 299-308.

Afuah, A., and Tucci, C. L. (2000). Internet Business Models and Strategies – Text and Cases McGraw Hill Irwin.

AG v Guardian Newspapers (No 2), 109 1990.

Agency for Healthcare Research and Policy, US. (n.d.). Retrieved September 13, 2007 from Agency for Healthcare Research and Policy, US.

Agrawal, S. K., Doucette, F., Gratton, R., Richardson, B., & Gagnon, R. (2003). Intrapartum computerized fetal heart rate parameters and metabolic acidosis at birth. *Obstet Gynecol, 102*(4), 731-738.

Agree Collaboration - http://www.agreecollaboration.org/

Agree Collaboration (n.d.). Retrieved September 8, 2007, from http://www.agreecollaboration.org/pdf/agreeinstrumentfinal.pdf

AHC Media LLC, freeCME.com (n.d.). Retrieved September 13, 2007 from http://www.freecme.com/gcourses1.php?specialty_id=41&specialty_name=OB/GYN

Alavi, M. A., and Leidner, D. E. (2001). Review: Knowledge Management and Knowledge Management Systems: Conceptual Foundations and Research Issues. MIS Quarterly, 25(1), 107-136.

Aletti, G. D., Dowdy, S. C., Gostout, B. S., Jones, M. B., Stanhope, R. C., Wilson, T. O., Podrzta, K. C., & Cliby, W. A. (2006). Aggressive surgical effort and improved survival in advanced-Stage Ovarian Cancer. *Obstet Gynecol, 107*(1), 1-11.

Alfirevic, Z., Devane, D., & Gyte, G. M. (2006). Continuous cardiotocography (CTG) as a form of electronic fetal monitoring (EFM) for fetal assessment during labour. *Cochrane Database Syst Rev, 3,* CD006066.

Allen, D. G., Baak, J., Belpomme, D., et al. (1993). Advanced epithelial ovarian cancer: 1993 consensus statements. *Ann Oncol, 4,* S83-S88.

Allen, D. G., Heinta, A. P. M., & Touw, F. W. M. M. (1995). A meta-analysis of residual disease and survival in stage 3 and 4 carcinoma of the ovary. *Eur J Gyn Oncol* 349-356.

Allen, E., Ollayos, C., Tellado, M., Butler, D., Buckner, S., Williams, B., et al. (2001). Characteristics of a telecytology consultation service. *Hum Pathol, 32,* 1323-1326.

Alli, P., Ollayos, C., Thompson, L., Kapadia, I., Butler, D., Williams, B., et al. (2001). Telecytology: Intraobserver and interobserver reproducibility in the diagnosis of cervical-vaginal smears. *Hum Pathol, 32,* 1318-1322.

Alvarez RC (2002), The promise of e-health - a Canadian perspective. eHealth International 1(4), 1-8.

Amaral, R., Zeferino, L., Hardy, E., Westin, M., Martinez, E., & Montemor, E. (2005). Quality assurance in cervical smears: 100% rapid rescreening vs 10% random rescreening. *Acta Cytol, 49*, 244-248.

Amatayjakul, M. (2005, November). Are you using an EHR – really? *Healthcare Financial Management, 59*(11), 126 .

American College Obstetricians and Gynecology, Obstetrics and Gynecology Journal (n.d.). Retrieved September 14, 2007 from http://www.acog.org/navbar/current/greenJournalLeader.cfm

American College of Nurse Midwives (n.d.). Retrieved September 13, 2007 from http://www.midwife.org

American College of Obstetricians and Gynecologists (n.d.). Retrieved August 17, 2007 from http://www.acog.org/postgrad/index.cfm

American College of Obstetricians and Gynecology, Today newsletter (n.d.). Retrieved September 15, 2007 from http://www.acog.org/member_access/lists/newslett.cfm

American College of Pathologists. (2000, 2000). About SNOMED. Retrieved January 11, 2002, from http://www.snomed.org/about_txt.html

Ammenwerth, E., & de Keizer, N. (2004). An inventory of evaluation studies of information technology in health care: Trends in evaluation research 1982 - 2002. Methods Inform Med.

Ammenwerth, E., Brender, J., Nykänen, P., Prokosch, U., Rigby, M., & Talmon, J. (2004). Visions and strategies to improve evaluations of health information systems - reflections and lessons based on the HIS-EVAL workshop in Innsbruck. Int J Med Inf.

Ammenwerth, E., Eichstädter, R., Haux, R., Pohl, U., Rebel, S., & Ziegler, S. (2001). A Randomized Evaluation of a Computer-Based Nursing Documentation System. Methods of Information in Medicine, 40(2), 61-8.

Ammenwerth, E., Iller, C., Mahler, C., Kandert, M., Luther, G., Hoppe, B., & Eichstädter, R. (2003a). Einflussfaktoren auf die Akzeptanz und Adoption eines Pflegedokumentationssystems - Studienbericht (2/2003). Innsbruck: Private Universität für Medizinische Informatik und Technik Tirol.

Ammenwerth, E., Mansmann, U., Iller, C., & Eichstädter, R. (2003). Factors Affecting and Affected by User Acceptance of Computer-Based Nursing Documentation:

Results of a Two-Year Study. Journal of the American Medical Informatics Association., 10(1), 69-84.

Anderson, S., & Wittwer, W. (2004). Using bar-code point-of-care technology for patient safety. *J Healthc Qual, 26*(6), 5-11.

Anon. (2008). Neonatology. *Merriam-Webster Online Dictionary.* Retrieved June 2008, from http://www.merriam-webster.com/dictionary/neonatology

Anonymous. (2007, 3rd October 2007). *Wikipedia - Hippocratic Oath*. Retrieved 16th October 2007, 2007, from http://en.wikipedia.org/wiki/Hippocratic_Oath

Antenatal Care-normal pregnancy - http://www.nice.org.uk

Aristotle. (1999). *Nicomachean Ethics*. Hackett Publishing Indianapolis.

ATHENS (n.d.). Retrieved September 13, 2007 from http://www.athens.ac.uk

Australian College of Midwives (n.d.). Retrieved September 14, 2007 from http://www.acmi.org.au/

Australian Department for Health and Ageing (n.d.). Retrieved September 14, 2007 from http://www.health.gov.au/

Ayres-de-Campos, D., & Bernardes, J. (2004). Comparison of fetal heart rate baseline estimation by SisPorto 2.01 and a consensus of clinicians. *Eur J Obstet Gynecol Reprod Biol, 117*(2), 174-178.

Balasubramanian, M., Capone, A., Jr., Hartnett, M., Pignatto, S., & Trese, M. (2006). The Photographic Screening for Retinopathy of Prematurity Study (Photo-ROP): Study design and baseline characteristics of enrolled patients. *Retina, 26*, S4-10.

Ball, M.J., Cortes-Comerer, N., Costin, M., Hudson, K. and Augustine B. (2004). HCA Inc.: standardization in action, *Journal of Healthcare Information Management*, 18(2),59-63.

Bangalore, A., Thorn, K. E., Tilley, C., & Peters, L. (2003). *The UMLS Knowledge Source Server: An Object Model For Delivering UMLS Data.* Paper presented at the AMIA Annual Symposium, Washington.

Bates, D. W., Cohen, M., Leape, L. L., Overhage, J. M., Shabot, M. M., & Sheridan, T. (2001). Reducing the Frequency of Errors in Medicine Using Information Technology. *J Am Med Inform Assoc, 8*(4), 299-308.

Battin, M. (2007). Health Informatics in Neonatology: What is the Potential to Further Improve Outcomes? *Health Care Informatics Review Online.*

Bayes, T. (1764). Essay Towards Solving a Problem in the Doctrine of Chances *Philosophical Transactions of the Royal Society of London.*

Beachamp, T. L., & Childress, J. F. (2001). *Principles of biomedical ethics 5th edition* Oxford University Press.

Beals, T. (2001). Digital imaging in Anatomic Pathology. *Lab Med, 32,* 327-330.

Becich, M., Gilbertson, J., Gupta, D., & et al. (2004). Pathology and patient safety: The critical role of pathology informatics in error reduction and quality initiatives. *Clin Lab Med, 24,* 913-943.

Beck, D. H., Taylor, B. L., Millar, B., & Smith, G. B. (1997). Prediction of outcome from intensive care: A prospective cohort study comparing Acute Physiology and Chronic Health Evaluation II and III prognostic systems in a United Kingdom intensive care unit. *Critical Care Medicine, 25*(1), 9-15.

Bell, K. N., & Oakley, G. P. (2006). Tracking the prevention of folic acid-preventable spina bifida and anencephaly. *Birth Defects Research. Part A, Clinical and Molecular Teratology, 76*(9), 654-7.

Benacerraf, B. R., Shipp, T. D., & Bromley, B. (2006). Three-dimensional US of the fetus: volume imaging. *Radiology, 238*(3), 988-996.

Bentham, J. (1789). *The principles of morals and legislation.*

Beolchi, Luciano (ed.) (2003). European Telemedicine Glossary of Concepts, Technologies, Standards and Users, 5th Edition, Brussels: European Commission.

Berg M (1999), Patient care information systems and health care work: A socio-technical approach. Int J Medical Informatics 55, 87-101

Berg M. & Toussaint, P. (2003). The Mantra of Modeling and the Forgotten Powers of Paper: A Sociotechnical View on the Development of Process-oriented ICT in Health Care. International Journal of Medical Informatics, **69**, 223-234.

Berg, M. (1994). Modeling Medical Work: On some Problems of Expert Systems in Medicine. *SIGBIO Newsletter of the ACM,* 2-6.

Berg, M. (1999). Patient care information systems and health care work: a sociotechnical approach. International Journal of Medical Informatics **55,** 87-101.

Berg, M., Aarts, J., & van der Lei, J. (2003). ICT in Health Care: Sociotechnical Approaches (Editorial). Methods Inf Med, 42, 297-301.

Berners-Lee, T., Hendler, J., & Lassila, O. (2001). The Semantic Web. *Scientific American,* (May 2001), 29-37.

Bibbo, M., Hawthorne, C., & Zimmerman, B. (1999). Does use of the AutoPap Assisted Primary Screener improve cytologic diagnosis? *Acta Cytol, 43,* 39622.

BioMedCentral (n.d.). Retrieved September 14, 2007 from http://www.biomedcentral.com/

Biomedical Informatics: Computer Applications in Health Care and Biomedicine (Health Informatics) by Edward H. Shortliffe and James J. Cimino

Biscotti, C., Dawson, A., Dziura, B., Galup, L., Darragh, T., Rahemtulla, A., et al. (2005). Assisted primary screening using the automated ThinPrep Imaging System. *Am J Clin Pathol, 123,* 281-287.

Bishop, E. H. (1964). Pelvic Scoring for Elective Induction. *Obstet. Gynecol., 24*(2), 266-268.

Bishop, J., Bigner, S., Colgan, T., Husain, M., Howell, L., McIntosh, K., et al. (1998). Multicenter masked evaluation of Autocyte PREP thinlayers with matched conventional smears: including initial biopsy results. *Acta Cytol, 42,* 189-197.

Blackwell Synergy E-journals Retrieved September 14, 2007 from http://www.blackwell-synergy.com/

BMC Pregnancy and Childbirth (n.d.). Retrieved September 14, 2007 from http://www.biomedcentral.com/bmcpregnancychildbirth/

BMC Women's Health (n.d.). Retrieved September 14, 2007 from http://www.biomedcentral.com/bmcwomenshealth/

BMC Women's Health Journal RSS (n.d.). Retrieved September 15, 2007 from http://www.biomedcentral.com/bmcwomenshealth/rss/

BNI (British Nursing Index) (n.d.). Retrieved September 13, 2007 from http://www.bniplus.co.uk/

Bolton, P., Douglas, K., Booth, B., & Miller, G. (1999). A relationship between computerisation and quality in general practice. *Australian Family Physician, 28*(9), 962-965.

Bomba, D. (1998). *A comparative study of computerised medical records usage among general practitioners in Australia and Sweden.* Paper presented at the Medinfo 9.

Bondy, S., Elit, L., Chen, Z., Law, C., & Paszat, L. (2006). Prognostic factors for women with Stage 1 ovarian cancer with or without adhesions. *Eur Journal Gyn Onc, 27*(6), 585-588.

Bonfiglio, T. (1989). Quality assurance in cytopathology. Recommendations and ongoing quality assurance activities of the American Society of Clinical Pathologists. *Acta Cytol, 33,* 431-433.

Bowman, G., Thompson, D., & Sutton, T. (1983). Nurses' attitudes towards the nursing process. Journal of Advanced Nursing, 8(2), 125-129.

Bracero, L. A., Roshanfekr, D., & Byrne, D. W. (2000). Analysis of antepartum fetal heart rate tracing by physician and computer. *J Matern Fetal Med, 9*(3), 181-185.

Brender, J. (2002). Methodological and Methodical Perils and Pitfalls within Assessment Studies Performed on IT-based solutions in Healthcare (ISSN 1397-9507). Aalborg: Virtual Centre for Health Informatics.

Bristow, R. E., Tomacruz, R. S., Armstrong, D. K., Trimble, E. L., & Montz, F. J. (2002). Survival effect of maximal cytoreductive surgery for advanced ovarian carcinoma during the platinum era: a meta-analysis. *J Clin Oncol, 20*(5), 1248-1259

Bristow, R. E., Zahurak, M. L., del Carmen, M. G., Gordon, T. A., Fox, H. E., Trimble, E. L. et al (2004) Ovarian cancer surgery in Maryland: volume-based access to care. *Gynecol Oncol, 93,* 353-360.

British Columbia Reproductive Care Program. BCRCP Obstetric Guideline 11 Hypertension in Pregnancy. 2006. Vancouver BC.

British Journal of Obstetrics and Gynaecology Journal, podcasts (n.d.). Retrieved September 15, 2007 from http://www.blackwellpublishing.com/podcast/bjog.asp

Bromley, S. E., Vries, C. S., & Farmer, R. D. T. (2004). Utilisation of hormone replacement therapy in the United Kingdom. A descriptive study using the general practice research database. *BJOG: An International Journal of Obstetrics and Gynaecology, 111*(4), 369-376.

Brownsword, R. (2004). Reproductive Opportunities and Regulatory Challenges. *Modern Law Review, 67*(2), 304-321.

Buchsbaum, H. J., Brady, M. F., Delgado, G., Miller, A., Hoskins, W., Manetta, A., et al. (1989). Surgical staging of carcinoma of the ovaries. *Surgery, Gynecology & Obstetrics, 169,* 226-32.

Budtz S & Witt K (2002), Consulting the Internet before visit to general practice. Patients' use of the Internet and other sources of health information. Scan J Primary Health Care 20(3), 174-176.

Campbell, D., & Fiske, D. (1959). Convergent and discriminant validity by the muli-trait, multi-method matrix. Psychological Bulletin, 56, 81-105.

Canada Health Infoway. 2015: Advancing the Next Generation of Health Care in Canada. 2006.

Canadian Association of Midwives (n.d.). Retrieved September 14, 2007 from http://www.canadianmidwives.org/

Canadian Charter of Rights and freedoms, Part 1 of the Constitution Act, 1982, Schedule B to the Canada Act 1982(United Kingdom) 11 (1982).

Canadian Partnership Against Cancer, Cancer Control Guidelines Action Group. (2007). *Opportunities for the Inter-Provincial Implementation of Synoptic Reporting Tools to Translate Standards and Guidelines into Practice for Cancer Surgery and Pathology.* Toronto, March 14, 2007.

Canadian Standards Association. Canadian Standards Association: Privacy Code. http://www.csa.ca/standards/privacy/code/Default.asp?language=english . 2007.

Cancer Care Ontario Web site for Quality Care

Cancer of the ovary. (1991). ACOG Technical Bulletin Number 141. *Int J Gynecol Obstet, 35,* 359-66.

Carey, T. S. et al. (2005). Developing Effective Interuniversity Partnerships and Community-Based Research to Address Health Disparities. *Academic Medicine, 80.11,* 1039-45.

Carney, M. E., Lancaster, J. M., Ford, C., Tsodikov, A., & Wiggins, C. L. (2002). A Population-based study of patterns of care for ovarian cancer: Who is seen by a gynecologic oncologist and who is not? *Gyn Onc, 84,* 36-42

Cartwright, D. (2004). Central venous lines in neonates: a study of 2186 catheters. *Arch Dis Child Fetal Neonatal Ed, 89*(6), F504-508.

CASP (n.d.). Retrieved September 6, 2007 from http://www.phru.nhs.uk/Pages/PHD/CASP.htm

CASP (the Critical Appraisal Skills Programme) - http://www.phru.nhs.uk/Pages/PHD/CASP.htm

CATmaker, Centre for Evidence-based Medicine (n.d.). Retrieved September 8, 2007 from http://www.cebm.net/index.aspx?o=1216

CEN, http://www.cenorm.be/cenorm/index.htm , accessed on February, 11 2005.

Centre for Disease Control CDC/ATSDR, US (n.d.). Retrieved September 15, 2007 from http://www.cdc.gov/women/pubs.htm

Centre for Evidence-Based Medicine http://www.cebm.net/

Centre for Health Evidence User Guides - http://www.cche.net/usersguides/main.asp

Chalmers, I., Enkin, M., & Kierse, M. J. N. C. (1989). *Effective Care in Pregnancy and childbirth.* Oxford: Oxford University Press.

Chan, J. K., Munro, E. G., Cheung, M. K., Husain, A., Teng, N. N., Berek, J. S., & Osann, K. (2007). Assocation of lymphadenectomy and survival in stage 1 ovarian cancer patients. *Obstet Gynecol, 109*(1)12-9.

Chard, T. (1987). Computerisation of Obstetric Records. In J. Studd (Ed.), *Progress in Obstetrics and Gynaecology: Volume Six* (1 ed., pp. 3-22). London: Chuchill Livingstone.

Chard, T. (1987). Computerisation of Obstetric Records. *Progress in Obstetrics and Gynaecology: Volume Six.* J. Studd (ed.). London: Chuchill Livingstone. **(pp** 3-22).

Chard, T., & Schreiner, A. (1990). Expert systems in obstetrics and gynaecology. Review. *Baillieres.Clinical. Obstetrics.&.Gynaecology., 4,* 815-840.

Chau, P.Y.K. & Hu, P.J.-H. (2002). Investigating Healthcare Professionals' Decisions to Accept Telemedicine Technology: an Empirical Test of Competing Theories. Information and Management, **39,** 297-311.

Chedoe, I., Molendijk, H., Dittrich, S., Jansman, F., Harting, J., Brouwers, J., et al. (2007). Incidence and nature of medication errors in neonatal intensive care with strategies to improve safety: a review of the current literature. *Drug Saf, 30*(6), 503-513.

Chief Nursing Officer, UK (n.d.). Retrieved September 13, 2007 from http://www.dh.gov.uk/en/Aboutus/Chief-professionalofficers/Chiefnursingofficer/index.htm

Chien, L. Y. et al. (2002). Variations in antenatal corticosteroid therapy: A persistent problem despite 30 years of evidence. *Obstet Gynecol, 99.3,* 401-08.

Chien, L., Macnab, Y., Aziz, K., Andrews, W., McMillan, D., Lee, S., et al. (2002). Canadian Neonatal Network Variations in central venous catheter-related infection risks among Canadian neonatal intensive care units. *Pediatr Infect Dis J, 2*(6), 505-511.

Childbirth Connection. (2006). A*bout This Book: A Guide to Effective Care in Pregnancy and* Childbirth. http://childbirthconnection.org/article.asp?ck=10014 .

Chin, J. (1988). Development of a tool measuring user satisfaction of the human-computer interface, Chi'88 Conf. Proceedings: Human factors in Computing (pp. 213-218). New York: Association for Computing Machinery.

Chivukula, M., Saad, R., Elishaev, E., White, S., Mauser, N., & Dabbs, D. (2007). Introduction of the ThinPrep Imaging System™ (TIS): Experience in a high volume academic practice. *CytoJournal, 4,* 6.

Choi, J., Starren, J., & Bakken, S. (2005). Web-based educational resources for low literacy families in the NICU. *AMIA Annu Symp Proc, 2005,* 922.

Cibas, E., Dean, B., Maffeo, N., & Allred, E. (2001). Quality assurance in gynecologic cytology.The value of cytotechnologist-cytopathologist discrepancy logs. *Am J Clin Pathol, 115,* 512-516.

Cinahl (Cumulative Index to Nursing and Allied Health Literature) (n.d.). Retrieved September 14, 2007 from http://www.cinahl.com/

Cleary, R. (1996). The standard primipara as a basis for inter-unit comparison of maternity care. *British Journal of Obstetrics & Gynaecology, 103,* 223-229.

Clinical guidelines - http://www.rcog.org.uk, http://www.ranzcog.edu.au, http://www.acog.org, Evidence based practice - http://www.cochrane.org

Clinical Trilas.gov (n.d.). Retrieved September 14, 2007 from http://clinicaltrials.gov/

COACH: Canada's Health Informatics Association. Guidelines for the Protection of Health Information. 16-12-0007. Toronto, Canada.

Cocchi, V., Sintoni, C., Carretti, D., Sama, D., Chiari, U., Segala, V., et al. (1996). External quality assurance in cervical/vaginal cytology: Interlaboratory agreement in the Emilia-Romagna region of Italy. *Acta Cytol, 40,* 480-488.

Cochrane Collaboration. (1997). Cochrane Pregnancy and Childbirth Database (Version III) [CD-Rom]. Oxford, UK: Update Software.

Cochrane Library (n.d.). Retrieved September 13, 2007 from http://www.thecochranelibrary.com/

Cochrane, A. L. *(1972). Effectiveness and Efficiency: Random Reflections on Health Services.* London: Nuffield Provincial Hospitals Trust.

Cochrane, A. L. (1979). *1931-1971: A critical review, with particular reference to the medical profession.* Retrieved from.

Coiera, E. (2004). Four Rules for the Reinvention of Healthcare. British Medical Journal, *328,* 1197-1199.

Coiera, E., & Tombs, V. (1998). Communication behaviours in a hospital setting: an observational study. *British Medical Journal, 316*(7132), 673-676.

Coiera, E., & Tombs, V. (1998). Communication behaviours in a hospital setting: An observational study. *British Medical Journal, 316*(7132), 673-676.

Colgan, T., Patten, S., & Lee, J. (1995). A clinical trial of the AutoPap 300 QC System for quality control of cervicovaginal cytology in the clinical laboratory. *Acta Cytol, 39,* 1191-1198.

Collaço, L., de Noronha, L., Pinheiro, D., & Bleggi-Torres, L. (2005). Quality assurance in cervical screening of a high risk population: A study of 65,753 reviewed cases in Parana Screening Program, Brazil. *Diagn Cytopathol, 33,* 441-448.

College of Family Physicians of Canada (n.d.). Retrieved September 15, 2007 from http://www.cfpc.ca/English/cfpc/clfm/critical/

Confidential enquiry into stillbirths and deaths in infancy (CESDI). Fourth Annual Report, 1 January - 31 December 1995. (1997). London: Maternal and Child Health Research Consortium.

Confidentiality NHS Code of Practice (2003).

Cooper, M. (1992). Should Physicians be Bayesian Agents? *Theoretical Medicine, 13,* 349-361.

Coory, M., & Cornes, S. (2005). Interstate comparisons of public hospital outputs using DRGs: Are they fair? *Australian and New Zealand Journal of Public Health, 29*(2), 143-148.

Cope, I., Greenwell, J., & Mather, B. S. (1971). An Obstetric Data Project- General Description. *Med J Aust, 1,* 12-14.

Covens, A., Carey, M., Bryson, P., Verma, S., Fung Kee Fung, M., Daya, D., DePetrillo, D., Eisenhauer E., Elit, L., Fyles, Kerr, I., Lukka, H., Malik, S., Rosen, B., Thomas, G., & Yoshida, S. (N/A). First-line chemotherapy for postoperative patients with Stage II, III, or IV epithelial ovarian cancer. *Cancer Care Ontario Practice Guideline,* 4-1-2.

Cowper, S. (2000). PathMax: A friendly guide to web pathology (abstract). *Arch Pathol Lab Med, 124,* 822.

Crawford, S. C., Vasey, P. A., Paul, J., Hay, A., Davis, J. A., Kaye, S. B. (2006). SCOTROC. Does aggressive surgery only benefit patients with less advanced ovarian cancer? Results from an international comparison within the SCOTROC-1 trial. SGO 2006. *Abstract 5003,* 455s.

Critical appraisal and using the literature (n.d.). Retrieved September 7, 2007 from www.shef.ac.uk/scharr/ir/units/critapp/websites

Croll, P. R., & Croll, J. (2007). Investigating risk exposure in e-health systems. *International Journal of Medical Informatics, 76,* 460-65.

Crowther, C. A., Hiller, J. E., & Doyle, L. W. (2002). Magnesium sulphate for preventing preterm birth in threatened preterm labour. *Cochrane. Database. Syst. Rev., 4,* CD001060.

Current Controlled Trials (n.d.). Retrieved September 14, 2007 from http://www.controlled-trials.com/

DARE database (Database of Abstracts of Reviews of Effects) (n.d.). Retrieved September 13, 2007 from http://www.york.ac.uk/inst/crd/crddatabases.htm#DARE

Darlow, B., Hutchinson, J., Henderson-Smart, D., Donoghue, D., Simpson, J., Evans, N., et al. (2005). Prenatal risk factors for severe retinopathy of prematurity among very preterm infants of the Australian and New Zealand Neonatal Network. *Pediatrics, 1*(4), 990-996.

Davis, F. (1993). User acceptance of information technology: System characteristics, user perceptions and behavioral impacts. International Journal of Man-Machine Studies, 38, 475-487.

Dawes, G. S., Moulden, M., & Redman, C. W. (1991). System 8000: Computerized antenatal FHR analysis. *J Perinat Med, 19*(1-2), 47-51.

Dawes, G. S., Rosevear, S. K., Pello, L. C., Moulden, M., & Redman, C. W. (1991). Computerized analysis of episodic changes in fetal heart rate variation in early labor. *Am J Obstet Gynecol, 165*(3), 618-624.

de Boo, H. A., & Harding, J. E. (2006). The developmental origins of adult disease (Barker) hypothesis. *Australian & New Zealand Journal of Obstetrics & Gynaecology, 46*, 4-14.

De Lusignan, S. et al. (2005). A knowledge audit of the managers of primary care organizations: Top priority is how to use routinely collected clinical data for quality improvement. *Medical Informatics & the Internet in Medicine, 30.1*, 69-80.

de Vries, H., Bakker, M. et al. (2006). The effects of smoking cessation counseling by midwives on Dutch pregnant women and their partners. *Patient Education and Counseling, 63*, 177-87.

de Vries, P. H., & P.F., d. V. R. (1985). An Overview of Medical Expert Systems. *Methods of Information in Medicine, 24*, 57-64.

De Wals, P., Tairou, F. et al. (2007). Reduction in neural-tube defects after folic acid fortification in Canada. *New England Journal of Medicine, 357*(2), 135-42.

de, C.-W., R. H., Wolfe, C., Fitzgerald, A., Spencer, M., Goodman, J., & Gamsu, H. (1995). Use of the CRIB (clinical risk index for babies) score in prediction of neonatal mortality and morbidity. *Arch Dis Child Fetal Neonatal Ed, 73*(1), F32-36.

de, W., S. N., Verzijden, R., van, D., Anker, J. N., & de, H. M. (2007). Information technology cannot guarantee patient safety. *BMJ, 334*, 851-852.

Deftereos, S., Lambrinoudakis, C., Andriopoulos, P., Farmakis, D., Aessopos, A. (2001). A Java-based electronic healthcare record software for beta-thalassaemia. Journal of Medical Internet Research, 3(4):E33.

Demeester, M. (1999). Cultural Aspects of Information Technology Implementation. International Journal of Medical Informatics, **56**, 25-41.

Denaro, T., Herriman, J., & Shapira, O. (1997). PAP-NET Testing System: Technical update. *Acta Cytol, 41*, 65-73.

Denzin, N. (1970). Strategies of multiple triangulation. In N. Denzin (Ed.), The Research Act (3rd ed., pp. 297-331). Chicago: Aldine.

DeOrio, J. K. Surgical templates for orthopedics operative reports. *Orthopedics, 25*(6), 639-42.

Department of Health and Human Services, US (n.d.). Retrieved September 13, 2007 from http://www.hhs.gov/index.html

Department of Health UK. (1998). *Information for Health.* Retrieved. from.

Department of Health, UK (n.d.). Retrieved September 13, 2007 from http://www.dh.gov.uk/

Devoe, L., Golde, S., Kilman, Y., Morton, D., Shea, K., & Waller, J. (2000). A comparison of visual analyses of intrapartum fetal heart rate tracings according to the new national institute of child health and human development guidelines with computer analyses by an automated fetal heart rate monitoring system. *Am J Obstet Gynecol, 183*(2), 361-366.

Dewan, N., & Lorenzi, N. (2000). Behavioral Health Information Systems: Evaluating Readiness and User Acceptance. MD Computing, 17(4), 50-52.

Dhillon, A., Albersheim, S., Alsaad, S., Pargass, N., & Zupancic, J. (2003). Internet use and perceptions of information reliability by parents in a neonatal intensive care unit. *J Perinatol, 2*(5), 420-424.

DiGiorgio, C., Richert, C., Klatt, E., & Becich, M. (1994). E-mail, the Internet, and information access technology in pathology. *Semin Diagn Pathol, 11*, 294-304.

Directory of Open Access Journals, health sciences section (n.d.). Retrieved September 14, 2007 from http://www.doaj.org/doaj?func=subject&cpid=20

DISCERN (n.d.). Retrieved September 6, 2007 from www.discern.org.uk

Dolin, R. H., Alschuler, L., Beebe, C., Biron, P. V., Boyer, S. L., Essin, D., et al. (2001). The HL7 Clinical Document Architecture. *J Am Med Inform Assoc, 8*(6), 552-569.

Donabedian, A. (1966). Evaluating the quality of medical care. *Milbanks Memorial Fund Quarterly, 44*, 166-206.

Donaldson, forewords by Sue, K. & Gerdin, U. (2000). *Nursing informatics: where caring and technology meet,* 3rd ed., Springer, New York ; London.

Dowie, J. (1996). 'Evidence-based', 'cost-effective' and 'preference-driven' medicine: decision analysis based medical decision making is the pre-requisite. *Journal of Health Services Research and Policy, 1*(2), 104-113.

DUETs database (Database of Uncertainties about the Effects Treatments) (n.d.). Retrieved September 13, 2007 from http://www.duets.nhs.uk/SearchResults.asp?T=5&TID=25

Dziura, B., Quinn, S., & Richard, K. (2006). Performance of an imaging system vs. manual screening in the detection of squamous intraepithelial lesions of the uterine cervix. *Acta Cytol, 50*, 309-311.

Earle, C. C., Schrag, D., Neville, B. A., Yabroff, K. R., Topor, M. Fahey, A. et al. (2006, February 1). Effect of surgeon specialty on processes of care and outcomes for ovarian cancer patients. *J Natl Cancer Inst, 98*(3), 172-80.

Edhemovic, I., Temple, W. J., de Gara, C. J., & Stuart, G. C. (2004, October). The computer synoptic operative report--A leap forward in the science of surgery. *Ann Surg Oncol, 11*(10), 941-947.

e-Health - making healthcare better for European citizens: An action plan for a European e-Health area (2004), Commission of the European Communities. COM (2004) 356, Brussels.

Eisenkop, S. M., Frieman, R. L., & Wang, H. J. (1998). Complete cytoreductive surgery is feasible and maximizes survival in patients with advanced epithelial ovarian cancer: A prospective study. *Gyn Onc, 69*, 103-108

Eisenkop, S. M., Spirtos, N. M., Montag, T. W., Nalick, R. H., & Wang, H. J. (1992). The impact of subspecialty training on the management of advanced ovarian cancer. *Gynecol Oncol, 47*, 203-209.

Electronic Health Records: A Practical Guide for Professional and Organizations, 3rd Edition by MBA, RHIA, CHPS, CPHIT, CPEHR, FHIMSS Margret K. Amatayakul

Electronic Health Records: Understanding and Using Computerized Medical Records by Richard W. Gartee

Elit, L. (2005). Outcomes for Surgery in Ovarian Cancer. *In Progress in Ovarian Cancer Research,*Bardos, A. P. (Ed.). NY: Nova Science Publishers Inc. ISBN 1-59454-241-4.

Elit, L., Bondy, S., Chen, Z., Law, C., & Paszat, L. (2006, October). The quality of Operative Reports for women with ovarian cancer. JOGC, *28*(10), 892-897.

Elit, L., Bondy, S., Paszat, L., Chen, Z., Hollowaty, E., Thomas, G., & Levine, M. (2006, October). Outcomes in Surgery for Ovarian Cancer. *Submitted to Canadian Journal of Surgery.*

Elit, L., Bondy, S., Paszat, L., Przybysz, R., & Levine, M. (2002). Outcomes in Surgery for ovarian cancer. *Gyn Onc, 87*, 260-267.

Elit, L., Cartier, C., Oza, A., Hirte, H., Levine, M., & Paszat, L. (2006, May). Outcomes for Systemic therapy in ovarian cancer. *Gyn Onc, 103*(2), 554-8.

Elit, L., Chambers, A., Fyles, A., Covens, A., Carey, M., & Fung Yee Fung, M. (2004). Systematic Review of Adjuvant Care for Newly diagnosed Stage 1 Ovarian Cancer. *Cancer, 101*(9), 1926-35

Elit, L., Oliver, T. K., Covens, A., Kwon, J., Fung, M. F., Hirte, H. W., & Oza, A. M. (2007). Intraperitoneal chemotherapy in the first-line treatment of women with stage III epithelial ovarian cancer: A systematic review with meta-analyses. Cancer, *109*(4), 692-702. Review.

Elit, L., Plante, M., Bessette, P., DePetrillo, D., Ehlen, T., Heywood, M., et al. (2000). Surgical management of an adnexal mass suspicious for malignancy. *J Soc Obstet Gynecol Can, 22*, 964-8.

Elsevier Science Direct (n.d.). Retrieved September 14, 2007 from http://www.sciencedirect.com/

Elson, J., Tailor, A., Banerjee, S., Salim, R., Hillaby, K., & Jurkovic, D. (2004). Expectant management of tubal ectopic pregnancy: prediction of successful outcome using decision tree analysis. *Ultrasound in Obstetrics and Gynecology, 23*(6), 552-556.

Embase (n.d.). Retrieved September 13, 2007 from http://www.embase.com/

Eng, T.R (2001), The eHealth Landscape: A Terrain Map of Emerging Information and Communication Technologies in Health and Health Care. Princeton, New Jersey, The Robert Wood Johnson Foundation, USA.

Engelen, M. J., Kos, H. E., Willemse, P. H., Aalders, J. G., de Bires, E. G., Schaapveld, M., Otter, R., & van der Zee, A. G. (2006). Surgery by consultant gynecologic oncologists improves survival in patients with ovarian carcinoma. *Cancer, 106*(3), 589-98.

Enkin, M. et al. (2000). *A Guide to Effective Care in Pregnancy and Childbirth.* 3 ed. London: Oxford University Press.

Enkin, M., Keirse, M., & Chalmers, I. (1989). *A Guide to Effective Care in Pregnancy and Childbirth.* 1 ed. London: Oxford Medical Publications.

Ensing, M., Paton, R., Speel, P. H., & Rada, R. (1994). An object-oriented approach to knowledge representation in a biomedical domain. *Artificial Intelligence in Medicine, 6*, 459-482.

EPIQ (n.d.). Retrieved September 8, 2007 from http://www.health.auckland.ac.nz/population-health/epidemiology-biostats/epiq/index.html

Espinoza, J., Romero, R., Kusanovic, J. P., Gotsch, F., Lee, W., Goncalves, L. F., et al. (2008). Standardised views of the fetal heart using four-dimensional sonographic and tomographic imaging. *Ultrasound in Obstetrics and Gynecology, 31,* 233-242.

European Court of Human Rights. (2007). The European Court of Human Rights. Retrieved 1st June 2008, 2008, from http://www.echr.coe.int/echr/en/bottom/contact/

Evans, N., Hutchinson, J., Simpson, J., Donoghue, D., Darlow, B., & Henderson-Smart, D. (2007). Prenatal predictors of mortality in very preterm infants cared for in the Australian and New Zealand Neonatal Network. *Arch Dis Child Fetal Neonatal Ed, 92*(1), F34-40.

Evidence-based medicine.co.uk, What is critical appraisal? (n.d.). Retrieved September 6, 2007 from www.evidence-based-medicine.co.uk

Eysenbach G (2001), What is e-health? Editorial. J Med Internet Res 1(2), e20.

Faculty of Sexual and Reproductive Healthcare, UK (n.d.). Retrieved August 17, 2007 from

Fallis D & Fricke M (2002), Indicators of accuracy of consumer health information on the Internet: a study of indicators relating to information for managing fever in children at home. JAMIA 9(1), 73-79.

Fayyad, U., Piatetsky-Shapiro, G., & Smyth, P. (1996). From Data Mining to Knowledge Discovery in Databases. *AI Magazine*(Fall), 37-53.

Feachem, R. G. A., Sekhri, N. K., White, K. L., Dixon, J., Berwick, D. M., & Enthoven, A. C. (2002). Getting more for their dollar: A comparison of the NHS with California's Kaiser Permanente. *BMJ, 324*(7330), 135-143.

Federal Privacy Act and Personal Information and Electronic Documents Act (PIPEDA) 2001., (1982).

Feeny, D. 2001 "Making Business Sense of the e-opportunity" MIT Sloan Management Review, Winter vol. 42, no. 2 p. 42.

Flegel, K. et al. (2008). Getting to the electronic medical record. *CMAJ, 178.5,* 531, 533.

Food and Drug Administration. (2007). *MonoPrepTM. Summary of safety and effectiveness data.* Retrieved Sept 14th, 2007, from http://www.fda.gov/cdrh/pdf4/p040052b.pdf.

Fowlie, P., & McHaffie, H. (2004). Supporting parents in the neonatal unit. *BMJ, 329*(7478), 1336-1338.

Frable, W. (2007). Error reduction and risk management in cytopathology. *Semin Diagn Pathol, 24,* 77-88.

Franco, A., Farr, F. L., King, J. D., Clark, J. S., & Haug, P. J. (1990). "NEONATE"--An expert application for the "HELP" system: comparison of the computer's and the physician's problem list. *J. Med. Syst., 14*(5), 297-306.

Frechtling, J. (1997). User-Friendly Handbook for Mixed Method Evaluation, [Ausdruck im Eval-Ordner]. Available: http://www.ehr.nsf.gov/EHR/REC/pubs/NSF97-153/start.htm [Feb. 2003].

Free Medical Journals (n.d.). Retrieved September 14, 2007 from http://freemedicaljournals.com/

Friedman, C., & Wyatt, J. C. (1997). Evaluation Methods in Medical Informatics. New York: Springer.

Gagnon, M., Inhorn, S., Hancock, J., Keller, B., Carpenter, D., Merlin, T., et al. (2004). Comparison of cytology proficiency testing: glass slides vs virtual slides. *Acta Cytol, 48,* 788-794.

Gagnon, M.-P. Godin, G. Gagne, C. Fortin, J.-P. Lamothe, L. Reinharz, D. & Cloutier, A. (2003). An Adaption of the Theory of interpersonal Behaviour to the Study fo Telemedicine Adoption by Physicians. International Journal of Medical Informatics, **71,** 103-115.

Gangliardi, A. R., Fung Kee Fung, M., Langer, B., Stern, H., & Brown, A. D. (2005). Development of Ovarian Cancer Surgery Quality Indicators Using a Modified Delphi Approach. *Gyn Onc, 97*(2), 446-456.

Gardner, M. (2003). Why clinical information standards matter. *BMJ, 326*(7399), 1101-1102.

Garg, A. X., Adhikari, N. K., McDonald, H., Rosas-Arellano, M. P., Devereaux, P. J., Beyene, J., et al. (2005). Effects of computerized clinical decision support systems on practitioner performance and patient outcomes: A systematic review. *Jama, 293*(10), 1223-1238.

Gargeya, V and D. Sorrell 2004 "Moving toward an e-hospital" pp.50-64 in Wickramasinghe, N., J. Gupta and S. Sharma Eds Creating Knowledge-Based Healthcare Organizations with IdeanGroup Publishers, Hershey.

Geneva Foundation for Medical Education and Research (GFMER) (n.d.). Retrieved September 14, 2007 from http://www.gfmer.ch/000_Homepage_En.htm

Geneva Foundation for Medical Education and Research (GFMER) http://www.gfmer.ch/000_Homepage_En.htm

Geneva Foundation for Medical Education and Research, Journal list (n.d.). Retrieved September 14, 2007 http://www.gfmer.ch/Medical_journals/Obstetrics_gynecology_reproductive_health.htm

Geneva Foundation for Medical Education and Research, Reproductive Health Journal (n.d.). Retrieved September 14, 2007 from http://www.reproductive-health-journal.com/home/

Geneva Foundation for Medical Education and Research, Research resources (n.d.). Retrieved September 14, 2007 from http://www.gfmer.ch/400_Publications_En.htm

Gerber BS & Eiser AR (2001), The patient-physician relationship in the Internet age: Future prospects and the research agenda. J Med Internet Res 3(2), e15.

Gibbs, D. D., & Gore, M. E. (2001). Pursuit of optimum outcomes in ovarian cancer. *Drugs, 61,* 1103-20.

Giede, K. C., Kieser, K., Dodge, J., & Rosen, B. (2005). Who should operate on patients with ovarian cancer? An evidence-based review. *Gyn Oncol.*

Giles, M. L., Mijch, A. M., Garland, S. M., Grover, S. R., & Hellard, M. E. (2004). HIV and pregnancy in Australia. *Australian & New Zealand Journal of Obstetrics & Gynaecology, 44*(3), 197-204.

Gillis, C. R., Hole, D. J., Still, R. M., & Kaye, S. B. (1991). Medical audit, cancer registration and survival in ovarian cancer. *Lancet, 337,* 611-612.

Gillon, R. (1986). *Philosophical Medical Ethics* (p. 108). Chichester: John Wiley.

Glaser, J. 2002 The Strategic Application of Information Technology in Health Care Organizations 2nd Ed. Jossey Bass, San Francisco.

Goff, B. A., Matthews, B. J., Larson, E. H., Andrilla, C. H., Wynn, M., Lishner, D. M., & Baldwin, L. M. (2007) Predictors of comprehensive surgical treatment in patients with ovarian cancer. *Cancer, 109*(10), 2031-42.

Goff, B. A., Matthews, B. J., Wynn, M., Muntz, H. G., Lishner, D. M., & Baldwin, L. M. Ovarian cancer: Patterns of surgical care across the United States. *Gyn Oncol, 103,* 383-399.

Goff, B., Larson, E., Mathews, B., Andrilla, H., Lishner, D., Baldwin, L., Lackey, M., & Muntz, H. (2006). What factors predict comprehensive surgical treatment of ovarian cancer patients? *Gyn Onc 101,* (S2), Abstract 1.

Goldstein, M.K. Coleman, R.W. Tu, S.W. Shankar, R.D. O'Connor, M.J. Musen, M.A. Martins, S.B. Lavori, P.W. Shilipak, M.G. Oddone, E. Advani, A. A. Gholami, P. & Hoffman, B.B. (2004). Translating Research into Practice: Organisational Issues in Implementing Automated Decision Support for Hypertension in Three Medical Centers. Journal of the American Medical Informatics Association, 11(5), 368-376.

Goodhue, D. (1995). Understanding user evaluations of information systems. Management Science, 41(12), 1827-44.

Gosling, A.S. Westbrook, J.I. & Braithwaite, J. (2003). Clinical Team Functioning and IT Innovation: A Study of the Diffusion of a Point-of Care Online Evidence System. Journal of the American Medical Informatics Association, 10(3), 244-251.

Grant, A. & Chalmers, I. (1981). Register of randomised controlled trials in perinatal medicine. *Lancet, 1.100.*

Grant, A., Plante, I., & Leblanc, F. (2002). The TEAM methodology for the evaluation of information systems in biomedicine. Comput Biol Med, 32(3), 195-207.

Grant, J. M. (1994). Induction of labour confers benefits in prolonged pregnancy. *Br. J. Obstet. Gynaecol., 101*(2), 99-102.

Gray, J., & Goldmann, D. (2004). Medication errors in the neonatal intensive care unit: Special patients, unique issues. *Arch Dis Child Fetal Neonatal Ed, 89*(6), F472-473.

Gray, J., Safran, C., Davis, R., Pompilio-Weitzner, G., Stewart, J., Zaccagnini, L., et al. (2000). Baby CareLink: Using the Internet and telemedicine to improve care for high-risk infants. *Pediatrics, 106*(6), 1318-1324.

Gray, J., Suresh, G., Ursprung, R., Edwards, W., Nickerson, J., Shiono, P., et al. (2006). Patient misidentification in the neonatal intensive care unit: quantification of risk. *Pediatrics, 117*(1), e43-47.

Greene, J., & McClintock, C. (1985). Triangulation in evaluation: Design and analysis issues. Evaluation Review, 9(5), 523-545.

Greenhalgh, T. Robert, G. MacFarlane, F. Bate, P. & Kyriakidou, O. (2004). Diffusion of Innovations in Service Organisations: Systematic Review and Recommendations. The Millbank Quarterly, 82(4), 581-629.

Grémy, F., & Degoulet, P. (1993). Assessment of health information technology: which questions for which systems? Proposal for a taxonomy. Medical Informatics, 18(3), 185-93.

Grigorenko, G. F., Zaiats, G. A., Kleshchev, A. S., Lifshits, A., & Samsonov, V. V. (1989). The outlook for introducing the Konsul'tant-2 expert medical system on board ships. *Voen Med Zh*(2), 49-50.

Grilli, R., Alexanian, A., Apolone, G., Fossati, R., Marsoni, S., Nicolucci, A. et al. (1990). The impact of cancer treatment guidelines on actual practice in Italian general hospitals: The case of ovarian cancer. *Annals of Oncology, 1,* 112-118.

Grimson J, Grimson W, Flahive M, Foley C, O'Moore R, Nolan J & Chadwick GA (2000), Multimedia approach to raising awareness of information and communications technology amongst health care professionals. Int J Medical Informatics 58-59, 297-305.

Groves, A., Kuschel, C., & Skinner, J. (Aug 2006). International Perspectives: The Neonatologist as an Echocardiographer. *NeoReviews,, 7,* e391 - e393.

Gruen J (1999), The Physician and the Internet: Observer or participant? MD Comput 16(6), 46-48.

Guidance index for Obstetrics and Gynecology - http://www.nice.org.uk/guidance/, index.jsp?action=byTopic

Guzman, E. R., Vintzileos, A. M., Martins, M., Benito, C., Houlihan, C., & Hanley, M. (1996). The efficacy of individual computer heart rate indices in detecting acidemia at birth in growth-restricted fetuses. *Obstet Gynecol, 87*(6), 969-974.

Gynaecologists, R. C. o. O. a. (2001). *The use of electronic fetal monitoring. The use and interpretation of of cardiotocography in intrapartum fetal surveillance.* London: RCOG Press.

Gynecologic Disease Site Group Program in Evidence-based Care. *Management of a Suspicious Ovarian Mass. Evidence Summary Report #4-15,* April 29, 2004

Hacker, N. F. (1995). Systematic pelvic and paraaortic lymphadenectomy for advanced ovarian cancer – Therapeutic advance or surgical folly? *Gyn Onc, 56,* 325-327.

Hacker, N. F., Berek, J. S., Lagasse, L. D., Nieberg, R. K., & Elashoff, R. M. (1983). Primary cytoreductive surgery for epithelial ovarian cancer. *Obstet Gynecol, 61,* 413.

Haglund H (2002), The significance of welfare services and their electronic applications for the business activities in the future. Presentation given in the eHealth - Tomorrow's eHealth services, Tampere, November 2002, www.etampere.fi, Feb 11, 2003

Hammond, W.E. and Cimino, J.J. (2001). Standards in Medical Informatics, *Medical Informatics – Computer Applications in Health Care and Biomedicine,* Edward H. Shortliffe and Leslie E. Perreault (eds.), New York: Springer, 212-255.

Hannah, M. E., Ohlsson, A., Farine, D., Hewson, S. A., Hodnett, E. D., Myhr, T. L., et al. (1996). Induction of labor compared with expectant management for prelabor rupture of the membranes at term. *N. Eng. Med. J., 334*(16), 1005-1010.

Harbour, R., & Miller, J. (2001). A new system for grading recommendations in evidence based guidelines. *British Medical Journal, 323*(11 August), 334-336.

Harlan, L. C., Clegg, L.X., & Trimble, E. L. (2003). Trends in surgery and chemotherapy for women diagnosed with ovarian cancer in the United States. *J Clin Oncol 21*(18), 3488-3494.

Harris, J. M. (1981). The hazards of bedside Bayes. *Journal of the American Medical Association, 246*(22), 2602-2605.

Haug, P. J., Gardner, R. M., & Tate, K. E. (1994). Decision Support in Medicine: Examples from the HELP System. *Computers & Biomedical Research, 27,* 396-418.

Hayter, M. A. et al. Variations in early and intermediate neonatal outcomes for inborn infants admitted to a Canadian NICU and born of hypertensive pregnancies. *JOGC* submitted July 2004; MS# pending (2004).

Health Canada (n.d.). Retrieved September 13, 2007 from http://www.hc-sc.gc.ca/index_e.html

Health Information Quality Assessment Tool (n.d.). Retrieved September 8, 2007 from http://hitiweb.mitretek.org/iq/

Health Level Seven Inc. (2001). HL7 Version 3 (Draft). Retrieved 11 January, 2002, from http://www.HL7.org/Library/standards_non1.htm

Health on the Net Foundation (n.d.). Retrieved September 7, 2007 from www.hon.ch

Healthcare Commission. (2007). *Heart surgery in the United Kingdom.* Retrieved June 2008, from http://heartsurgery.healthcarecommission.org.uk

Heathfield, H., Hudson, P., Kay, S., Mackay, L., Marley, T., Nicholson, L., Peel, V., Roberts, R., & Williams, J. (1999). Issues in the multi-disciplinary assessment of healthcare information systems. Assessment of Healthcare Information Technology & People, 12(3), 253-75.

Heathfield, H., Pitty, D., & Hanka, R. (1998). Evaluating information technology in health care: barriers and challenges. British Medical Journal, 316, 1959-61.

Heavy Menstrual Bleeding - http://www.nzgg.org.nz

Heckerman, D., & Wellman, M. P. (1995). Bayesian Networks. *Communications of the ACM, 38*(3), 27-30.

Heermann, L., & Thompson, C. (1997). Prototype expert system to assist with the stabilization of neonates prior to transport. *Proc AMIA Annu Fall Symp, 0,* #VALUE!

Heintz, A. P., Hacker, N. F., Berek, J. S., Rose, T. P., Munoz, A. K., & Lagsse, L. D. (1986). Cytoreductive Surgery in Ovarian Carcinoma: Feasibility and morbidity. *Obstet Gynecol, 67,* 783

Heller, G., Misselwitz, B., & Schmidt, S. (2000). Early neonatal mortality, asphyxia related deaths, and timing of low risk births in Hesse, Germany, 1990-8: observational study. *Bmj, 321*(7256), 274-275.

Heller, G., Schnell, R., Misselwitz, B., & Schmidt, S. (2003). Why are babies born at night at increased risk of early neonatal mortality?. *Z Geburtshilfe Neonatol, 207*(4), 137-142.

Hendersen, J and N. Venktraman 1992 "Strategic Alignment: A model for organizational transformation through information technology," in T. Kochan & M. Unseem, eds, Transforming Organisations, Oxford University Press, NY,

Henderson-Smart, D., Hutchinson, J., Donoghue, D., Evans, N., Simpson, J., Wright, I., et al. (2006). Prenatal predictors of chronic lung disease in very preterm infants. *Arch Dis Child Fetal Neonatal Ed, 9*(1), F40-45.

Herbert, A., Bergeron, C., Wiener, H., Schenck, U., Klinkhamer, P., Bulten, J., et al. (2007). European guidelines for quality assurance in cervical cancer screening: Recommendations for cervical cytology terminology. *Cytopathology, 18,* 213-219.

Heritage Foundation for Medical Research Alberta (n.d.). Retrieved September 8, 2007, from http://www.ihe.ca/documents/hta/HTA-FR13.pdf

Heuchan, A., Evans, N., Henderson, S., D. J., & Simpson, J. (2002). Perinatal risk factors for major intraventricular haemorrhage in the Australian and New Zealand Neonatal Network, 1995-97. *Arch Dis Child Fetal Neonatal Ed, 8*(2), F86-90.

Hewson, M., & Hewson, P. (2008). *NICU Tools. A free source of browser-based neonatal and infant calculators.* Retrieved June 2008, from http://www.nicutools.org/

Highwire (n.d.). Retrieved September 14, 2007 from http://highwire.stanford.edu/lists/freeart.dtl

HL 7 Web site: www.hl7.0rg

Ho, L., McGhee, S., Hedley, A., & Leong, J. (1999). The application of a computerized problem-oriented medical record system and its impact on patient care. *International Journal of Medical Informatics, 55*(1), 47-59.

Hofer, C 1975 "Toward a Contingency Theory of Business Strategy" Academy of Management, vol 18, no.4 pp.784-810.

Hole, D. J., & Gillis, C. R. (1993). Use of cancer registry data to evaluate the treatment of ovarian cancer on a hospital basis. Health Reports, 5(1), 117-119.

Holliday I & Tam W (2004), eHealth in the East Asian tigers. Int J Medical Informatics (article in press).

Honey, M., Øyri, K., Newbold, S., Coenen, A., Park, H., Ensio, A., et al. (2007). *Effecting change by the use of emerging technologies in healthcare: A future vision for u-nursing in 2020.* Paper presented at the Health Informatics New Zealand (HINZ), 6th Annual Forum., Rotorua.

Hong Kong College of Obstetricians and Gynaecologists (n.d.). Retrieved September 14, 2007 from http://www.hkcog.org.hk/

Horbar, J. D., Rogowski, J., Plsek, P. E. et al. (2001). Investigators of the Vermont, Oxford Network, Collaborative quality improvement for neonatal intensive care, NIC/Q Project. *Pediatrics, 10*(1), 14-22.

Horwood, A., & Richards, F. (1988). Implementing a Maternity Computer System. *Mid Chron Nurs Notes,* (11), 356-357.

Horwood, A., & Richards, F. (1988). Implementing a Maternity Computer System. *Mid Chron Nurs Notes*(11), 356-357.

Hoskins, W. (1993). Surgical staging and cytoreductive surgery of epithelial ovarian cancer. *Cancer, 71,* 1534-40.

Hoskins, W., Rice, L., & Rubin, S. (1997). Ovarian cancer surgical practice guidelines. *Oncology, 11,* 896-904.

http://www.cancercare.on.ca/pdf/ovarianIndicatorsSummary.pdf (7 July 2007)

http://www.fsrh.org/Default2.asp?Section=Publications&SubSection=FACTS

http://www.nsu.govt.nz/Health-Professionals/1060.asp

Huff, S. M., Rocha, R. A., McDonald, C. J., De Moor, G. J. E., Fiers, T., Bidgood, W. D., Jr., et al. (1998). Development of the Logical Observation Identifier Names and Codes (LOINC) Vocabulary. *J Am Med Inform Assoc, 5*(3), 276-292.

Hunter, R. W., Alexander, N. D. E., & Soutter, W. P. (1992). Meta-analysis of surgery in advanced ovarian carcinoma: Is maximum cytoreductive surgery an independent determinant of prognosis? *AJOG, 166,* 504-11.

Hutchinson, M. (1996). Assessing the costs and benefits of alternative rescreening strategies. *Acta Cytol, 40*, 39664.

Hutchinson, M., Zahniser, D., Sherman, M., Herrero, R., Alfaro, M., Bratti, M., et al. (1999). Utility of liquid-based cytology for cervical carcinoma screening. *Cancer, 87*, 48-55.

IHTSDO Web site: www.ihtsdo.org/

Ikemba, C., Kozinetz, C., Feltes, T., Fraser, C., Jr., McKenzie, E., Shah, N., et al. (2002). Internet use in families with children requiring cardiac surgery for congenital heart disease. *Pediatrics, 10*(3), 419-422.

Iliakovidis I, Wilson P & Healy JC (2004), eHealth. Current situation and examples of implemented and beneficial e-health applications. IOS Press, Studies in Health Technology and Informatics, Amsterdam, The Netherlands.

ImagesMD (n.d.). Retrieved September 14, 2007 from http://www.images.md/

Implementing an Electronic Health Record System (Health Informatics) by James M. Walker, Eric J. Bieber, Frank Richards, and Sandra Buckley

Institute of Medicine. (2001). Crossing the Quality Chasm: A New Health System for the 21st Century. Washington: National Academy Press.

International Breastfeeding Journal (n.d.). Retrieved September 14, 2007 from http://www.internationalbreast-feedingjournal.com/

International Midwifery - http://www.internationalmidwives.org

International Society for the Study of Vulvovaginal Diseases (n.d.). Retrieved September 14, 2007 from http://www.issvd.org/

International Society for the Study of Women's Sexual Health (n.d.). Retrieved September 14, 2007 from http://www.isswsh.org/

International Views - http://who.int/en/

Intute, medicine section (n.d.). Retrieved September 14, 2007 from http://www.intute.ac.uk/healthandlifesciences/medicine/

Intute, nursing and midwifery section (n.d.). Retrieved September 14, 2007 from http://www.intute.ac.uk/healthandlifesciences/nursing/

Ioka, A., Tsukuma, H., Ajiki, W., & Oshima, A. (2004). Influence of hospital procedure volume on ovarian cancer survival in Japan, a country with low incidence of ovarian cancer. *Cancer Sci, 95*(3), 233-237.

ISO, Why standards matter? http://www.iso.org/iso/en/aboutiso/introduction/index.html#one, accessed on February, 11 2005.

Johanson, R., Newburn, M., & Macfarlane, A. (2002). Has the medicalisation of childbirth gone too far? *Bmj, 324*(7342), 892-895.

Johnston, H. R., & Vitale, M. R. (1988). Creating Competitive Advantage with Interorganizational Information Systems. *MIS Quarterly, 12*(2), 153-165.

Johnston, M. E., Langton, K. B., Haynes, R. B., & Mathieu, A. (1994). Effects of computer-based clinical decision support systems on clinician performance and patient outcome. A critical appraisal of research. *Ann Intern Med, 120(2)*, 135-142.

Johnston, M., Langton, K., Haynes, R., & Mathieu, A. (1994). Effects of Computer-based Clinical Decision Support Systems on Clinician Performance and Patient Outcome - A Critical Appraisal of Research. Annuals of Internal Medicine, 120, 135-42.

Jones R, Balfour F, Gillies M, Stobo D, Cawsey AJ & Donaldson K (2001), The accessibility of computer-based health information for patients: Kiosks and the Web. Medical Information 10, 1469-73.

Jones, B., Peake, K., Morris, A., McCowan, L., & Battin, M. (2004). Escherichia coli: A growing problem in early onset neonatal sepsis. *Aust N Z J Obstet Gynaecol, 44*(6), 558-561.

Jones, B., Valenstein, P., & Steindel, S. (1999). Gynecologic cytology turnaround time. A College of American Pathologists Q-Probes Study of 371 laboratories. *Arch Pathol Lab Med, 123*, 682-686.

Jones, R. W., Coughlan, E., Reid, J. S., Sykes, P., Watson, P. D., & Cook, C. (2007). Human papilloma virus vaccines and their role in cancer prevention. *Journal of the New Zealand Medical Association, 120*(1266), U2829.

Joste, N., Crum, C., & Cibas, E. (1995). Cytologic/histologic correlation for quality control in cervicovaginal cytology. Experience with 1,582 paired cases. *Am J Clin Pathol, 103*, 32-34.

Journal - Artificial Intelligence in Medicine

Junor, E. (2000). The impact of specialist training for surgery in ovarian cancer. *Int J Gynecol Cancer, 10*(Supp 1), 16-18.

Junor, E. J., Hole, D. J., & Gillis, C. R. (1994). Management of ovarian cancer: Referral to a multidisciplinary team matters. *Br J Cancer, 70,* 363-370.

Junor, E. J., Hole, D. J., McNulty, L., Mason, M., & Young, J. (1999). Specialist gynecologists and survival outcome in ovarian cancer: a Scottish national study of 1866 patients. *Br J Obstet Gynecol, 106,* 1130-1136.

Junor, E. J., Hole, D. J., McNulty, L., Mason, M., & Young, J. (1999). Specialist gynecologists and survival outcome in ovarian cancer: A Scottist national study of 1866 patients. *Br J Obstet Gynecol, 106*(11), 1130-6.

Kant, I. (1785). *Groundwork of the metaphysics of morals*

Kantor, G. S., Wilson, W. D., & Midgley, A. (2003). Open-source software and the primary care EMR. *Journal of the American Medical Informatics Association, 10*(6), 616.

Kaplan, B. (2001). Evaluating informatics applications - clinical decision support systems literature review. International Journal of Medical Informatics, 64, 15-37.

Kaplan, B. (2001). Evaluating informatics applications-some alternative approaches: theory, social interactionism, and call for methodological pluralism. International Journal of Medical Informatics 64, 39-56.

Kaplan, B., & Shaw, N. (2002). People, Organizational and Social Issues: Evaluation as an exemplar. In R. Haux & C. Kulikowski (Eds.), Yearbook of Medical Informatics 2002 (pp. 91 - 102). Stuttgart: Schattauer.

Katz, N. Lazer, D. Arrow, H. & Contractor, N. (2004). Network Theory and Small Groups. Small Group Research, **35**(3), 307-332.

Kawamoto, K., Houlihan, C. A., Balas, E. A., & Lobach, D. F. (2005). Improving clinical practice using clinical decision support systems: A systematic review of trials to identify features critical to success. *BMJ, 330*(7494), 765-.

Kayongo, M., Rubardt, M. et al. (2006). Making EmOC a reality--CARE's experiences in areas of high maternal mortality in Africa. *International Journal of Gynaecology and Obstetrics, 92*(3), 308-19.

Keene, R., & Cullen, D. (1983). Therapeutic Intervention Scoring System: Update 1983. *Critical Care Medicine 11*(1), 1-3.

Kehoe, S., Powell, J., Wilson, S., & Woodman, C. (1994). The influence of the operating surgeon's specialization on patient survival in ovarian carcinoma. *Br J Cancer, 70,* 1014-1017.

Keith, R. D., Beckley, S., Garibaldi, J. M., Westgate, J. A., Ifeachor, E. C., & Greene, K. R. (1995). A multicentre comparative study of 17 experts and an intelligent computer system for managing labour using the cardiotocogram. *Br J Obstet Gynaecol, 102*(9), 688-700.

Kennedy, J., Kennedy, J., & Eberhart, R. (1995). *Particle swarm optimization*

Kenney, N., & Macfarlane, A. (1999). Identifying problems with data collection at a local level: survey of NHS maternity units in England. *BMJ, 319*(7210), 619-622.

Kerbrat, P., Lhomme, C., Fervers, B., Guastalla, J. P., Thomas, L., Tournemaine, N., et al. (2001). Ovarian cancer. *British Journal of Cancer, 84*(Suppl2), 18-23.

Khoshdel, A., Attia, J., & Carnery, S. L. (2006). Basic concepts in meta-analysis: a primer for clinicians. *International Journal of Clinical Practice, 60.10,* 1287-94.

Kikkawa, F., Ishikawa, H., Tamakoshi, K., Suganuma, N., Mizuno, K., Kawai, M. et al. (1995). Prognostic evaluation of lymphadenectomy for epithelial ovarian cancer. *J Surg Oncol, 60,* 227-231.

Kirchner, L., Weninger, M., Unterasinger, L., Birnbacher, R., Hayde, M., Krepler, et al. (2005). Is the use of early nasal CPAP associated with lower rates of chronic lung disease and retinopathy of prematurity? Nine years of experience with the Vermont Oxford Neonatal Network. *J Perinat Med, 33*(1), 60-66.

Kirshbaum, M. N. (2004). Are we ready for the Electronic Patient Record? Attitudes and perceptions of staff from two NHS trust hospitals. *Health Informatics Journal, 10*(4), 265-276.

Kleiner KD, Akers R, Burke BL & Werner EJ (2002), Parent and physician attitudes regarding electronic communication in pediatric practices. Pediatrics 109 (5), 740-744 Larner AJ (2002), Use of the Internet medical websites and NHS Direct by neurology outpatients before consultation. Int J Clin Pract 56(3), 219-221.

Klimek, J., Morley, C., Lau, R., & Davis, P. (2006). Does measuring respiratory function improve neonatal ventilation? *J Paediatr Child Health, 42,* 140-142.

Kline, T. (1997). The challenge of quality improvement with the Papanicolaou smear. *Arch Pathol Lab Med, 121,* 253-255.

Knafl, K., & Breitmayer, B. (1991). Triangulation in qualitative research: Issues of conceptual clarity and purpose. In J. Morse (Ed.), A contemporary dialogue (pp. 226-239). Newbury Park, California: Sage.

Kohlenberg, C. F. (1994). Computerization of Obstetric Antenatal Histories. *Aust NZ J Obstet Gynaecol, 34*(5), 520-524.

Kohlenberg, C. F. (1994). Computerization of Obstetric Antenatal Histories. *Aust NZ J Obstet Gynaecol, 34*(5), 520-524.

Kramer, M. S. et al. (2001). A new and improved population-based Canadian reference for birth weight for gestational age. *Pediatrics, 108.2*, E35.

Kumar, D., Super, D., Fajardo, R., Stork, E., Moore, J., & Saker, F. (2004). Predicting outcome in neonatal hypoxic respiratory failure with the score for neonatal acute physiology (SNAP) and highest oxygen index (OI) in the first 24 hours of admission. *J Perinatol, 24*(6), 376-381.

Kumar, N., & Jain, S. (2004). Quality control and automation in cervical cytology. *J Indian Med Assoc, 102*, 372, 374.

Kumpulainen, S., Grenman, S., Kyyronen, P., Pukkala, E., & Sankila, R. (2002). Evidence of benefit from centralized treatment of ovarian cancer: A nationwide population-based survival analysis in Finland. *Int J Cancer, 102*, 541-544.

La Monica, M. (October 2000). "Building trust into e-business models," InfoWorld, 22(28): 3.

Laflamme, M. R., Dexter, P. R., Graham, M. F., Hui, S. L., & McDonald, C. J. (2005). Efficiency, comprehensiveness and cost-effectiveness when comparing dictation and electronic templates for operative reports. *AMIA Annu Symp Proc.*, 425-9.

Land, R., Parry, E., Rane, A., & Wilson, D. (2001). Personal preferences of obstetricians towards childbirth. *Aust N Z J Obstet Gynaecol, 41*(3), 249-252.

Lau, T. K. (2007). *3D Aids Biometry Skills*. Paper presented at the ISUOG.

Lauer, J. A., & Betran, A. P. (2007). Decision aids for women with a previous caesarean section. *BMJ, 334*(7607), 1281-1282.

Laughon, M., Bose, A., & Clark, R. (2007). Treatment strategies to prevent or close a patent ductus arteriosus in preterm infants and outcomes. *Journal of Perinatology, 27*, 164-170.

Le, T., Adolph, A., Krepart, G. V., Lotocki, R., Heywood, M. S. (2002). The benefits of comprehensive surgical staging in the management of early-stage epithelial ovarian carcinoma. *Gynecologic Oncology, 85*, 351-5.

Leblanc, E., Querleu, D., Narducci, F., Chauvet, M. P., Chevalier, A., Lesoin, A., et al. (2000). Surgical staging of early invasive epithelial ovarian tumors. *Seminars in Surgical Oncology, 19*, 36-41.

Lee, E., Kim, I., Choi, J., & et al. (2003). Accuracy and reproducibility of telecytology diagnosis of cervical smears. A tool for quality assurance programs. *Am J Clin Pathol, 119*, 356-360.

Lee, J., Kuan, L., Oh, S., Patten, F., & Wilbur, D. (1998). A feasibility study of the AutoPap System Location-Guided Screening. *Acta Cytol, 421*, 221-226.

Lee, K., Ashfaq, R., Birdsong, G., Corkill, M., McIntosh, K., & Inhorn, S. (1997). Comparison of conventional Papanicolaou smears and a fluid-based, thin-layer system for cervical cancer screening. *Obstet Gynecol, 90*, 278-287.

Lee, S. K. et al. (2000). Variations in practice and outcomes in the Canadian NICU network: 1996-1997. *Pediatrics, 106.5*,1070-79.

Lee, S. K. et al. (2001). Evidence for changing guidelines for routine screening for retinopathy of prematurity. *Arch. Pediatr.Adolesc.Med., 155.3*, 387-95.

Lee, S., Lee, D., Andrews, W., Baboolal, R., Pendray, M., Stewart, S., et al. (2003). Higher mortality rates among inborn infants admitted to neonatal intensive care units at night. *J Pediatr, 1*(5), 592-597.

Lee, W., Deter, R. L., McNie, B., Goncalves, L. F., Espinoza, J., Chaiworapongsa, T., et al. (2004). Individualized growth assessment of fetal soft tissue using fractional thigh volume. *Ultrasound in Obstetrics and Gynecology, 24*(7), 766-774.

Lehmann, C., Conner, K., & Cox, J. (2004). Preventing provider errors: online total parenteral nutrition calculator. *Pediatrics, 113*(4), 748-753.

Leonard, M. Graham, S. Bonacum, D. (2004). The Human Factor: The Critical Importance of Effective Teamwork and Communication in Providing Safe Care, Quality and Saftey in Health Care, **13**(Suppl 1), i85-i90.

Leslie, K. O., & Rosai, J. (1994, November). Standardization of the Surgical Pathology Report: formats, templates and synoptic reports. *Sem Diag Pathology, 11*(4), 253-257.

Lewin, K. (1947). Frontiers in group dynamics: concepts, methods, and reality of social sciences: Social equalization and social change. Human Relations, 1, 5-14.

Liberati, A., Mangioni, C., Bratina, L., Carinelli, G., Marsoni, S., Parazzini, F. et al. (1885). Process and outcome of care for patients with ovarian cancer. *Br M J 291*, 1007-1012/

Liggins, G. C., & Howie, R. N. (1972). A controlled trial of antepartum glucocorticoid treatment for prevention of the respiratory distress syndrome in premature infants. *Pediatrics, 50*(4), 515-525.

Lilford, R. J., & Chard, T. (1981). Microcomputers in antenatal care: a feasibility study on the booking interview. *B Med J, 283*, 533-536.

Lilford, R. J., & Chard, T. (1981). Microcomputers in antenatal care: A feasibility study on the booking interview. *B Med J, 283*, 533-536.

Linder, J., & Zahniser, D. (1997). The ThinPrep test: A review of clinical studies. *Acta Cytol, 41*, 30-38.

Lindsey, E., & Hartrick, G. (1996). Health-promoting nursing practice: the demise of the nursing process? Journal of Advanced Nursing, 23(1), 106-112.

Littlejohns, P., Wyatt, J. C., & Garvican, L. (2003). Evaluating computerised health information systems: Hard lessons still to be learnt. *British Medical Journal, 326*(7394), 860-863.

Llewelyn, H., & Hopkins, A. (1993). *Analysing how we reach clinical decisions.* London: Royal College of Physicians

Lloyd, D., Kalra, D. (2003). EHR requirements. *Studies in Health Technology and Informatics*, 96, 231-237.

Lolock, L. Dopson, S. Chambers, D. & Gabbay, J. (2001). Understanding the role of opinion leaders in improving clinical effectiveness. Social Science and Medicine, **53**, 745-757.

Lorenzato, M., Bory, J., Cucherousset, J., Nou, J., Bouttens, D., Thil, C., et al. (2002). Usefulness of DNA ploidy measurement on liquid-based smears showing conflicting results between cytology and high-risk human papillomavirus typing. *Am J Clin Pathol, 118*, 708-713.

Lorenzi, N., & Riley, R. (1995). Organizational Aspects of Health Informatics - Managing Technological Change. New York: Springer.

Lorenzi, N.M. & Riley, R.T. (2000). Managing Change: An Overview. Journal of the American Medical Informatics Association, 7(2), 116-124.

Lorenzi, N.M. (2004). Beyond the Gadgets: Non-technological barriers to information systems need to be overcome. British Medical Journal **328**, 1146-1147.

Lorenzi, N.M. Riley, R.T. Blythe, A.J.C. Southon, G. & Dixon, B.J., (1997). Antecedents of the People and Organizational Aspects of Medical Informatics: Review of the Literature. Journal of the American Medical Informatics Association, **4**(2), 79-93.

Loudon, I. (2000). Maternal mortality in the past and its relevance to developing countries today. *American Journal of Clinical Nutrition, 72(suppl)*, 241S–246S.

Louwerse, K. (2002). Demonstration results for the standard ENV 12924. *Studies in Health Technology and Informatics*, 69,111-139; discussion 229-237.

Love, D. et al. Data Sharing and Dissemination Strategies for Fostering Competition in Health Care. *Health Services Research, 36.1*, 277-90.

Lowry, C. (1994). Nurses' attitudes toward computerised care plans in intensive care. Part 2. Intensive and Critical Care Nursing, 10, 2-11.

Lozano, R. (2007). Comparison of computer-assisted and manual screening of cervical cytology. *Gynecol Oncol, 104*, 134-138.

Lyytinen, K., and Rose, G. M. (2003). The Disruptive Nature of Information Technology Innovations: The Case of Internet Computing in Systems Development Organizations. MIS Quarterly, 27(4), 557-595.

Macdonald, D., Grant, A., Sheridan-Pereira, M., Boylan, P., & Chalmers, I. (1985). The Dublin randomized controlled trial of intrapartum fetal heart rate monitoring. *American Journal of Obstetrics and Gynecology, 152*, 524-539.

MacDowell, M., Somoza, E., Rothe, K., Frye, R., Brady, K., & Bocklet, A. (2001). Understanding Birthing Mode Decision Making Using Artificial Neural Networks. *Med Decis Making, 21*(6), 433-443.

MacIntyre, A. (1985). *After Virtue, 2nd edition.* Duckworth Press

Magee, L. A., Cote, A. M., & von Dadelszen, P. (2005). Nifedipine for severe hypertension in pregnancy: Emotion or evidence? *J. Obstet. Gynaecol. Can., 27.3*, 260-62.

Magrabi, F. Westbrook, J.I. Coiera, E. W. & Gosling, A.S. (2004). Clinicians' Assessments of the Usefulness of Online Evidence to Answer Clinical Questions. Proceedings of the 11th World Congress on Medical Informatics, 297-300.

Mählck, C. G., Jonsson, H. et al. (1994). Pap smear screening and changes in cervical cancer mortality in

Sweden. *International Journal of Gynaecology and Obstetrics, 44*(3), 267-72.

Main, D. S., Quintela, J., Araya-Guerra, R., Holcomb, S., & Pace, W. D. (2004). Exploring Patient Reactions to Pen-Tablet Computers: A Report from CaReNet. *Ann Fam Med, 2*(5), 421-424.

Maldonado, J.A., Crespo, P., Sanchis, A., Robles, M. (2004). Pangea: a mediator for the integration of distributed electronic healthcare records. *Medinfo 2004,* (CD),1738.

Mango, L., & Valente, P. (1998). Neural-network-assisted analysis and microscopic rescreening in presumed negative cervical cytologic smears A comparison. *Acta Cytol, 42,* 227-232.

Manrique, E., Amaral, R., Souza, N., Tavares, S., Albuquerque, Z., & Zeferino, L. (2006). Evaluation of 100% rapid rescreening of negative cervical smears as a quality assurance measure. *Cytopathology, 17,* 116-120.

Marcelo, A., Fontelo, P., Farolan, M., & Cualing, H. (2000). Effect of image compression on telepathology. A randomized clinical trial. *Arch Pathol Lab Med, 124*(11), 1653-1656.

Marchevsky, A., Khurana, R., Thomas, P., Scharre, K., Farias, P., & Bose, S. (2006). The use of virtual microscopy for proficiency testing in gynecologic cytopathology: A feasibility study using ScanScope. *Arch Pathol Lab Med, 130,* 349-355.

Marchevsky, A., Wan, Y., Thomas, P., Krishnan, L., Evans-Simon, H., & Haber, H. (2003). Virtual microscopy as a tool for proficiency testing in cytopathology: A model using multiple digital images of Papanicolaou tests. *Arch Pathol Lab Med, 127,* 1320-1324.

Marley, T. (2002). Standards supporting interoperability and EHCR communication--a CEN TC251 perspective. *Studies in Health Technology and Informatics,* 87,72-77.

Marrett, L., Dryer, D., Logan, H. et al. (2007). *Canadian Cancer Statistics 2007.*

Marsan, C. (1995). Quality control in cytopathology applied to screening for cervical carcinoma. *Pol J Pathol, 46,* 245-248.

Martin, P., & Kauser, A. (2001). An informaticist working in primary care: A descriptive study. *Health Informatics Journal, 7*(2), 66-70.

Martins, E., & Morse, L. (2005). Evaluation of internet websites about retinopathy of prematurity patient education. *Br J Ophthalmol, 8*(5), 565-568.

Masood, S., Cajulis, R., Cibas, E., Wilbur, D., & Bedrossian, C. (1998). Automation in cytology: a survey conducted by the New Technology Task Force, Papanicolaou Society of Cytopathology. *Diagn Cytopathol, 18,* 47-55.

Mayer, A. R., Chambers, S. K., Graves, E., Holm, C., Tseng, P. C., Nelson, B. E. et al. (1992). Ovarian cancer staging: Does it require a gynecologic oncologist? *Gyn Oncol, 47,* 223-227

Mayring, M. (1993). Einführung in die qualitative Sozialforschung. Weinheim: Psychologie-Verlag-Union.

McDonald, C. J., Schadow, G., Barnes, M., Dexter, P., Overhage, J. M., Mamlin, B., et al. (2003). Open Source software in medical informatics--why, how and what. *International Journal of Medical Informatics, 69*(2-3), 175-184.

Mcgilchrist, M., Sullivan, F., & Kalra, D. Assuring the confidentiality of shared electronic health records. *British Medical Journal, 335,* 1223-24.

McIntosh, N., Becher, J., Cunningham, S., Stenson, B., Laing, I., Lyon, A., et al. (2000). Clinical diagnosis of pneumothorax is late: use of trend data and decision support might allow preclinical detection. *Pediatr Res, 48*(3), 408-415.

Medical University of South Carolina, podcasts (n.d.). Retrieved September 15, 2007 from http://www.muschealth.com/multimedia/Podcasts/index.aspx?type=topic&groupid=3

Medline/Pubmed(n.d.).RetrievedSeptember13,2007from http://www.ncbi.nlm.nih.gov/sites/entrez?db=PubMed

Menzies, J. et al. Instituting surveillance guidelines and adverse outcomes in preeclampsia. *Obstet.Gynecol., 110.1,*121-27.

Michnikowski, M., Rudowski, R., Siugocki, P., Grabowski, J., & Rondio, Z. (1997). Evaluation of the expert system for respiratory therapy of newborns on archival data. *Int J Artif Organs, 20*(12), 678–680.

Miller, F., Nagel, L., & Kenny-Moynihan, M. (2007). Implementation of the ThinPrep imaging system in a high-volume metropolitan laboratory. *Diagn Cytopathol, 35,* 213-217.

Mills, J. S. (1861). *Utilitarianism.*

Mitchell, E., & Sullivan, F. (2001). A descriptive feast but an evaluative famine: systematic review of published articles on primary care computing during 1980-97. *BMJ, 322*(7281), 279-282.

Moehr, J. R. (2002). Evaluation: salvation or nemesis of medical informatics? Comput Biol Med, 32(3), 113-25.

Montgomery, A. A., Emmett, C. L., Fahey, T., Jones, C., Ricketts, I., Patel, R. R., et al. (2007). Two decision aids for mode of delivery among women with previous caesarean section: randomised controlled trial. *BMJ, 334*(7607), 1305-.

Moore's law: past, present and future. *Spectrum, IEEE, 34*(6), 52-59.

Morgan, R. J., Copeland, L., Gershenson, D., et al. (1996). NCCN Ovarian Cancer Practice Guidelines. *Oncology, 10*, 293-310.

Muir Gray, J. A. (2006). Best Current Evidence: Concepts and Plans (pp. 5-28). National Health Services.

Mulford, D. (2006). Telepathology education: reaching out to cytopathology progrmas throughout the country. *ASC Bulletin, 43*, 25-30.

Munoz, K. A., Harlan, L. C., & Trimble, E. L. (1997). Patterns of care for women with ovarian cancer in the United States. *JCO,15*(11), 3408-3415.

Munro, E. G., Cheung, M. K., Husain, A., Teng, N. N., Chan, J. K., Leiserowitz, G. S., & Osann, K. (2006). The survival benefit of lymph node dissection in stage 1 epithelial ovarian cancer. *Gyn Onc 101*(S27), Abstract 59.

Musen, M. (2001). *Creating and using Ontologies: What informatics is all about.* Paper presented at the Medinfo 2001, London.

National Health and Medical Research Council, Australia (n.d.). Retrieved September 13, 2007 from http://www.nhmrc.gov.au/publications/subjects/women.htm

National Institute of Health. (1994). *Ovarian cancer: screening, treatment and follow-up,12*, 1-30.(Abstract).

National Library of Medicine, US (n.d.). Retrieved September 13, 2007 from www.nlm.nih.gov

National Screening Unit, New Zealand (n.d.). Retrieved September 13, 2007 from

Nelson, S., Schopen, M. J. S. & N., A. (2001). *An Interlingual Database of MeSH Translations.* Retrieved October, 2003, from http://www.nlm.nih.gov/mesh/intlmesh.html

New Zealand Guidelines Group (n.d.). Retrieved August 18, 2007 from http://www.nzgg.org.nz

New Zealand Privacy Commissioner. (1994). Health Information Privacy Code 1994. Retrieved June 2008, from http://www.privacy.org.nz/health-information-privacy-code-1994/

Nguyen, H. N., Averette, H. E., Hoskins, W., Penalver, M., Sevin, B. U., & Steren, A. (1993). National Survey of ovarian carcinoma Part V. *Cancer, 72*, 3663-70.

NHS Airdale Trust v Bland 1993).

NHS Information Authority, The Consumers association, & Health Which. (2002). *Share and Care! Peoples views on consent and confidentiality of patient information.*

Nickell, G., & Pinto, J. (1986). The Computer Attitude Scale. Computers in Human Behaviour, 2, 301-306.

Nicoll, A., Hutchinson, E., Soldan, K., McGarrigle, C., Parry, J. V., Newham, J., et al. (1994). Survey of human immunodeficiency virus infection among pregnant women in England and Wales: 1990-93. *Communicable Disease Report. CDR Review, 4*(10), R115-120.

NIH Consensus Development Panel on Ovarian Cancer. (1995). Ovarian cancer: screening, treatment, and follow-up. *JAMA, 273*, 491-497.

NIH. (2003). Guidance on the use of paclitaxel in the treatment of ovarian cancer.

NLH Women's Health Specialist Library - www.library.nhs.uk/womenshealth

Noone, J., Warren, J., & Brittain, M. (1998). *Information overload: opportunities and challenges for the GP's desktop.* Paper presented at the Medinfo 9.

Norris, A. C., & Brittain, J. M. (2000). Education, training and the development of healthcare informatics. *Health Informatics Journal, 6*(4), 189-195.

Noy, N., Sintek, M., Decker, S., Crubézy, M., Ferguson, R., & Musen, M. (2001). Creating Semantic Web Contents with Protégé-2000. *IEEE Intelligent Systems*(March/April), 60-71.

Nykänen P & Karimaa E (2004), Success and failure factors during development of a regional health information system - results from a constructive evaluation study. Submitted for Methods of Information in Medicine.

O'Connor, R. A. (1994). Induction of labour - not how but why? *British. Journal. of. Hospital. Medicine., 52*(11), 559-563.

O'Leary, T., Tellado, M., Buckner, S., Ali, I., Stevens, A., & Ollayos, C. (1998). PAPNET-assisted rescreening of cervical smears: cost and accuracy compared with a 100% manual rescreening strategy. *JAMA, 279*, 235-279.

O'Neil, M. P., & Read, C. J. (1995). Read Codes Version 3: A User Led Terminology. *Methods of Information in Medicine, 34*(1/2), 187-192.

Oates, M. (2003). Suicide: the leading cause of maternal death. *British Journal of Psychiatry, 183*, 279-81.

Oberaigner, W., & Stuhlinger, W. (2006). Influence of department volume on cancer survival for gynecological cancers-A population-based study in Tyrol, Austria. *103*, 527-534.

Odd, D., Battin, M., & Kuschel, C. (2004). Variation in identifying neonatal percutaneous central venous line position. *J Paediatr Child Health, 40*(39730), 540-543.

Office for Civil Rights. (2006). Office for Civil Rights - Privacy of Health Records. Retrieved June 2008, from http://www.hhs.gov/ocr/hipaa/privacy.html

Ohmann, C., Boy, O., & Yang, Q. (1997). A systematic approach to the assessment of user satisfaction with health care systems: constructs, models and instruments. In C. Pappas (Ed.), Medical Informatics Europe ,97. Conference proceedings (Vol. 43 Pt B, pp. 781-5). Amsterdam: IOS Press.

Oksefjell, H., Sandstad, B., & Trope, C. (2006). Ovarian cancer stage 3C. Consequences of treatment level on overall and progression-free survival. *Eur J Gynecol Oncol, 27*(3), 209-14.

Olaitin, A., Weeks, J., Mocroft, A., Smith, J., Howe, K., & Murdoch, J. (2001, December 14). The surgical management of women with ovarian cancer in the south west of England. *Br J Cancer, 85*(12), 1824-30.

Oliver, K. B., & Roderer, N. K. (2006). Working towards the informationist. *Health Informatics Journal, 12*(1), 41-48.

openEHR Foundation. (2007). Welcome to openEHR. Retrieved 1st April 2008, from http://www.openehr.org/home.html

Oxford University Press E-journals (n.d.). Retrieved September 14, 2007 from http://www.oxfordjournals.org/

Ozols, R. F., Morgan, R. J., Copeland, L., & Gershenson, D. (1997). Update of the NCCN Ovarian Cancer Practice Guidelines. *Oncology, 11*, 95-100.

PACS and Imaging Informatics: Basic Principles and Applications by H. K. Huang - 2004

Palcic, B., Sun, X., & Wang, J. (2007). Automated screening for cervical cancer in developing countries (abstract). *Acta Cytologica, 51*(suppl 2), 265.

Palvia, S., Sharma, R., & Conrath, D. (2001). A socio-technical framework for quality assessment of computer information systems. Industrial Management & Data Systems, 101(5), 237-251.

Pantanowitz, L., Henricks, W., & Beckwith, B. (2007). Medical laboratory informatics. *Clinics in Laboratory Medicine, 77*, In press.

Papillo, J., Zarka, M., & St., J., TL. (1998). Evaluation of the ThinPrep Pap test in clinical practice. *Acta Cytol, 42*, 203-208.

Pardey, J., Moulden, M., & Redman, C. W. (2002). A computer system for the numerical analysis of nonstress tests. *American Journal of Obstetrics and Gynecology, 186*(5), 1095-1103.

Park, R. (2007). Picturing change – enhancing every pathology report with images. *ASC Bulletin, 44*, Sep-22.

Parker, M., & Lucassen, A. (2004). Genetic information: A joint account? *BMJ, 329*, 165-167.

Parliamentary reporter. (2007). Three million records lost in another government data scandal. *Computing, 18*, Dec. 2007.

Parry, D. T. (2006). Evaluation of a fuzzy ontology based medical information system. *International journal of Health Information Systems and Informatics, 1*(1), 40-49.

Parry, D. T., Parry, E. C., Chebi, A., Dorji, P., & Stone, P. (2008 (in press)). Open source software – a key component of E-Health in Developing nations. *International Journal of Health Information Systems and Informatics.*

Parry, D. T., Yeap, W. K., & Pattison, N. (1998). Using Rough Sets to study expert behaviour in induction of labour. *Australian Journal of Intelligent Information Processing Systems, 5*(3), 219-225.

Parry, E. C., Parry, D. T. et al. (1998). Induction of Labour for post term pregnancy: An observational study. *Aust NZ J Obstet Gynaecol, 38*(3), 275-279.

Parry, E. C., Parry, D. T., & Pattison, N. (1999). Induction of labour for post-term pregnancy: an observational study. *Australian and New Zealand Journal of Obstetrics and Gynaecology, 38*(3), 275-279.

Parry, E. C., Parry, D. T., & Pattison, N. (1999). Induction of labour for post-term pregnancy: an observational study. *Australian and New Zealand Journal of Obstetrics and Gynaecology, 38*(3), 275-279.

Parry, E. C., Sood, R., & Parry, D. T. (2006). Investigation of optimization techniques to prepare ultrasound images for electronic transfer [Abstract]. *Ultrasound in Obstetrics and Gynecology, 28*(4), 487-488(482).

Parry, G., Gould, C., McCabe, C., & Tarnow-Mordi, W. (1998). Annual league tables of mortality in neonatal intensive care units: longitudinal study - International Neonatal Network and the Scottish Neonatal Consultants and Nurses Collaborative Study Group. *BMJ, 316*(7149), 1931-1935.

Parry, G., Tucker, J., & Tarnow-Mordi, W. (2003). Neonatal Staffing Study Collaborative Group, CRIB, II: An update of the clinical risk index for,babies score. *Lancet, 361*(9371), 1789-1791.

Particle swarm optimization. Paper presented at the Neural Networks, 1995. Proceedings IEEE International Conference

Patrick, J., Wang, Y., & Budd, P. (2007). *An automated system for conversion of clinical notes into SNOMED clinical terminology.* Paper presented at the Conference Name|. Retrieved Access Date|. from URL|.

Patrick, J., Wang, Y., & Budd, P. (2007). *An automated system for conversion of clinical notes into SNOMED clinical terminology.* Paper presented at the Conference Name|. Retrieved Access Date|. from URL|.

Patten Jr., S., Lee, J., & Nelson, A. (1996). NeoPath AutoPap 300 Automatic Screener System. *Acta Cytol, 40,* 45-52.

Patterson, E.S. Nguyen, A.D. Halloran, J.P. & Asch, S.M. (2004) Human Factors Barriers to the Effective Use of Ten HIV Clinical Reminders. Journal of the American Informatics Association, **11**(1), 50-59

Peleg, M., & Tu, S. (2006). Decision support, knowledge representation and management in medicine. *Methods Inf Med, 45*(Suppl 1), 72-80.

Peleg, M., Tu, S., Bury, J., Ciccarese, P., & al., e. (2003). Comparing computer-interpretable guideline models: A case-study approach. Journal of the American Medical Informatics Association 52. *Journal of the American Medical Informatics Association,, 10*(1), 52-69.

Pello, L. C., Rosevear, S. K., Dawes, G. S., Moulden, M., & Redman, C. W. (1991). Computerized fetal heart rate analysis in labor. *Obstet Gynecol, 78*(4), 602-610.

Pena-Reyes, C. A., & Sipper, M. (2000). Evolutionary computation in medicine: an overview. *Artificial Intelligence in Medicine, 19*(1), 1-23.

Penn, D. L., Burns, J. R., Georgiou, A., Davies, P. G. P., & Harris, M. F. (2004). Evolution of a register recall system to enable the delivery of better quality of care in general practice. *Health Informatics Journal, 10*(3), 165-176.

Penz, J. F., Carter, J.S., Elkin, P.L., Nguyen, V.N., Sims, S.A., & Lincoln, M. J. (2004). *Evaluation of SNOMED coverage of Veterans Health Administration terms.* Paper presented at the Medinfo. Amsterdam.

Personal Information and Electronic Documents Act (PIPEDA), (2001).

Petignat, P., Vajda, D., Joris, F., & Obrist, R. (2000). Surgical management of epithelial ovarian cancer at community hospitals: A population-based study. *Journal of Surgical Oncology, 75,* 19-23

Petru, E., Lahousen, M., Tamussino, K., Pickel, H., Stranzl, H., Stettner, H. et al. (1994). Lymphadenectomy in stage 1 ovarian cancer. *AJOG, 170,* 656-62.

Picture Archiving and Communications System (PACS) - NHS www.connectingforhealth.nhs.uk/systemsandservices/pacs

Piver, N., & Baker, T. (1986). The potential for optimal (<2cm) cytoreductive surgery in advanced ovarian carcinoma at a tertiary medical center; a prospective study. *Gyn Onc, 24,* 1-8.

Poissant, L., Pereira, J., Tamblyn, R., & Kawasumi, Y. (2005). The Impact of Electronic Health Records on Time Efficiency of Physicians and Nurses: A Systematic Review. *Journal of the American Medical Informatics Association, 12*(5), 505-516.

Poissant, L., Perira, J., Tamblyn, R., & Kawasumi, Y. (2005). The impact of electronic health record on time efficiency of physicians and nurses: A Systematic Overview. *Journal of the American Medical Informatics Association, 12,* 505-516.

Porter, M and E. Teisberg 2004 "Redefining Competition in Healthcare" Harvard Business Review pp. 65-76 June.

Porter, M. 1980 Competitive Strategy New York Free Press

Porter, M. 1985 Competitive Advantage, New York free Press.

Potts HWW & Wyatt JC (2002), Survey of doctors' experience of patients using the Internet. J Med Internet Res 4(1), e5.

Powell J & Clarke A (2002), The WWW of the World Wide Web: Who, what and why. J Med Internet Res 18, 4(1), e4.

Prendiville, W. J., Elbourne, D., & McDonald, S. (2001). Active versus expectant management in the third stage of labour *Journal,* (Issue 4),

Pritt, B., Gibson, P., & Cooper, K. (2003). Digital imaging guidelines for pathology: a proposal for general and academic use. *Adv Anat Pathol, 10,* 96-100.

PsychInfo (n.d.). Retrieved September 14, 2007 from http://www.apa.org/psycinfo/

Puls, C, R., Morrow, M. S., & Blackhurst, D. (1997, November). Stage I ovarian carcinoma: Specialty-related differences in survival and management. *South Med J., 90*(11), 1097-100.

Raab, S., , Z., MS., , T., PA., , N., TH., , I., C., & , J., CS. (1996). Telecytology: diagnostic accuracy in cervical-vaginal smears. *Am J Clin Pathol, 105,* 599-603.

Raab, S., Grzybicki, D., Zarbo, R., Meier, F., Geyer, S., & Jensen, C. (2005). Anatomic pathology databases and patient safety. *Arch Pathol Lab Med, 129,* 1246-1251.

Reid, P. R., Mirowski, M., Mower, M. M., Platia, E. V., Griffith, L. S., Watkins, L., Jr., et al. (1983). Clinical evaluation of the internal automatic cardioverter- defibrillator in survivors of sudden cardiac death. *Am J Cardiol, 51*(10), 1608-1613.

Reproductive Biology and Endocrinology (n.d.). Retrieved September 14, 2007 from http://www.rbej.com/

Reproductive Health Library - www.rhlibrary.com

Reuss, E., Menozzi, M., Buchi, M., Koller, J., & Krueger, H. (2004). Information access at the point of care: What can we learn for designing a mobile CPR system? *International Journal of Medical Management, 73,* 363-369.

Reynolds, P., Dale, R., & Cowan, F. (2001). Neonatal cranial ultrasound interpretation: A clinical audit. *Arch Dis Child Fetal Neonatal Ed, 8*(2), F92-95.

Ribbert, L. S., Snijders, R. J., Nicolaides, K. H., & Visser, G. H. (1991). Relation of fetal blood gases and data from computer-assisted analysis of fetal heart rate patterns in small for gestation fetuses. *Br J Obstet Gynaecol, 98*(8), 820-823.

Richards, A., Farnsworth, A., Davey, E., Irwig, L., Macaskill, P., & Chan, S. (2007). The impact of automation on a large Australian cytology laboratory (abstract). *Acta Cytologica, 51*(suppl 2), 264-265.

Rigby, M. (2001). Evaluation: 16 Powerful Reasons Why Not to Do It - And 6 Over-Riding Imperatives. In V. Patel, R. Rogers, & R. Haux (Eds.), Proceedings of the 10th World Congress on Medical Informatics (Medinfo 2001) (Vol. 84, pp. 1198-202). Amsterdam: IOS Press.

Rigby, M., Forsström, J., Roberts, R., & Wyatt, W. (2001). Verifying quality and safety in health informatics services. BMJ, 323(8 September 2001), 552-556.

Ritterband, L., Borowitz, S., Cox, D., Kovatchev, B., Walker, L., Lucas, V., et al. (2005). Using the Internet to provide information prescriptions. *Pediatrics, 11*(5), e643-647.

Roberts, C. (1998). Quality assurance in primary care with information management and technology. *Health Informatics Journal, 4*(2), 101-105.

Roberts, D., & Dalziel, S. (2006). Antenatal corticosteroids for accelerating fetal lung maturation for women at risk of preterm birth. *Cochrane. Database. Syst. Rev., 3,* CD004454.

Robson, M. S., Scudamore, I. W. et al. (1996). Using the medical audit cycle to reduce cesarean section rates. *American Journal of Obstetrics and Gynecology, 174*(1 Pt 1), 199-205.

Rocher, A., Gonzalez, A., Palaoro, L., & Blanco, A. (2006). Usefulness of AgNOR technique and CEA expression in atypical metaplastic cells from cervical smears. *Anal Quant Cytol Histol, 28,* 130-136.

Rodrigues RJ & Risk A (2003), eHealth in Latin America and the Caribbean: Development and policy issues. J Med Internet Res, 5(1), e4.

Rodrigues, J.M., Trombert Paviot, B., Martin, C., Vercherin. P., Samuel, O. (2002). Co-ordination between clinical coding systems and pragmatic clinical terminologies based on a core open system: the role of ISO/TC215/WG3 and CEN/TC2511/WG2 standardisation?, *Studies in Health Technology and Informatics,* 90,401-405.

Roger, F., De Plaen, J., Chatelain, A., Cooche, E., Joos, M., & Haxhe, J. (1978). Problem-oriented medical records according to the Weed model. *Medical Informatics, 3*(2), 113-129.

Rohr, L. (1990). Quality assurance in gynecologic cytology What is practical? *Am J Clin Pathol, 94,* 754-758.

Rojo, M., Garcia, G., Mateos, C., & et al. (2006). Critical comparison of 31 commercially available digital slide systems in pathology. *Int J Surg Pathol, 14,* 285-230.

Rosen, B., Le, T., Elit, L., Goubanova, E., Fung Kee Fung, M., & Sadovy, B. (2007, May 23-24). Provincial synoptic Operative reporting. *Celebrating Innovations in Health Care Expo 2007.*

Rosenberg, W., & Donald, A. (1995). Evidence based medicine: an approach to clinical problem-solving. *British Medical Journal, 310,* 1122-1126.

Rosenfeld, R. (2000). Two decades of statistical language modeling: where do we go from here? *Proceedings of the IEEE, 88*(8), 1270-1278.

Rousseau, N. McColl, E. Newton, J. Grimshaw, J. & Eccles, M. (2003). Practice-based, Longitudinal, Qualitative Interview Study of Computerised Evidence Based Guidelines in Primary Care. British Medical Journal, **326,** 314-321.

Royal Australia and New Zealand College of Obstetricians and Gynaecologists, Australia and New Zealand Journal of Obstetrics and Gynaecology (n.d.). Retrieved September 14, 2007 from http://www.ranzcog.edu.au/publications/anzjog.shtml

Royal Australia and New Zealand College of Obstetricians and Gynaecologists (n.d.). Retrieved August 18, 2007 from http://www.ranzcog.edu.au/flp/index.shtml

Royal College of Midwives, RSS (n.d.). Retrieved September 15, 2007 from http://www.rcm.org.uk/news/rss/rss.php

Royal College of Midwives, UK (n.d.). Retrieved September 14, 2007 from http://www.rcm.org.uk/

Royal College of Obstetricians and Gynaecologists, UK (n.d.). Retrieved September 14, 2007 from http://www.rcog.org.uk/

Royal College of Obstetricians and Gynaecologists, UK, British Journal of Obstetrics and Gynaecology (n.d.). Retrieved September 14, 2007 from http://www.rcog.org.uk/index.asp?PageID=554

Royal College of Obstetricians and Gynaecologists, UK, webcasts (n.d.). Retrieved September 15, 2007 from http://rcog.mediaondemand.net/login.aspx?ReturnUrl=http%3A%2F%2Frcog%2Emediaondemand%2Enet%2Fplayer%2Easpx%3FEventID%3D325

Royal college of Physicians, Royal College of Pathologists, & British society for Human Genetics. (2006). *Consent and confidentiality in genetic practice: Guidance on genetic testing and sharing genetic information. Report of the Joint Committee on Medical Genetics.* London: RCP, RCPath, BSHG.

Ruotsalainen P, Nykänen P, Doupi P, Cheshire P, Pohjonen H, Kinnunen J, Keskisaari-Kajaste L, Hirvonen-Kari M, Moisio I & Tripovsky T (2003), The state of eHealth in Europe. Report D1 of the MEDITRAV-project, EU IST 1999-11490, Stakes, Helsinki.

safe abortion - http://www.figo.org/

Safe motherhood - http://www.unfpa.org/

Safran C & Goldberg H (2000), Electronic patient records and the impact of the Internet. Int J Medical Informatics 60, 77-83.

Salomon, L. J., Bernard, J. P., Perl, B., Hamon, H., Calla, M., Auger, M., et al. (2007). An internet based tool for quality assessment of fetal ultrasound examination. *Ultrasound in Obstetrics and Gynecology, 30*(4), pp. 532-532(531).

Salomon, L. J., Nasr, B., Beoist, G., Bouhanna, P., Bernard, J. P., & Ville, Y. (2007). Implementation of quality control for standard gynaecological examination. Feasibility and reproducibility of an image scoring method for gynaecological ultrasound examination in the emergency room. *Ultrasound in Obstetrics and Gynecology, 30*(4), 512.

Salomon, L. J., Poercher, R., Bernard, J. P., Rozenberg, P., & Ville, Y. (2007). Cumulative sum (CUSUM) charts and tests: A simple method to assess the quality of fetal biometry. *Ultrasound in Obstetrics and Gynecology, 30*(4), 480-481.

Salomon, L. J., Porcher, R., Bernard, J. P., Rozenberg, P., & Ville, Y. (2007). Quantitative quality assessment of nuchal translucency measurements at 11-14 weeks: A role for cumulative sum (CUSUM) charts and tests. *Ultrasound in Obstetrics and Gynecology, 30*(4), 391.

Salomon, L. J., Winer, N., Bernard, J. P., & Ville, Y. (2007). Feasibility and reproducibility of an image scoring method for quality assessment of standard ultrasound planes at second trimester examination. *Ultrasound in Obstetrics and Gynecology, 30*(4), 370.

Salvetto, M., & Sandiford, P. (2004). External quality assurance for cervical cytology in developing countries. Experience in Peru and Nicaragua. *Acta Cytol, 48,* 23-31.

Schaller, R. R., & Schaller, R. R. (1997). Moore's law: past, present and future

Schenck, U. (2007). Web-based training in cytology (abstract). *Acta Cytologica, 51*(suppl 2), 260-261.

Schledermann, D., Hyldebrandt, T., Ejersbo, D., & Hoelund, B. (2007). Automated screening versus manual screening: A comparison of the ThinPrep imaging system and manual screening in a time study. *Diagn Cytopathol, 35*, 348-352.

Schloendorff v New York Hospitals. (105 NE 92 1914).

Schrag, D., Earle, C., Xu, F., Panageas, K. S., Yabroff, K. R., Bristow, R. E., Trimble, E. L., & Warren, J. L. (2006). Associations between hospital and surgeon procedure volumes and patient outcomes after ovarian cancer resection. *J Natl Cancer Inst, 98*(3), 163-71.

Science citation index (n.d.). Retrieved September 14, 2007 from http://scientific.thomson.com/products/sci/

Scottish Intercollegiate Guidelines Network. (2003). *Epithelial ovarian cancer.*

See Tai, S., Donegan, C., & Nazareth, I. (2000). Computers in general practice and the consultation: the health professionals' view. *Health Informatics Journal, 6*(1), 27-31.

Sengupta, P. S., Jayson, G. C., Slade, R. J., Eardley, A., & Radford, J. A. (1999). An audit of primary surgical treatment for women with ovarian cancer referred to a cancer center. *Br J Cancer, 80*(3/4), 444-447.

Shah, P., Shah, V., Qiu, Z., Ohlsson, A., & Lee, S. (2005). Neonatal Network. Improved outcomes of outborn preterm infants if admitted to perinatal centers versus freestanding pediatric hospitals. *J Pediatr, 14*(5), 626-631.

Shahar, Y. (2002). Medical Informatics: Between Science and Engineering, Between Academia and Industry. Methods Inf Med, 41, 8-11.

Sharma, S. and N. Wickramasinghe, 2004 "e-health with Knowledge Management: areas for Tomorrow" pp. 110-124 in Wickramasinghe, N., J. Gupta and S. Sharma Eds Creating Knowledge-Based Healthcare Organizations with IdeanGroup Publishers, Hershey.

Sharma, S. N. Wickramasingeh, B. Xu and N. Ahmed , 2006 "Electronic Healthcare :Issues and Challenges" Int. J. Electronic Healthcare vol 2 no. 1 pp. 50-65

Shaw, M., Wolfe, C., Raju, K. S., & Papadopoulos, A. (2003). National Guidance on gynecological cancer management; an audit of gynecological cancer services and management in the South East of England. *Eur J Gynecol Oncol, 24*(2-4), 246-50.

Shaw, N. (2002). ,CHEATS': a generic information communication technology (ICT) evaluation framework. Computers in Biology and Medicine, 32, 209-200.

Sherman, M., Dasgupta, A., Schiffman, M., Nayar, R., & Solomon, D. (2007). The Bethesda Interobserver Reproducibility Study (BIRST): A Web-based assessment of the Bethesda 2001 System for classifying cervical cytology. *Cancer, 111*, 15-25.

Shipton, H. W. (1979). The microprocessor, a new tool for the biosciences. *Annual Review of Biophysics and Bioengineering, 8*, 269-286.

Shirata, N., Gomes, N., Garcia, E., & Longatto, F., A. (2001). Nuclear DNA content analysis by static cytometry in cervical intraepithelial lesions using retrospective series of previously stained PAP smears. *Adv Clin Path, 5*, 87-91.

Shirata, N., Longatto, F., A., Roteli-Martins, C., Espoladore, L., Pittoli, J., & Syrjänen, K. (2003). Applicability of liquid-based cytology to the assessment of DNA content in cervical lesions using static cytometry. *Anal Quant Cytol Histol, 25*, 210-214.

Shortliffe, E. H. (1997). Computer Programs to Support Clinical Decision Making. *Journal of the American Medical Association, 258*(1), 61-66.

Shortliffe, E., & Cimino, J. (Eds.). (2006). *Biomedical Informatics: Computer Applications in Health Care and Biomedicine (Health Informatics)* (Third ed.): Springer.

Shoultz, J. et al. Reducing health disparities by improving quality of care: Lessons learned from culturally diverse women. *Journal of Nursing Care Quality, 21.1*, 86-92.

Shylasree, T. S., Howells, R. E., Lim, K., Jones, P. W., Flander, A., Adams, M. et al. (2006). Survival in ovarian cancer in WalesL Prior to introduction of all Wales guidelines. *Int J Gyn Onc, 16*(5),1770-6.

Silber D (2003), The case for ehealth. European Commission, Information Society, eHealth Conference 2003, Atlanta, Belgium.

Silber, J. H., Rosenbaum, P. R., Polsky, D., Ross, R. N., Even-Shoshan, O., Schartz, J. S. et al. (2007, April 1). Does ovarian cancer treatment and survival differ by the specialty providing chemotherapy? *J Clin Oncol., 25*(10),1169-75.

Silfen, E. (2006). Documentation and coding of ED patient encounters: An evaluation of the accuracy of an electronic medical record. *The American Journal of Emergency Medicine, 24*(6), 664-678.

Sim, J., & Sharp, K. (1998). A critical appraisal of the role of triangulation in nursing research. Int J Nurs Stud, 35(1-2), 23-31.

Sim, N., Kitteringham, L., Spitz, L., Pierro, A., Kiely, E., Drake, D., et al. (2007). Information on the World Wide Web--how useful is it for parents? *J Pediatr Surg, 42*(2), 305-312.

Simpson, J., Evans, N., Gibberd, R., Heuchan, A., & Henderson-Smart, D. (2003). New Zealand Neonatal, Network. Analysing differences in clinical outcomes between hospitals. *Qual Saf Health Care, 12*(4), 257-262.

Simpson, J., Lynch, R., Grant, J., & Alroomi, L. (2004). Reducing medication errors in the neonatal intensive care unit. *Arch Dis Child Fetal Neonatal Ed, 89*(6), F480-482.

Singer, L., Salvator, A., Guo, S., Collin, M., Lilien, L., & Baley, J. (1999). Maternal psychological distress and parenting stress after the birth of a very low-birth-weight infant. *JAMA, 281*(9), 799-805.

Sittig, D. F., Gardner, R. M., Pace, N. L., Morris, A. H., & Beck, E. (1989). Computerized management of patient care in a complex, controlled clinical trial in the intensive care unit. *Comput Methods Programs Biomed, 30*(2-3), 77-84.

Skirnisdottir, E., & Sorbe, B. (2007). Prognostic factors for surgical outcome and survival in 447 women treated for advanced (FIGO stages 3-4) epithelial ovarian carcinoma. Int J Oncol, (3), 727-34

Skov, B., & Th. Hoegh. (2006). Supporting information access in a hospital ward by a context-aware mobile electronic patient record. *Personal Ubiquitous Comput., 10*(4), 205-214.

Smart, J., & Williams, B. (1973). *Utilitarianism: for and against.* Cambridge University Press.

Smith, J. H., Anand, K. J., Cotes, P. M., Dawes, G. S., Harkness, R. A., Howlett, T. A., et al. (1988). Antenatal fetal heart rate variation in relation to the respiratory and metabolic status of the compromised human fetus. *Br J Obstet Gynaecol, 95*(10), 980-989.

SNOMED. www.update-software.com/history/clibhist. htm . 2007.

SNOMED_Clinical_Terms_Fundamentals.pdf (http:// www.ihtsdo.org/fileadmin/user_upload/Docs_01/ SNOMED_Clinical_Terms_Fundamentals.pdf)

Snowden, S., Brownlee, K., & Dear, P. (1997). An expert system to assist neonatal intensive care. *J Med Eng Technol, 2*(2), 67–73.

Society of Obstetricians and Gynaecologists of Canada (n.d.). Retrieved August 18, 2007 from http://www.sogc. org/cme/online_e.asp

Society of Obstetricians and Gynaecologists of Canada, podcasts (n.d.). Retrieved September 15, 2007 from http://sogc.medical.org/media/podcasts_e.asp

Sodhani, P., Singh, V., Das, D., & Bhambhani, S. (1997). Cytohistological correlation as a measure of quality assurance of a cytology laboratory. *Cytopathology, 8,* 103-107.

Solomon, D., Davey, D., Kurman, R., Moriarty, A., O'Connor, D., Prey, M., et al. (2002). The 2001 Bethesda System: Terminology for reporting results of cervical cytology. *JAMA, 287,* 2114-2119.

South, J., & Rhodes, P. (1971). Computer Service for Obstetric Records. *B Med J, 4,* 32-35.

South, J., & Rhodes, P. (1971). Computer Service for Obstetric Records. *B Med J, 4,* 32-35.

Spanjers, R., & Feuth, S. (2002). Telebaby videostreaming of newborns over Internet. *Stud Health Technol Inform, 90,* 195-200.

Speroff, T., & O'Connor, G. T. (2004). Study designs for PDSA quality improvement research. *Qual. Manag. Healthcare, 13.1,* 17-32.

Spink A, Yang Y, Jansen J, Nykänen P, Lorence D, Ozmutlu S & Ozmutlu HC (2004), A study of medical and health queries to web search engines. Health Information and Libraries Journal 21, 44-51

Sribnick, R. L., & Sribnick, W. B. (1994). *Smart Patient, Good Medicine: Working With Your Doctor to Get the Best Medical Care.* New York: Walker and Company.

Starr, M., & Chalmers, I. (2003). *The evolution of The Cochrane Library,* 1988-2003. www.update-software. com/history/clibhist.htm . 2003.

Stauch, M., Wheat, K., & Tingle, J. (2006a). *Text, cases and materials on medical law 5th Edition* Routledge Cavendish .

Stauch, M., Wheat, K., & Tingle, J. (2006b). Chapter 5. In *Text, cases and materials on medical law chapter 5th Edition 2006*: Routledge Cavendish.

Steinberg, D., & Ali, S. (2001). Application of virtual microscopy in clinical cytopathology. *Diagn Cytopathol, 25,* 389-396.

Stenson, B. (1996). Promoting attachment, providing memories. *BMJ, 313*(7072), 1615.

Stevens, M., Garland, S., Rudland, E., Tan, J., Quinn, M., & Tabrizi, S. (2007). Comparison of the Digene Hybrid Capture 2 assay and Roche AMPLICOR and LINEAR

ARRAY human papillomavirus (HPV) tests in detecting high-risk HPV genotypes in specimens from women with previous abnormal Pap smear results. *J Clin Microbiol, 45*, 2130-2137.

Stewart, J. H., Andrews, J., & Cartlidge, P. H. (1998). Numbers of deaths related to intrapartum asphyxia and timing of birth in all Wales perinatal survey, 1993-5. *Bmj, 316*(7132), 657-660.

Stewart, J., 3rd., Miyazaki, K., Bevans-Wilkins, K., Ye, C., Kurtycz, D., & Selvaggi, S. (2007). Virtual microscopy for cytology proficiency testing: are we there yet? *Cancer, 111*, 203-209.

Stoll, B., Hansen, N., Fanaroff, A., Wright, L., Carlo, W. et al. (2002). Changes in pathogens causing early-onset sepsis in very-low-birth-weight infants. *N Engl J Med, 347*(4), 240-247.

Street, P., Dawes, G. S., Moulden, M., & Redman, C. W. (1991). Short-term variation in abnormal antenatal fetal heart rate records. *Am J Obstet Gynecol, 165*(3), 515-523.

Strong, D. F., & Leach, P. B. (2005). *National Concultation on Access to Scientific Research Data: Final Report.* 31-1-2005. Ottawa, Canada, Canada Institure for Scientific and Technical Information.

SUMSearch (n.d.). Retrieved September 9, 2007 from http://sumsearch.uthscsa.edu/

Suresh, G., Horbar, J., Plsek, P., Gray, J., Edwards, W., Shiono, P., et al. (2004). Voluntary anonymous reporting of medical errors for neonatal intensive care. *Pediatrics, 113*(6), 1609-1618.

Synnes, A. R. et al. (2001). Variations in intraventricular hemorrhage incidence rates among Canadian neonatal intensive care units. *J Pediatr., 138.4*, 525-31.

Synnes, A., Macnab, Y., Qiu, Z., Ohlsson, A., Gustafson, P., Dean, C., et al. (2006). Neonatal intensive care unit characteristics affect the incidence of severe intraventricular hemorrhage. *Med Care, 4*(8), 754-759.

Tabor, A., Philip, J., Madsen, M., Bang, J., Obel, E. B., & Nørgaard-Pedersen, B. (1986). Randomised controlled trial of genetic amniocentesis in 4606 low-risk women. *Lancet, 1*(8493), 1287-1293.

Talmon, G., & Abrahams, N. (2005). The Internet for pathologists: A simple schema for evaluating pathology-related Web sites and a catalog of sites useful for practicing pathologists. *Arch Pathol Lab Med, 129*, 742-746.

Talmon, J., & Hasmann, A. (2002). Medical Informatics as a Discipline at the Beginning of the 21th Century. Methods Inf Med, 41, 4-7.

Tapscott, D., & Williams, A. (2008). *Wikinomics: How Mass Collaboration Changes Everything.*

Taylor, R. (2003). Changes in thresholds for prescribing postnatal corticosteroids between 2000 and 2002: are we better educated? *Ped Res, 53*(4), 103A.

Thakkar, M., & O' Shea, M. (2006). The role of neonatal networks. *Semin Fetal Neonatal Med, 11*(2), 105-110.

Thatcher, R. A. (1968). A package deal for computer processing in Obstetric records. *Med J Aust, 2*, 766-768.

The (Commonwealth) Privacy Act 1988 (as amended by the Privacy Amendment (Private Sector) Act 2000 . (1998).

The Cochrane Collaboration. (1997). Cochrane Pregnancy and Childbirth Database (Version III) [CD-Rom]. Oxford, UK: Update Software.

The Data Protection Act. (1998). from http://www.opsi. gov.uk/acts/acts1998/ukpga_19980029_en_1

The health on the net foundation www.hon.ch

The Knowledge basket. (2002). The Privacy Act 1993. Retrieved June 2008, from http://gpacts.knowledge-basket.co.nz/gpacts/public/text/2002/an/073.html

Thede, L. Q. (2003). *Informatics and nursing: Opportunities & challenges,* 2nd ed., Lippincott Williams & Wilkins, Philadelphia ; London.

This presentation gives an introduction to SNOMED CT: What is SNOMED CT, what is it for, how is it organized, etc.

Thornton, C., Hennessy, A., von Dadelszen, P., Nishi, C., Makris, A., & Ogle, R. An international benchmarking collaboration: measuring outcomes for the hypertensive disorders of pregnancy. *J Obstet Gynaecol Can., 29.10* (7 A.D.), 794-800.

Thornton, J. G., & Lilford, R. J. (1989). Basic reference gambles recommended for utility assessment. *Am.J.Obstet.Gynecol., 161*(1), 256-257.

Thornton, J., & Lilford, R. (1989). The caesarean section decision: patients' choices are not determined by immediate emotional reactions. *J.Obs.Gyn., 9*, 283-288.

Tilley, S. & Chambers, M. (2004). The process of implementing evidence-based practice- the curates egg. Journal of Psychiatric and Mental Health Nursing, **11**, 117-119.

Tilyard, M., Munro, N., Walker, S., & Dovey, S. (1998). Creating a general practice national minimum data set: Present possibility or future plan? *New Zealand Medical Journal, 111*(1072), 317-318, 320.

Timmons, S. 2003, Nurses Resisting Information Technology. Nursing Inquiry, **10**(4), 257-269.

Tingay, D., Mills, J., Morley, C., Pellicano, A., & Dargaville, P. (2007). New Zealand Neonatal, Network. Trends in use and outcome of newborn infants treated with high frequency ventilation in Australia and New Zealand, 1996-2003. *J Paediatr Child Health, 4*(3), 160-166.

Tingulstad, S., Skjeldestad, F. E., & Hagen, B. (N/A). The effect of centralization of primary surgery on survival in ovarian cancer patients. *Ob Gyn, 102*, 499-505.

Tingulstad, S., Skjeldestad, F. E., Halvorsen, T. B., & Hagen, B. (2003). Survival and prognostic factors in patients with ovarian cancer. *Obstet Gynecol, 101*(5Pt1), 885-91

Tong, R. (1998). The ethics of care: A feminist virtue ethics of care for healthcare practitioners. *Journal Medicine and Philosophy, 23*, 131-152.

Trimbos, J. B., & Bolis, G. (1994). Guidelines for surgical staging of ovarian cancer. *Obstetrical and Gynecological Survey, 49*, 814-816.

Trimbos, J. B., Schueler, J. A., van der Burg, M., Hermans, J., van Lent, M., Heintz, A. P. M., et al. (1991). Watch and wait after careful surgical treatment and staging in well-differentiated early ovarian cancer. *Cancer, 67*, 597-602

Trimbos, J. B., Schueler, J. A., van Lent, M., Hermans, J., & Fleuren, G. J. (1990). Reasons for incomplete surgical staging in early Ovarian Carcinoma. *Gynecol Oncol, 37*, 374-377.

Trimbos, J. B., Schueler, J. A., van Lent, M., Hermans, J., & Fleuren, G. J. (1990). Reasons for incomplete surgical staging in early ovarian carcinoma. *Gynecologic Oncology, 37*, 374-7.

Trimbos, J. B., Vergote, I., Bolis, G., Vermorken, J. B., Mangioni, C., Madronal, C., Franchi, M., Tateo, S., Zanetta, G., Scarfone, G., Giurgea, L., Timmers, P., Coens, C., & Pecorelli, S. (2003). EORTC-ACTION collaborators. European Organisation for Research and Treatment of Cancer-Adjuvant ChemoTherapy in Ovarian Neoplasm. Impact of adjuvant chemotherapy and surgical staging in early-stage ovarian carcinoma: European Organisation for Research and Treatment of Cancer-Adjuvant ChemoTherapy in Ovarian Neoplasm trial. J Natl Cancer Inst., 15, *95*(2), 113-125.

TRIP (Turning Research into Practice) (n.d.). Retrieved September 14, 2007 from http://www.tripdatabase.com/index.html

Tsuchihashi, Y., Okada, Y., Ogushi, Y., & et al. (2000). The current status of medicolegal issues surrounding telepathology and telecytology in Japan. *J Telemed Telecare, 6*(Suppl 1), S143-145.

U.S. National Library of Medicine. (2001, 15 November 2001). *Medical Subject* Headings. Retrieved 11 January, 2002, from http://www.nlm.nih.gov/mesh/

U.S. National Library of Medicine. (2001, 15 November 2001). Medical Subject Headings. Retrieved 11 January, 2002, from http://www.nlm.nih.gov/mesh/

University of Michigan, Department of Pediatrics (n.d.). Retrieved September 8, 2007 from http://www.med.umich.edu/pediatrics/ebm/Cat.htm

Van De Ven, A., Angle, H. and Poole, S. (2000). Research on the Management of Innovation, Oxford: Oxford University Press.

van der Loo, R. (1995). Overview of Published Assessment and Evaluation Studies. In E. M. S. J. van Gennip & J. S. Talmon (Eds.), Assessment and evaluation of information technologies (pp. 261-82). Amsterdam: IOS Press.

Van Gorp, T., Amant, F., Neven, P., Berteloot, P., Leunen, K., & Vergote, I. (2006). The position of neoadjuvant chemotherapy within the treatment of ovarian cancer. *Minerva Ginecol, 58*(5), 393-403

Various. (2006). *Clinical Guidelines Index. Newborn Services, Auckland City Hospital*. Retrieved June 2008, from http://www.adhb.govt.nz/newborn/Guidelines.htm

VATAM. (2000). The VATAM Websites. Validation of Health Telematics Applications (VATAM). Available: http://www-vatam.unimaas.nl/html/aboutvalidation.shtml [January 2004].

Vaughan, N.J., Cashman, S.J., Cavan, D.A., Gallego, M.R., Kohner, E., Benedetti, M.M., Sando, S.H., Sonksen, P.H., Storms, G.E., Vermeij, D. (2000). A detailed examination of the clinical terms and concepts required for communication by electronic messages in diabetes care. Diabetes, Nutrition and Metabolism, 13(4), 201-209.

Vergote, I., & Stuart, G. *Phase 3 study: Upfront debulking surgery versus neo-adjuvant chemotherapy, stage 3c or 4 epithelial ovarian cancer EORTC #55971, NCIC OV13*

Vernooij, F., Peter, A., Heintz, M., Witteveen, E., & van der Graff, Y. (2007, April 11). The outcomes of ovarian cancer treatment are better when provided by gynecologic oncologists and in specialized hospitals: A systematic review. *Gynecol Oncol.*

Von Lubitz, D and N. Wickramasinghe,. 2006 "Healthcare and Technology: The Doctrine of Networkcentric Healthcare" in press Intl. J Electronic Healthcare (IJEH).

Walley, P., & Gowland, B. (2004). Completing the circle: from PD to PDSA. *Int. J. Health Care Qual. Assur. Inc. Leadersh. Health Serv., 17.6*, 349-58.

Walley, T., & Mantgani, A. (1997). The UK General Practice Research Database. *The Lancet, 350*(9084), 1097-1099.

Wang, S. J., Middleton, B., Prosser, L. A., Bardon, C. G., Spurr, C. D., Carchidi, P. J., et al. (2003). A cost-benefit analysis of electronic medical records in primary care. *The American Journal of Medicine, 114*(5), 397-403.

Ward, R., & Scrivener, R. (2002). The development of NMAP - the UK's gateway to high quality Internet resources in nursing, midwifery and allied health. *Health Informatics Journal, 8* (3), 122-126.

Watanabe, S., Iwasaka, T., Yokoyama, M., Uchiyama, M., Kaku, T., & Matsuyama, T. (2004). Analysis of nuclear chromatin distribution in cervical glandular abnormalities. *Acta Cytol, 48*, 505-513.

Webster, J., Forbes, K., Foster, S., Thomas, I., Griffin, A., & Timms, H. (1996). Sharing antenatal care: Client satisfaction and use of the 'patient-held record'. *Aust N Z J Obstet Gynaecol, 36*(1), 11-14.

Weed, L. (1971). The problem-oriented record as a basic tool in medical education, patient care and clinical research. . *Annals of Clinical Research, 3*, 131-134.

Weed, L. (1975). The problem-oriented record-its organizing principles and its structure. *League Exchange, 103*, 3-6.

Weed, L. L. (1968). Medical records that guide and teach. *New England Journal of Medicine, 278*(11+12), 593–600 + 652–597.

Weed, L., & Zimny, N. (1989). The problem-oriented system, problem-knowledge coupling, and clinical decision making. *Physical Therapy, 69*(7), 565-568.

Weerasinghe, S., Mirghani, H., Revel, A., & Abu-Zidan, F. M. (2006). Cumulative sum (CUSUM) analysis in the assessment of trainee competence in fetal biometry measurement. *Ultrasound in Obstetrics and Gynecology, 28*(2), 199-203.

Weinstein, R. (2005). Innovations in medical imaging and virtual microscopy. *Hum Pathol, 36*, 317-319.

Weiser, M. (1993). Some computer science issues in ubiquitous computing. *Communications of the ACM, 36*(7), 75-84.

Westgate, J. A., Gunn, A. J., & Gunn, T. R. (1999). Antecedents of neonatal encephalopathy with fetal acidaemia at term. *Br J Obstet Gynaecol, 106*(8), 774-782.

Westgate, J., & Gunn, A. (2001). Early neonatal mortality and timing of low risk births. Data suggest that difficulties in fetal monitoring are magnified at night. *Bmj, 322*(7283), 433-434.

Wheeler, D. (2006). Google as a pathology portal. *Adv Anat Pathol, 13*, 275-276.

Whiddett, R., Hunter, I., Engelbrecht, J., & Handy, J. (2006). Patients' attitudes towards sharing their health information. *International Journal of Medical Informatics, 75*(7), 530-541.

Whiddett, R., Hunter, I., Engelbrecht, J., & Handy, J. (2006). Patients' attitudes towards sharing their health information. *International Journal of Medical Informatics, 75*(7), 530-541.

WHO – Making pregnancy safer initiative: http://www.who.int/making_pregnancy_safer/en/index.html

WHO Reproductive Health and Research - http://www.who.int/reproductive-health/

WHO reproductive health data http://www.who.int/reproductive-health/

Wickramasinghe, N. A. Fadlalla, E. Geisler, and J. Schaffer, 2005 "A Framework For Assessing E-Health Preparedness" International J. Electronic Healthcare (IJEH) vol. 1 no. 3 pp. 316-334

Wickramasinghe, N. and J. Silvers 2003 "IS/IT The Prescription To Enable Medical Group Practices To Manage Managed Care" Health Care Management Science vol. 6 no 2 pp-75-86

Wickramasinghe, N. and R. Lamb 2002 "Enterprise-wide systems enabling physicians to manage care", International Journal Healthcare Technology and Management vol 4 Nos. 3/4 pp.288-302

Widrow, B., Widrow, B., & Lehr, M. A. (1990). 30 years of adaptive neural networks: perceptron, Madaline, and backpropagation

Wikipedia contributors. 2007 UK child benefit data scandal. Wikipedia, The Free Encyclopedia . 29-2-2008.

Wikipedia www.wikipedia.org

Wilbur, D., Cibas, E., Merritt, S., James, J., Berger, G., & Bonfiglio, T. (1994). ThinPrep processor clinical trials demonstrate an increased detection rate of abnormal cervical cytology specimens. *Am J Clin Pathol, 101,* 209-214.

Wilbur, D., Prey, M., Miller, W., Pawlick, G., & Colgan, T. (1998). The AutoPap System for primary screening in cervical cytology: comparing the results or a prospective, intended-use study with routine manual practice. *Acta Cytol, 42,* 214-220.

Wiley InterScience (n.d.). Retrieved September 14, 2007 from http://www3.interscience.wiley.com/

Williams, S. D., Goulet, R., & Thomas, G. (1996). Early ovarian cancer: A review of its genetic and biologic factors, detection, and treatment. *Curr Probl Cancer, 20,* 83-137.

Wilson P (2002), How to find the good and avoid the bad or ugly: a short guide to tools for rating quality and health information on the Internet. BMJ 9 (324), 598-602

Wilson P, Leitner C & Moussalli A (2004), Mapping the potential of eHealth. Empowering the citizen through eHealth tools and services. eHealth Conference 2004. European Institute for Public Administration. Maastricht, The Netherlands.

Wilson, R. G., Purves, I. N., & Smith, D. (2000). Utilisation of computerised clinical guidance in general practice consultations. *Studies in health technology and informatics, 77,* 229-233.

Wilson, R. G., Purves, I. N., & Smith, D. (2000). Utilisation of computerised clinical guidance in general practice consultations. *Studies in health technology and informatics, 77,* 229-233.

Wimberger, P., Lehmann, N., Kimmig, R., Burges, A., Meier, W., & Du Bois, A. (2007). For the AGO-OVAR. Prognostic factors for complete debulking in advanced ovarian cancer and its impact on survival. An exploratory analysis of a prospectively randomized phase 3 study of the Arbeitsgemeinschaft Gynaekologische Onkologie Ovarian cancer study group (AGO-OVAR). *Gynecol Oncol, Ma3 28.*

Winter, A., Ammenwerth, E., Bott, O., Brigl, B., Buchauer, A., Gräber, S., Grant, A., Häber, A., Hasselbring, W., Haux, R., Heinrich, A., Janssen, H., Kock, I., Penger, O.-S., Prokosch, H.-U., Terstappen, A., & Winter, A.

(2001). Strategic Information Management Plans: The Basis for Systematic Information Management in Hospitals. International Journal of Medical Informatics, 64(2-3), 99-109.

Winter, W. E., Kucera, P. R., Rodgers, W., McBroom, J. W., Olsen, C., & Maxwell, G. L. (2002). Surgical staging in patients with ovarian tumors of low malignant potential. *Obstetrics & Gynecology, 100,* 671-6.

Witten, I., & E., F. (2005). *Data Mining: Practical machine learning tools and techniques* (2 ed.). San Francisco: Morgan Kaufmann.

Wolfe, C. D., Tilling, K., & Raju, K. S. (1997). Management and survival of ovarian cancer patients in southeast England. *Eur J Cancer, 33*(11), 1835-40.

Women's health Specialist library GBS Teaching Package, UK (n.d.). Retrieved August 17, 2007 from http://www.whsl.org.uk/gbs/

Women's Health Specialist Library Update, RSS (n.d.). Retrieved September 15, 2007 from http://www.library.nhs.uk/womenshealth/SearchResults.aspx?catID=10394

Women's Health Specialist Library, UK (n.d.). Retrieved August 18, 2007 from www.library.nhs.uk/womenshealth

Woodman, C., Baghdad, A., Collins, S., & Clyma, J-A. (1997). What changes in the organization of cancer services will improve the outcome for women with ovarian cancer? *Br J Ob Gyn, 104,* 135-139.

Woolery, L. K., & Grzymala-Busse, J. (1995). Machine learning for development of an expert system to predict premature birth. *Biomedical. Sciences. Instrumentation., 31,* 29-34.

World Health Organisation (n.d.). Retrieved September 13, 2007 from http://www.who.int/en/

World Health Organisation, Gender, Women and Health (n.d.). Retrieved September 13, 2007 from http://www.who.int/gender/en/

World Health Organisation, Making Pregnancy Safer (n.d.). Retrieved September 13, 2007 from http://www.who.int/making_pregnancy_safer/en/

World Health Organisation, Pregnancy in the European region (n.d.). Retrieved September 13, 2007 from http://www.euro.who.int/healthtopics/HT2ndLvlPage?HTCode=pregnancy

World Health Organisation, Reproductive Health and Research (n.d.). Retrieved September 13, 2007 from http://www.who.int/reproductive-health/

World Health Organisation, Reproductive Health Library (n.d.). Retrieved August 17, 2007 from www.rhlibrary.com

World Health Organization. (2001, 14 November 2001). ICD-10: The International Statistical Classification of Diseases and Related Health Problems, tenth revision. Retrieved 11 January, 2002, from http://www.who.int/whosis/icd10/

Wyatt, J. (1994). Clinical data systems, part 3: development and evaluation. The Lancet, 344, 1682-8.

Wyatt, J., & Spiegelhalter, D. (1992). Field trials of medical decision-aids: potential problems and solutions. In P. Clayton (Ed.), 15th Annual Symposium on Computer Applications in Medical Care (pp. 3-7). New York: McGraw-Hill.

Yagi, Y., & Gilbertson, J. (2005). Digital imaging in pathology: The case for standardization. *J Telemed Telecare, 11*, 109-116.

Yang, C.-M., & Reinke, W. (2006). Feasibility and validity of International Classification of Diseases based case mix indices. *BMC Health Services Research, 6*(1), 125.

Z V Finland, 371 (EHRR 1998).

Zanetta, G., Chiari, S., Rota, S., Bratina, G., Maneo, A., Torri, V., et al. (2007). Conservative surgery for stage I ovarian carcinoma in women of childbearing age. *British Journal of Obstetrics & Gynaecology, 104*, 1030-5.

Zanstra, P., Rector, A., Ceusters, W., & de Vries Robbe, P. (1998). Coding systems and classifications in healthcare: the link to the record. *International Journal of Medical Informatics., 48*(1-3), 103-109.

Zhao, L., Lee, K., & Hu, J. (2005). Generating XML schemas for DICOM structured reporting templates. *Journal of the American Medical Informtics Association, 12*(1), 72-83.

Zimmerman, J.E. Shortell, S.M. Rousseau, D.M. Duffy, J. Gillies, R.R. Knaus, W.A. Devers, K. Wagner, D.P. & Draper, E.A. (1993). Improving Intensive Care: Observations based on organisational case studies in nine intensive care units: A prospective multicenter study. Critical Care Medicine, 21(10), 1143-1451.

About the Contributors

David Parry is a senior lecturer in the Auckland University of Technology School of Computing and Mathematical Sciences, New Zealand. His PhD thesis was concerned with the use of fuzzy ontologies for medical information retrieval. He holds degrees from Imperial College and St. Bartholomew's Medical College, London, Auckland University of Technology and the University of Otago, New Zealand. His research interests include internet-based knowledge management and the Semantic Web, health informatics, the use of radio frequency ID in healthcare and information retrieval.

Emma Parry's (FRANZCOG CMFM senior lecturer in obstetrics and gynaecology, The University of Auckland) main interests over the last few years have been induction of labour rates and the techniques used to achieve labour induction. Her MD thesis is titled 'Induction of labour: How, why and when?' She has also been involved in looking at obstetricians views on induction of labour and caesarean section. She is a trained sub-specialist in maternal-fetal medicine.

* * *

J. Mark Ansermino is an assistant professor in University of British Columbia's Department of Anesthesiology, Pharmacology and Therapeutics. Dr. Ansermino holds the position of director of research for the Department of Anesthesia at BC Children's Hospital. He has formal training in health informatics from City University, London, UK. He holds a scholar award from the Michael Smith Research Foundation. His research focuses on the use of information and technology to improve patient care.

Malcolm Battin is a senior lecturer in neonatology at The University of Auckland. He trained in paediatrics and neonatology in the UK and Canada and has worked as a specialist neonatologist in New Zealand since 1997. His research interests in neonatal outcome and neonatal neurology led to pioneering work with "new technologies" such as neonatal MRI, selective cerebral cooling and bedside EEG monitoring. More recently he has turned his focus to the use of neonatal networks, large databases and medical informatics for both quality improvement and research purposes.

Susan Bondy (PhD) is an associate scientist, clinical epidemiology, Sunnybrook Research Institute, adjunct scientist, Institute for Clinical Evaluative Sciences, assistant professor, public health sciences, University of Toronto and principal investigator, Ontario Tobacco Research Unit.

Peter von Dadelszen is an associate professor of obstetrics and gynaecology (maternal-fetal medicine) at the University of British Columbia and consultant in maternal-fetal medicine, Children's and Women's Health Centre of BC. A New Zealander, he studied medicine at the University of Otago, Dunedin. He completed an intercalated research degree in anatomy in 1981, his medical degree (Bachelor of Medicine, Bachelor of Surgery) in 1984, and gained a postgraduate Diploma in Obstetrics and Gynaecology in 1987. He moved to the UK in 1990, to continue his specialty training in obstetrics and gynaecology and undertake a DPhil project with Professor Chris Redman in Oxford. He gained his Membership of the Royal College of Obstetricians and Gynaecologists in 1991 (Fellowship, 2003), and began his DPhil project in 1993, whilst continuing part-time clinical training. With the DPhil benchwork completed in 1996, he moved to Toronto, to undertake subspecialty training in maternal-fetal medicine (1996-8), was admitted to Fellowship of the newly amalgamated Royal Australian and New Zealand College of Obstetricians and Gynaecologists in 1998. Subsequent to the MFM fellowship, he undertook an additional year of residency training for the Royal College of Physicians and Surgeons of Canada (1998-9). His appointment at UBC is that of a clinician-scientist, with 80% protected time for research; his research interests are focussed on the area of pre-eclampsia and pregnancy hypertension, from basic science to clinical epidemiology and health services research. He is currently the president of the North American Society for the Study of Hypertension in Pregnancy and editor (non-Europe) of *Hypertension in Pregnancy*. Peter is married to Laura Magee, an obstetric and general internist at UBC and CWHCBC. They share the leadership of the pregnancy hypertension research group at UBC. Peter is a CIHR new investigator and Michael Smith Foundation for Health Research senior scholar. He is currently investigating the mechanisms involved in the development of pre-eclampsia, outcome prediction, a possible disease-modifying therapy, and the impact of introducing standardised care for the hypertensive diseases of pregnancy in the Province of British Columbia. Peter has published over 50 peer-reviewed papers since his appointment to UBC 7 years ago.

Laurie Elit (MD MSc FRCS(C)) is an associate professor with the Department of Obstetrics and Gynecology, McMaster University and gynecologic oncologist at the Hamilton Health Sciences Centre and Juravinski Cancer Centre, Hamilton, Canada

Premila Fade (BSc MB BS MA FRCP) graduated from London in 1992 and gained her MRCP in 1995. She interrupted her higher specialist training in geriatrics to study for a Master in Medical Ethics and Law (King's College London) in 2001. Prem is now a consultant geriatrician at Poole Hospital NHS Foundation Trust Dorset UK appointed 2003. Prem set up (in 2004) and chairs the Poole Hospital Clinical Ethics Group. She has spoken at regional and national meetings on ethical topics and is currently co authoring a guideline on advance directives for the British Geriatrics Society and the Royal College of Physicians London. She has published on consent and capacity.

Michael Fung-Kee-Fung (MD FRCS(C)) is a professor with the Department of Obstetrics and Gynecology at the University of Ottawa and gynecologic oncologist at the Ottawa Hospital, head of the division of surgical oncology, Ottawa, Canada.

Prafull Ghatage (MB ChB FRCS(C)) Department of Obstetrics and Gynecology at the University of Calgary and gynecologic oncologist at the Tom Baker Cancer Centre and Foothills Hospital, Calgary, Canada.

Robert A. Goulart (MD) is medical director of the division of cytopathology and the Cytopathology Fellowship Program at Baystate Medical Center - Tufts University School of Medicine, Springfield, Massachusetts, USA. Dr. Goulart received his medical degree from the University of Massachusetts, followed by a residency in anatomic and clinical pathology and a fellowship in cytopathology, all at Boston's Beth Israel Hospital and Harvard Medical School. He is active in the leadership of the American Society for Clinical Pathology and the American Society of Cytopathology, with research interests in the fields of diagnostic cytopathology, breast pathology, quality assurance and medical education.

Maryanne Hornish is a compliance cytotechnologist for the Cytology Department at Baystate Medical Center in Springfield, Massachusetts, USA. Ms. Hornish was awarded a Master of Business Administration (*summa cum laude*) from Western New England College in Springfield, Massachusetts, USA. She holds cytotechnologist certifications from the American Society for Clinical Pathology and the International Academy of Cytology. Ms. Hornish received her Certificate in Cytotechnology from the University of Connecticut Health Center in Farmington, Connecticut, USA after obtaining a Bachelor of Science in pathobiology from the University of Connecticut in Storrs, Connecticut, USA. She is a member of the American Society of Cytopathology and has served as a laboratory inspector for the College of American Pathologists. Her research interests include pathology informatics, statistics, quality assurance, and database management. Although at the beginning of her career as an academic author, Kiran Angelina Massey, has proved to be someone to watch for in the future. Her work not only addresses current issues in knowledge translation but the impact it will have on the future of medicine and the patients it supports. After she completed her undergraduate degree at Queen's University in Life Sciences she migrated to the west coast. Now she can be found at the University of British Columbia in Vancouver doing graduate work in the Department of Obstetrics and Gynecology. Her work focuses on the concept of the dissemination of knowledge though translation and interaction especially within surveillance programs such as the Canadian Perinatal Network with which she is affiliated. This is the first book chapter publication for Kiran and she is extremely thrilled to be a part of process.

Jamila Abd Al-Rahman Abu Idhail earned her BSc in nursing from Jordan University of Science and Technology (1996) and an MSc in critical care nursing from Jordan University (2003). Then recently she gained her PhD in the field of maternal and child health care from Glasgow Caledonian University (2008). Through working in a variety of staff nurses roles, her clinical experience was built in ICU / CCU over four years. However, the academic experience has been started with working at The Hashemite University/ Faculty of Nursing in Jordan as research and teaching assistant since 2000-2004. Now after gaining a PhD, she is teaching at The Hashemite University/ Faculty of Nursing as an assistant professor.

Tien Le (MD FRCS(C) DABOG) is associate professor with the Department of Obstetrics and Gynecology at the University of Ottawa and gynecologic oncologist at the Ottawa Hospital. He is the post graduate training program director and chair of the resident research committee at the University of Ottawa, Canada,

Shona Kirtley has an MA (Hons) from the University of St Andrews and an MSc in Information and Library Studies from the University of Strathclyde. Shona is currently project co-ordinator for the NHS Women's Health Specialist Library based at Oxford University. She has a very keen interest in electronic resource provision, in particular women's health online resources, and in raising awareness of the wealth of resources available to health professionals to both support and improve evidence-based clinical practice.

David Knight is director of neonatology at the Mater Mother's in Brisbane. David completed his medical training in the UK and qualified as a neonatal specialist in New Zealand after emigrating. He was director of neonatology at one of the largest maternity units in Australasia: National Women's Hospital in Auckland, New Zealand. He developed the neonatal database whilst in this position. More recently he has been in a larger management role as clinical leader of paediatrics and women's health in Auckland prior to his recent move to Australia.

Carl Kuschel (MBChB FRACP) is a neonatologist who undertook his training in New Zealand, Australia and Canada. He returned to National Women's Hospital, Auckland, New Zealand, in 1998 as a neonatal specialist and moved to Melbourne, Australia, in 2008 to take up a position as medical director (neonatal services) at the Royal Women's Hospital. Carl's neonatal research interests include nutrition, ventilation strategies, haemodynamic assessment, and substance use in pregnancy. Other clinical interests include the impact of the neonatal intensive care unit design on the outcomes for staff, babies and families. He has had a long-standing interest in the use of information technologies to improve clinical care, and has designed or contributed to a number of websites.

Tien Le (MD FRCS(C) DABOG) is associate professor with the Department of Obstetrics and Gynecology at the University of Ottawa and gynecologic oncologist at the Ottawa Hospital. He is the post graduate training program director and chair of the resident research committee at the University of Ottawa, Canada,

Rob Liston is professor and head of the Department of Obstetrics and Gynecology UBC and head of the Department of Obstetrics and Gynecology BC Women's, Vancouver Hospital and Health Sciences Centre, and Providence Hospitals. Dr. Rob Liston received his MB, ChB from the University of St. Andrews, Scotland in 1971 and training in obstetrics and gynecology at the University of Edinburgh and the University of Dundee. He received his membership in the Royal College of Obstetricians and Gynecologists in 1977 and subsequently his FRCSC, FRCOG (London) and American Boards. He came to North America in 1978 as an assistant professor at the University of Pennsylvania and then moved to Dalhousie in 1981 where he became associate professor in 1988 and professor in 1996. He was director of the Division of Maternal Fetal Medicine, and chief of obstetrics at IWK Grace Hospital. In addition, he served as a consultant to the Nova Scotia Reproductive Care Program where he developed a keen insight into the obstetrical needs of the whole community. He came to Vancouver in 1998 to take on the responsibility of head of obstetrics and gynecology at the Children's & Women's Health Centre of BC and was appointed Head of the Department of Obstetrics and Gynaecology at UBC in July 2000. He is well known in the Canadian obstetrics and gynecology community, particularly for his interest in fetal surveillance, labour management, post dates pregnancy and induction. He has been active in the Society of Obstetrics and Gynecology of Canada where, as chairman of the Maternal Fetal Medicine Committee, he took an active role in the development of clinical practice guidelines. He brings an exciting and progressive vision to the Department of Obstetrics and Gynecology which encompasses all of the Vancouver teaching hospitals and has an outlook throughout the Province of British Columbia and beyond. Rob and his wife Leslie have four children. He is well aware of the issues facing academic, clinical departments and believes that a collaborative approach to those issues is the key to improving the health of women and their families.

Laura Magee, internationally renowned researcher in maternal medicine who has a practice based at BC en's Hospital, has been the driving force behind Kiran's work. After completing her residency, clinical pharmacology fellowship and an MSc in community health at the University of Toronto she completed Detweiler Traveling and Duncan Gordon Fellowships, at Oxford University and the University of London, UK. She is currently a clinical associate professor of medicine at the University of British Columbia, section head in maternal medicine at BC Women's Hospital, a Michael Smith Foundation for Health Research Scholar and practices out of BC Women's Hospital, St. Paul's Hospital and Vancouver General Hospital. Her academic and clinical interests lie in medical complications of pregnancy, hypertensive disorders of pregnancy and meta-analysis of clinical trials.

Anne-Marie McMahon (RCN DPSN LLB) is lead nurse for Chronic Obstructive Pulmonary Disease (COPD) at Poole Hospital Foundation Trust. She has 20 years experience in acute health care within the UK including intensive and coronary care nursing. She has studied law as a part-time student since 2000 and holds an LLB (Hons). In July 2007 she completed a part-time Bar Vocational Course and was called to the Bar in 2007. She is a non-practising Barrister and a member of Lincolns Inn. Anne-Marie has been a member of Poole Hospital Clinical Ethics Group since 2005. She has a special interest in human rights and ethics in medical and healthcare law. She is currently undertaking a Master in Law (LLM) which she hopes to complete at the end of 2008.

Tara Morris received her Bachelor of Science in molecular biology in 2004 from Simon Fraser University (Burnaby, British Columbia, Canada). After graduating, she worked as a laboratory technician for the Department of Pathology and Laboratory Medicine at B.C. Children's Hospital in Vancouver, where she was worked on several research projects including a project examining carrier testing for Tay-Sachs Disease (Common HEXB polymorphisms reduce serum HexA and HexB enzymatic activities, Molecular Genetics & Metabolism, Feb;87(2):122-7) and a molecular study involving a family with hereditary hemochromatosis (A novel ferroportin mutation in a Canadian family with autosomal dominant hemochromatosis, Blood Cells, Molecules & Diseases, Nov-Dec;35(3):309-14). Since 2005, Tara has worked as a clinical research co-ordinator for the Department of Obstetrics & Gynaecology at B.C. Women's Hospital in Vancouver, co-ordinating several projects in the area of high-risk obstetrics. She is currently the National Co-ordinator for the Canadian Perinatal Network, and is concurrently completing her Masters degree in Health Administration from the University of British Columbia.

Liron Pantanowitz (MD) is medical director of pathology informatics for Baystate Health, Massachusetts, USA. He is assistant professor of pathology at Tufts University School of Medicine and assistant professor of biology at the University of Massachusetts, Amherst. Dr. Pantanowitz received his medical degree from the University of the Witwatersrand in South Africa, followed by a residency in anatomic and clinical pathology at Boston's Beth Israel Deaconess Medical Center, Harvard Medical School. He has fellowships in Cytopathology and Haematopathology. He serves on the informatics committee of the College of American Pathologists, is a member of the International Academy of Cytology and Association of Pathology Informatics, and has research interests in the fields of informatics, diagnostic cytopathology, and HIV/AIDS.

Gareth Parry (MBBS MRCGP DRCOG MSC) is a general practitioner principal (family doctor) in Dartford Kent UK. He trained at Guy's Hospital. London and holds a MBBS degree from London University along with a BSc in medical physics and a master's degree in medical informatics. His interests include the use of IT in primary healthcare.

Graham Parry is a consultant obstetrician who now spends his days doing obstetric ultrasound instead of delivering babies. He first became interested in ultrasound in the late 1970s when working with Prof. Stuart Campbell, one of the pioneers of obstetric scanning. Since that time he has used ultrasound in his everyday practise as an obstetrician and gynaecologist. The computer has revolutionised the techniques of imaging as well as the management of an imaging department in a way that could not have been dreamt of by the early pioneers. He now feels privileged to use modern informatic technology for imaging, storing of images as well as teaching and research.

Barry Rosen (MD FRCS(C)) is associate professor with the Department of Obstetrics and Gynecology and divisional head of gynecologic oncology at the University of Toronto and a gynecologic oncologist at Princess Margaret Hospital, Toronto, Canada

Bohdan Sadovy (MHSc CHE) Information Technology, Princess Margaret Hospital, Toronto, Canada

Peter Stone is professor of maternal fetal medicine in The University of Auckland and currently head of the Department in Obstetrics and Gynaecology. His postgraduate training was in Britain, gaining an Doctor of Medicine based on Doppler studies in fetal growth restriction from the University of Bristol. After working in Wellington at the University of Otago for 11 years, where he set up the maternal fetal medicine service he moved to Auckland in 1998. He has been involved in obstetrics, maternal and fetal medicine and women's health throughout his professional career. He has been a member of a number of ministerial advisory groups most recently on the screening advisory groups for HIV and Down syndrome as well as being a member of the National Screening Advisory Group for the Director General of Health He is part of the ISTAR group which brought Mifepristone into New Zealand. He is a councillor for the RANZCOG and is currently chair of the New Zealand Training and Accreditation Committee of RANZCOG. Research interests include fetal welfare assessment, ultrasound studies of the cervix in pregnancy, and early pregnancy development including implantation and trophoblast deportation. Other research interests include teaching quality improvement. Currently he is developing an ultrasound teaching programme for the Pacific in association with the RANZCOG and the Pacific Women's Health Research Development unit set up in his Department in Middlemore Hospital.

Jenny Westgate (MBChB, MD, MRCOG, FRANZCOG) is associate professor in obstetrics and gynaecology, The University of Auckland. She is chair of the NZ Training and Accreditation Committee of the Royal Australian and New Zealand College of Obstetricians and Gynaecologists and an examiner for the MRANZCOG. Her primary research interests are in the areas of fetal responses to hypoxia and fetal heart rate monitoring. She is also involved in a two year study of South Auckland pregnant women with gestational or type II diabetes looking at a metabolic profile of the baby and relationship with maternal glycaemia and fetal size.

Index